Sclerotherapy

Chinese Association of Phlebology (CHINA)

Vascular Surgery Branch of Guangdong Medical Doctor Association (CHINA)

Egyptian Venous Forum (EGYPT)

Georgian Association of Angiologists and Vascular Surgeons (GEORGIA)

Indonesian Society for Vascular and Endovascular Surgery - PESBEVI (INDONESIA)

Morocco Society of Internal Medicine (MOROCCO)

Morocco Society of Vascular Medicine (MOROCCO)

Italian Society of Phlebology and Lymphology (ITALY)

French Society of Phlebology (FRANCE)

Thai Venous Forum (THAILAND)

Spanish Chapter of Phlebology & Lymphology (SPAIN)

Japanese Society of Phlebology (JAPAN)

Venous-lymphatics World International Network (v-WIN) foundation (GLOBAL)

Sergio Gianesini • Yung Wei Chi
Editors

Sclerotherapy

From Basic Science to Clinical Practice

Springer

Editors
Prof. Sergio Gianesini, MD, PhD
Department of Translational Medicine
University of Ferrara
Ferrara, Italy

Department of Surgery
Uniformed Services University
of Health Sciences
Bethesda, MD, USA

Prof. Yung Wei Chi, MD
Department of Cardiovascular Medicine
University of California,
Davis Vascular Center
Sacramento, CA, USA

ISBN 978-3-032-32793-2 ISBN 978-3-032-32794-9 (eBook)
https://doi.org/10.1007/978-3-032-32794-9

This Springer imprint is published by the registered company Springer Nature Switzerland AG
The registered company address is: Gewerbestrasse 11, 6330 Cham, Switzerland

The textbook is in memory of the beloved Dr. Pauline Raymond-Martimbeau, global example of professionalism and passion in Sclerotherapy and beyond. Her teachings remain in the following pages, as well as in the related everyday best clinical actions of the colleagues who will follow proper Sclerotherapy practice.

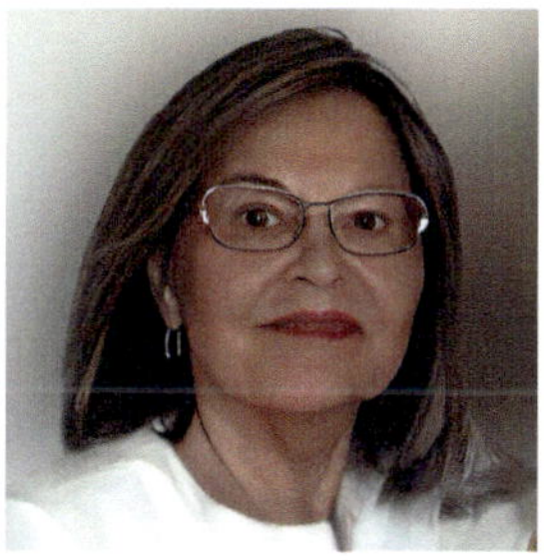

Foreword

Sclerotherapy has evolved from a largely empirical technique into a sophisticated, evidence-informed therapeutic discipline grounded in vascular biology, hemodynamics, physics, and translational medicine. The authors' clear presentation of the principles of venous and lymphatic disease illustrates the convergence of basic science, technological innovation, and clinical pragmatism of sclerotherapy. This work represents an unbelievable compendium of knowledge presented by a who's who of international experts. This outstanding faculty represents the unique ability of Professor Gianesini to gather people from the far corners of the world to present many opinions and elaborate discussion focused, in this case, on the evolving world of sclerotherapy.

The contributions assembled in this volume reflect the full intellectual and practical breadth of modern sclerotherapy. Beginning with a historical perspective that traces the origins and evolution of the technique, the issue progresses logically through venous pathophysiology, sclerosant pharmacology, foam production methodologies, and the complex physical and biochemical behavior of sclerosant bubbles. These foundational chapters establish a scientific framework that supports the clinical sections that follow. Particular emphasis is placed on foam science and its translation into daily practice—an area that has reshaped treatment paradigms across chronic venous disease, pelvic venous disorders, vascular malformations, and telangiectatic disease. The detailed discussions of indications, contraindications, safety profiles, and complication management provide clinicians with practical, experience-based guidance while remaining firmly anchored in current evidence. Equally valuable are the chapters addressing catheter-based sclerotherapy, cryo-laser cryo-sclerotherapy, and advanced technical tips and procedural refinements, which collectively highlight how innovation continues to expand both efficacy and safety. The inclusion of chapters on medical technology advancement, regulatory considerations, and international guideline similarities and controversies underscores an important reality: sclerotherapy does not exist in a vacuum but is shaped by healthcare systems, regulatory environments, and evolving global consensus. This issue represents a truly international and multidisciplinary collaboration, bringing together leading clinicians, scientists, and educators who have shaped—and continue to shape—the field. Their collective expertise offers readers not only a comprehensive reference but also a forward-looking vision of where sclerotherapy is headed.

The authors conclude that even though sclerotherapy is widely used with proven effectiveness, global standardization is lacking in technical protocols along with specific success criteria and post-treatment follow-up. High-quality prospective randomized clinical trials are needed to evaluate occlusion rates, outcomes using validated instruments, and standardized ultrasound protocols. Much work remains to be done. But this outstanding treatise lays the foundation for moving into the future.

I am thrilled that the authors chose to dedicate this outstanding volume to the memory of Pauline Raymond-Martimbeau who was a pillar of knowledge, research, and most notably, continued to search for the truth by enlisting members of the world community to contribute their scientific and clinical expertise to the treatment of venous disease. It is very fitting that the authors described her as a "global example of professionalism and passion in Sclerotherapy and beyond." Her sudden and untimely death was a shock to all of us, but through the creation of this incredible resource her memory will live forever.

It is our hope that this volume will serve as a definitive resource for practitioners at all stages of experience, stimulate thoughtful discussion, and ultimately contribute to improved patient care in venous and vascular disease.

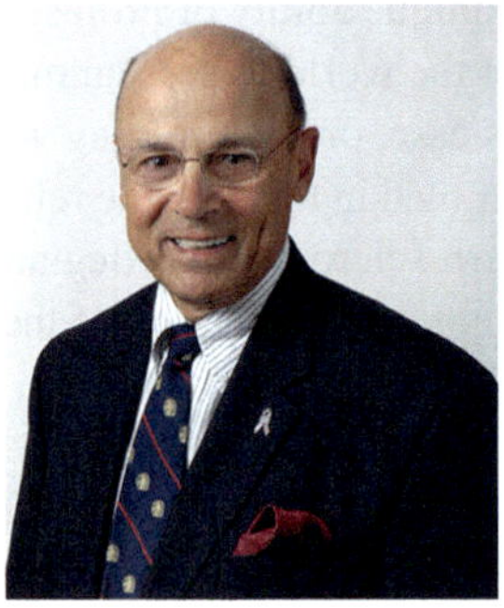

NorthWestern University
Chicago, IL, USA

Joseph Caprini

Preface

Sclerotherapy is an ART that found its SCIENCE

Sclerotherapy is practiced *Wherever* in the world and *Whenever* (every single day in large amount), therefore it is fundamental not to practice it in a "*Whatever*" way.

At first glance, sclerotherapy may appear deceptively simple. The injection of a sclerosant into a vein is often perceived as little more than "just" poking a vein. This misconception has probably been responsible for one of the greatest mistakes in the history of the procedure: underestimating its complexity. Such an oversimplified approach may expose both the physician and the patient to unnecessary risks, leaving the outcome to chance rather than to sound clinical judgment.

In reality, high-quality sclerotherapy requires a comprehensive understanding of vascular biology and pathology. The operator must master venous anatomy and hemodynamics, endothelial biology and histopathology, sclerosant pharmacology, foam physics, ultrasound imaging, patient selection, and complication management. Every injection represents the culmination of a complex interaction between science, technology, and clinical decision-making.

Technical proficiency, refined through experience, together with countless practical nuances acquired over years of clinical practice, constitutes the *Art of Sclerotherapy*. The biological principles, physical laws, pharmacological mechanisms, and evidence supporting each therapeutic decision constitute its *Science*. Neither can exist without the other.

Modern phlebology clearly demonstrates that, despite the remarkable evolution of endovenous technologies, appropriately performed sclerotherapy continues to be highly competitive in terms of anatomical success, patient satisfaction, patient-reported outcomes, recovery, versatility, and potentially cost-effectiveness. Rather than being replaced by newer technologies, sclerotherapy has continued to evolve alongside them, also because the real "battle" to venous reflux sits in the tributaries more than in the saphenous trunks.

The recent introduction of semi-automated and fully automated foam-generation systems has opened an entirely new chapter in the field. These technological advances require a deeper understanding of what may be defined as *sclero-pharmacology*: the complex interaction between sclerosant concentration, gas composition, bubble characteristics, foam stability, vascular response, and device-specific performance. The challenge is no longer simply producing foam, but producing the most appropriate foam for each clinical scenario, with the lowest nitrogen possible.

Emerging evidence already suggests the magnitude of this evolution. Recent meta-analyses indicate that fully automated foam produced with ultra-low nitrogen concentrations (below 0.8%) may achieve saphenous vein occlusion rates approaching those of endovenous thermal ablation, while potentially reducing some of the limitations traditionally associated with foam sclerotherapy. Although further high-quality research is still required, these findings signal the beginning of a new era in which technological innovation must be interpreted through rigorous scientific evidence rather than enthusiasm alone.

This textbook was conceived precisely within this rapidly evolving landscape. It brings together internationally recognized experts from every continent, representing both basic scientists and experienced clinicians, with the shared objective of guiding the reader from the fundamental mechanisms underlying sclerotherapy to the practical, step-by-step techniques required for safe and effective daily clinical practice. Throughout the book, equal emphasis is placed on understanding *why* each intervention works and *how* it should be performed according to the best available evidence.

Upon completing this volume, readers will hopefully appreciate that the traditional statement describing sclerotherapy as "*an art still searching for its science*" is not accurate. Today, well-performed sclerotherapy is unquestionably an *Art*, but it is an art *that found its Science*.

Ultimately, this is the philosophy underpinning the entire book: transforming knowledge into competence, competence into excellence, and excellence into better patient care.

University of Ferrara, Italy
Uniformed Services University of Health Sciences, Bethesda, USA
Prof. Sergio Gianesini

University of California Davis, USA
Prof. Yung Wei Chi

Acknowledgments

Together Forward

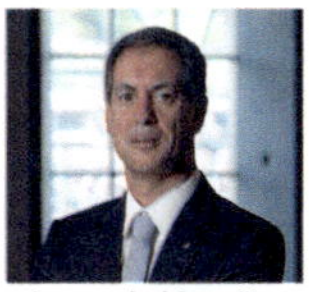
Armando Mansilha
(PORTUGAL)

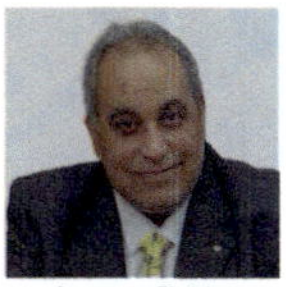
Ayman Fakhry
(EGYPT)

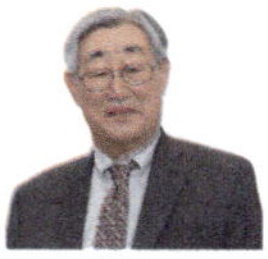
BB Lee
(USA)

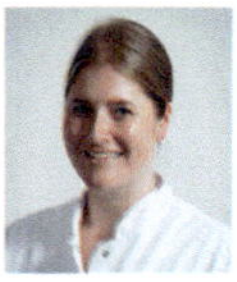
Celine Eggen
(NETHERLANDS)

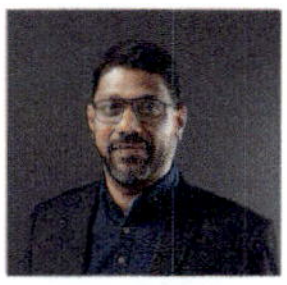
Danny Pratama
(INDONESIA)

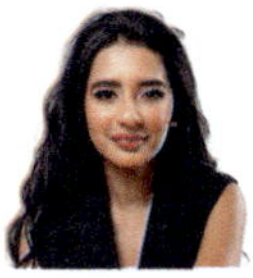
Gisele Peron
(BRAZIL)

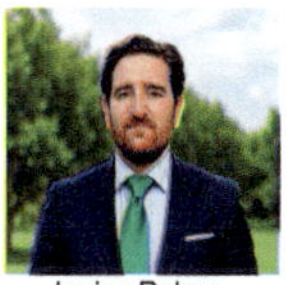
Javier Palma
(SPAIN)

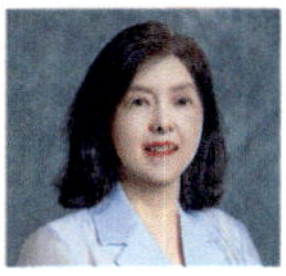
Jinsong Wang
(CHINA)

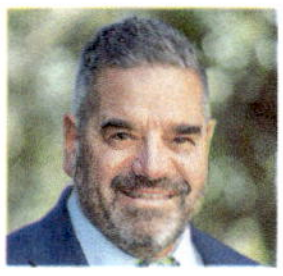
Jospeh Dante Raffetto
(USA)

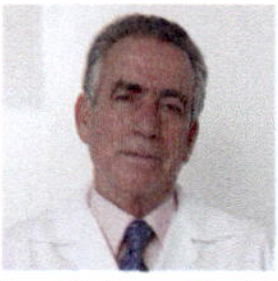
Juan Cabrera Garrido
(SPAIN)

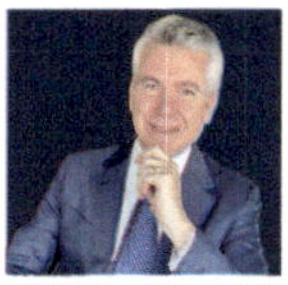
Juan Cabrera García Olmedo
(SPAIN)

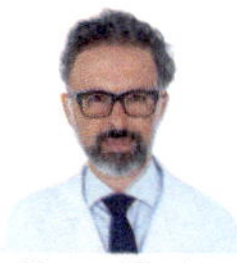
Kasuo Miyake
(BRAZIL)

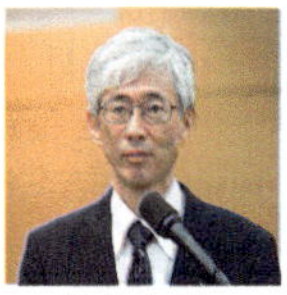
Makoto Mo
(JAPAN)

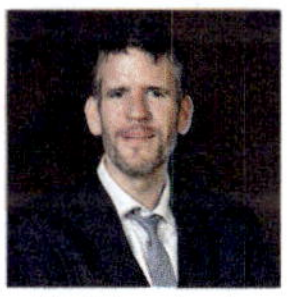
Matthieu Josnin
(FRANCE)

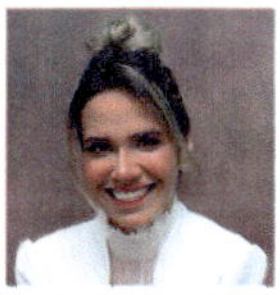
Nathalia Cardoso Oliveira
(BRAZIL)

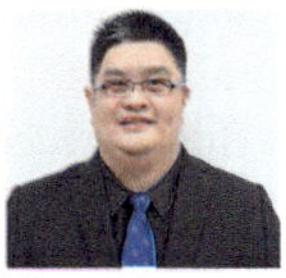
N. Sermsathanasawadi
(THAILAND)

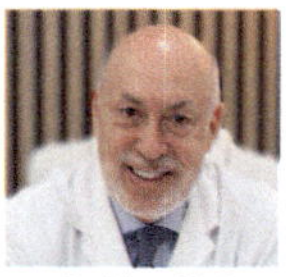
Rodrigo Rial
(SPAIN)

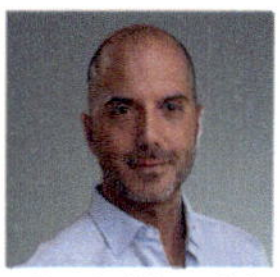
Sergio Gianesini
(ITALY)

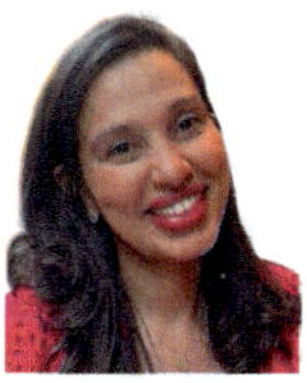
Yasmina Chhih
(MOROCCO)

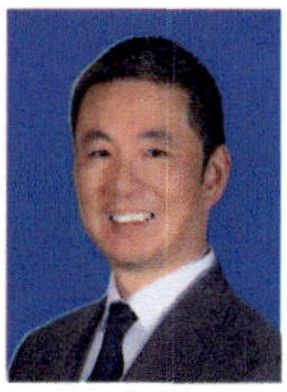
Yung Wei Chi
(USA)

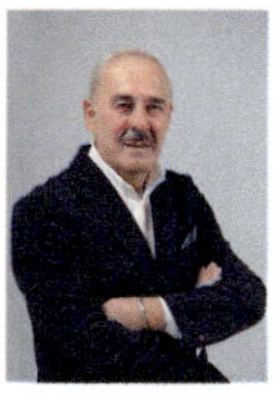
Zaza Lazarashvili
(GEORGIA)

Traditionally, only the Editors of the textbooks appear with their headshots.

In appreciation of the outstanding Authors who joined this teamwork from All Contnents, we are delighted in representing all of them herein, in alphabetical order.

A sign that "pictures" how the only way truly forward in vein-lymphatic care is "together."

Contents

About the Editors

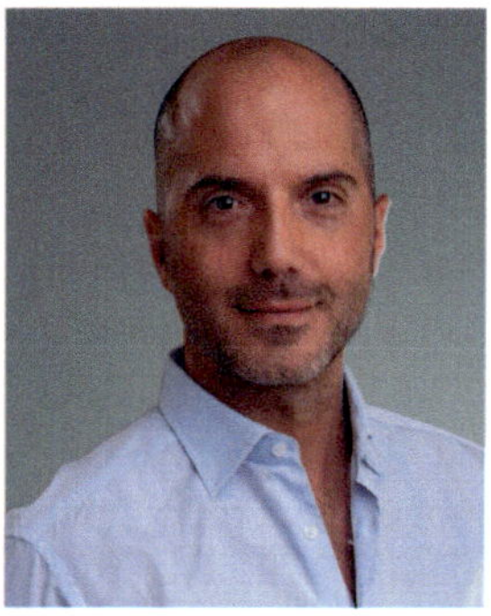

Prof. Sergio Gianesini, MD, PhD Prof. Sergio Gianesini is a surgeon of the University of Ferrara (ITALY) and of the Uniformed Services University of Health Sciences (Bethesda, USA). He is president of the World Union of International Phlebolymphology (WUIP) and emeritus president of the venous-lymphatic World International Network (v-WIN) foundation. He is a licensed surgeon in Italy, United Arab Emirates, and Switzerland. He is Associate Editor of *International Angiology Journal* and editorial board member of nine international scientific journals dedicated to vein and lymphatic care. He is the principal investigator of the global v-REGISTRY project on vein-lymphatic global real-world data. He has authored more than 100 scientific publications in Phlebology and Lymphology and he has given more than 700 invited lectures in all continents. He holds a PhD in molecular vascular pathophysiology, and he has been involved in several translational medicine research projects on biosignaling and venous hemodynamics. He serves as advisor in the development of medical devices and he developed the university spin-off Science Per Aquam dedicated to standardized hydrotherapic protocols for vein-lymphatic patients and vein-lymphatic scientific and educational activities. He is the project lead of the first clinical governance document on vein-lymphatic care (V.A.L.I.D. project). He is the founder of Le.G.athering multi-specialty global project for appropriate vein-lymphatic holistic care.

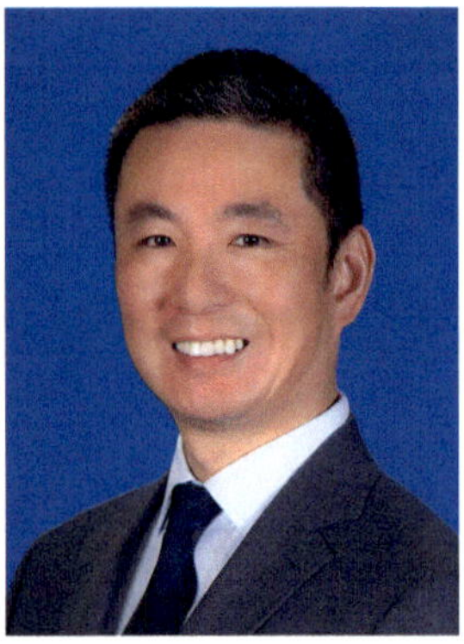

Prof. Yung Wei Chi, MD Prof. Chi is an internationally recognized authority on venous and lymphatic disease, and is a Professor of Medicine at the University of California, Davis, Vascular Center. He is widely published in the field of venous and lymphatic disease with over 60 peer-reviewed publications, and lectures globally. He sits on the editorial board of *Phlebology*, *Vascular Medicine*, *Veins and Lymphatic*, *Advanced Interventional Materials*, and the *Chinese Medical Journal*, and is the Chinese Language Editor for *International Angiology*, the Associate Editor for *Vascular Investigation and Therapy*, and the Associate Editor for *Journal of Vascular and Endovascular Research*. As the President of the Venous-lymphatic World International Network (v-WIN) foundation, the Vice President of the Asian Pacific Angiology Academic Alliance, and the World Union of International Phlebolymphology, Prof. Chi currently holds an H-Index of 19. His recent research had been funded by the University of California Science and Innovation Grant as well as the American Vein and Lymphatic Society. He holds patents in various healthcare wearable device innovations.

1 Sclerotherapy: Past, Present, and Future

Sergio Gianesini and Juan Cabrera Garrido

1 Historical Background

Lower limb varicose veins' treatment description can be found in the dawn of humankind, as testified for example by the famous Ebers Papyrus, dated around 1550 BC [1]. Yet, we have to wait until the seventeenth century for proper documentation of a sclerotherapy injection. Interestingly, Dr. Elsholtz injected an alkaloid plant extract in a patient affected by a venous ulcer (Fig. 1.1) [2]. Up to our knowledge though there is no report related to the outcome of this procedure.

In 1682, in Switzerland, the narrative reports Dr. Zollikofer performing an injection of an acid into a vein to induce a thrombotic/occlusive process, yet solid evidence in support of this fact is lacking too [3]. The ground of the sclerotherapy global ascent begins in the nineteenth century with the appearance of the hypodermic needles and the use of irritant solutions such as iron perchlorate and tannin/iodine. In 1815, Joseph Hodgson was the first reporting in a textbook how a superficial venous thrombosis could cure the varicosity, therefore paving the way toward the modern concept of therapy based on the

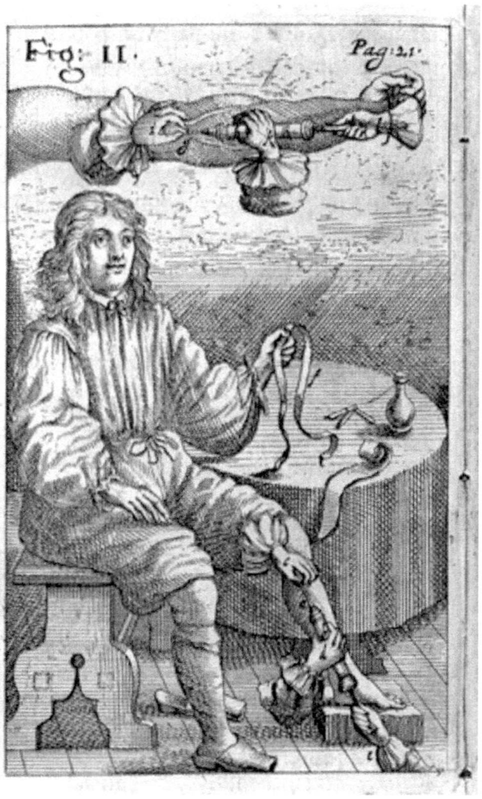

Fig. 1.1 Representation of the first reported sclerotherapy injection by Dr. Elsholtz in 1665. (Picture from https://wellcomecollection.org/ (query: "Elsholtz, Johann Sigismund, 1623–1688."))

S. Gianesini (✉)
Department of Translational Medicine, University of Ferrara, Ferrara, Italy

Department of Surgery, Uniformed Services University of Health Sciences, Bethesda, MD, USA
e-mail: gnssrg@unife.it

J. C. Garrido
Phlebology Department, International Institute of Phlebology, Granada, Spain
e-mail: juan@drjuancabrera.com

S. Gianesini, Y. W. Chi (eds.), *Sclerotherapy*, https://doi.org/10.1007/978-3-032-32794-9_1

sclerosis of the target vein [4]. The aggressiveness of the sclerosing agents and the lack of experience in their management led to frequent severe complications, among which necrosis, thrombosis, ulceration, without successful therapeutic lasting outcomes. For these reasons, varicose veins' surgery remained dominant over the injection methods along the century. Yet, in the early-twentieth century, prominent vein experts began to use less aggressive drugs like hypertonic saline and phenol and then detergents like polidocanol and sodium tetradecyl sulfate. Historic pioneers of this era are Sigg in Switzerland, Tournay in France, Fegan in Ireland, and Bassi in Italy. The first doctor mentioning the term "sclerotherapy" appears to be Biegeleisen from the USA in 1936, almost 300 years after the 1665 first injection with sclerosing purposes performed by Johann Sigismund Elsholtz, before the famous Dr. Pravaz modern times syringe [5]. This last one appeared in 1835, simultaneously with a similar proposal by Dr. Alexander Wood from Edinburgh. While the latter was injecting morphine for neuralgia treatment, Pravaz was using iron chloride for varicose veins treatment, offering a treatment that became very popular in France, together with the use of different sclerosing agents (acetic acid, iodine-tannin, ferric chloride). Sclerotherapy by these agents was such an intense procedure for the patients to require more than 10 days of hospitalization, in antithesis to modern mini-invasiveness of the same act [6].

The high complication rates and the poor clinical results led to even ban sclerotherapy in France, as reported by the 1894 Lyon Congress extracts [3]. In 1904 the concern linked to the possible complications led Dr. Tavel to propose to ligate the saphenofemoral junction to avoid thrombo-embolic complications. It was in 1932 in Madrid, during the International Society of Surgery meeting, that, considering the invasiveness, the recurrences, and the complication rates of varicose veins surgery, the experts expressed the need to go back in focusing more on possible mini-invasive sclerotherapic approaches [7]. That's when three main sclerotherapic centers flourished in Europe: the one of Tournay in France, of Fegan in Ireland, and of Sigg in Switzerland. In the same period, the advantages of the foam use were then reported by Orbach in 1950, after 6 years of its famous "air-block" technique for its production [8]. The concept of emptying the vein before the injection was first proposed by Thornill in 1929, while foam was first produced by McAusland simply shaking sodium morrhuate with air in a bottle in 1939, changing then to lithium salicylate and quinine [9]. In the same years, Dr. Foote used ethanolamine oleate shaken in a 2 ml syringe for producing a froth that was then used by Sigg and slightly modified by Dr. Ree from Norway.

In 1962, Fluckiger from Switzerland described a method to produce the finer froth from ethanolamine oleate, basically pumping in and out air and sclerosant from a syringe to a drug vial. He initiated the narrative of the bubbles' capacity to increase the contact surface of the sclerosant, therefore reducing the concentration need [10]. An alternative foam production method was proposed by Gillesberger in 1969 by creating a negative pressure inside a glass syringe, yet with the limit of no possible standardization of the amount of gas involved, considered that the technique was based on the suction of air into the syringe through the piston that was moved back and forth [11]. The first real foam sclerotherapy production is to be possibly attributed to the German physicians Mayer and Brucke, who IN the late 50s used ethanolamine oleate in a double-piston syringe with a fenestrated plunger [12]. Approaching the modern times, Hobbs published the first randomized trial of sclerotherapy vs. varicose veins' surgery in 1974, reporting how at 1-year follow-up, sclerotherapy performed better, yet losing its competitiveness against surgery at 6 years' observation [13]. In the following decades, many attempts to improve and simplify the foam production were done. In 1984, in Germany, Hauer proposed a twin-syringe system (one with air, the other with the sclerosant) to produce foam [14]. Two years later, in Australia, Grigg connected two syringes by a tube and pumped gas and sclerosant back and forth [3]. The following historical jump in sclerotherapy advancement happened in 1993 by means of the microfoam standardized production by Cabrera, obtained using biocompatible gases, optimizing the safety profile thanks to highly soluble gas use, enhancing the mechanical efficacy of the bubbles displacing blood and increasing the drug-contact surface. By eliminating nitrogen and reducing bubble size, larger injectable volumes became clinically tolerable, allowing effective blood displacement while maintaining safety. This shift enabled a fundamental transition in therapeutic decision-making: Indication was no longer determined by vein caliber, but by foam behavior. As a consequence, the traditional paradigm was replaced by a unified approach in which both small and large varicose veins became amenable to treatment using microfoam [15].

In 1997, Monfreux showcased how to produce foam by closing a glass syringe outlet and pulling back the piston to allow air entrance, similarly to what previously proposed by Gillesberger [16]. In the same year Tessari proposed to connect two disposable syringes and a 3-way stopcock, mixing liquid sclerosant and air in a $\frac{1}{4}$ or $\frac{1}{5}$ ratio, using multiple passes between the two syringes to produce the foam (Fig. 1.2) [17].

Along the first decade of the twenty-first century, different biocompatible gas mixtures were proposed to improve safety and performance, yet the literature showcased just a mild possible evidence on the improvement of dizziness, chest tightness, and visual disturbances [18]. It's an evidence-based fact that appropriate material and methods must be applied in order to obtain a physician-compounded safe and effective foam [19]. For this reason, different kits have been proposed along the years, providing the appropriate low-silicon syringes, bidirectional connectors, needles, and, in some cases, also sterile air prefilled in the syringe. Indeed, even the same needle can impact the foam stability [20]. Along those years, catheters of different types have been proposed to deliver sclerotherapy, with the rationale of enhancing its efficacy. While preliminary evidence seems to support the use of such devices, both in terms of safety and efficacy, a significant heterogeneity has been clearly highlighted, therefore limiting the certainty of the finding [21]. Around 2010 more elaborated devices have then been proposed with the aim of performing a so called "mechano-chemical" ablation in the saphenous trunk, combining the endothelial lesion induced by the device with the one obtained by the sclerosant agent chemical properties. Literature related to the topic has demonstrated a lack of competitiveness in the comparison with laser and radiofrequency techniques in the mid-term follow-up as well as in the large calibers' vein treatment [22, 23]. Another category of sclerotherapy catheter was proposed back in 2008 in the form of a double-balloon device, by J. Leu and R. Inderbitzi, from Switzerland (Fig. 1.3). The device allows to isolate a segment of vein in between the two inflated balloons, allowing the injection of a sclerosant agent in an empty bloodless tract, and moreover, aspirating the residual sclerosant once the treatment is completed. While reported in the literature, no large publications can be found for the validation of this device [24].

In 2013, after 18 years of investigations for FDA validation, a canister based on the 1995 Cabrera microfoam was approved for the US market under the name of Varithena. It consists in a mix of 1% polidocanol with carbon dioxide/oxygen 35/65% nitrogen-free mix. In comparison with the physician compound method of Tessari, it demonstrated smaller bubble sizes,

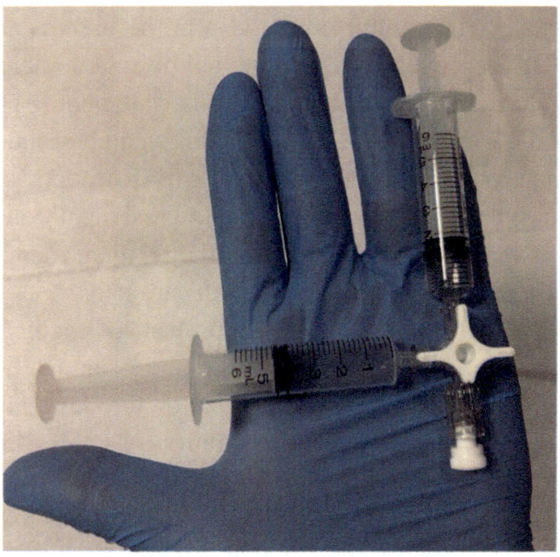

Fig. 1.2 Tessari method (drug/gas = $\frac{1}{4}$)

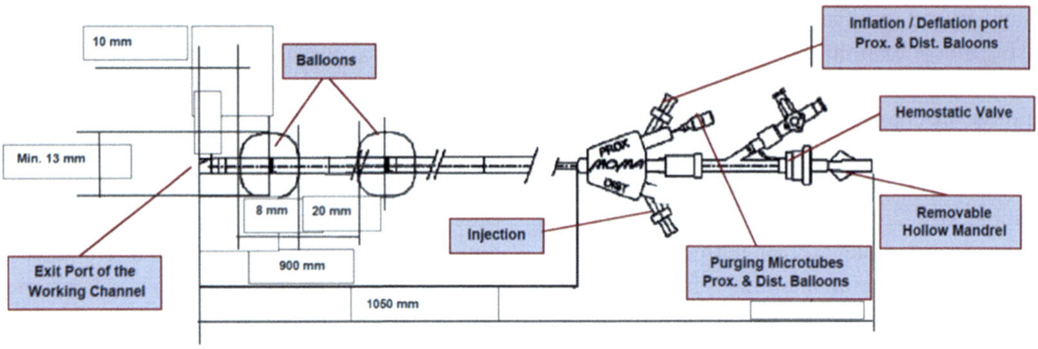

Fig. 1.3 Double balloon catheter for sclerotherapy. (Picture from Leu and Inderbitzi [24]. Used with permission of © 2008 by Verlag Hans Huber, Hogrefe AG, Bern)

bigger homogeneity, and more stability. The device offers a <0.8% nitrogen content, allowing the FDA validation [25]. A recent network meta-analysis reported its possible competitiveness with thermal tumescent gold-standard techniques (laser and radiofrequency) [26]. In 2021 a magnetic stirrer called Varixio entered the market, offering single-use sterile capsules containing air or low nitrogen gas (2–10% nitrogen, the remaining being 2/3 oxygen and 1/3 carbon dioxide), to be then combined with the manually injected sclerosant agent introduced by the healthcare professional. The stirring process produces the foam that is then aspirated by the same professional [27].

Up to our knowledge, at the moment there is no randomized trial comparing it with physician-compounded methods, while there is a one single-center retrospective investigation reporting a great saphenous vein recanalization rate of 26.8% at 3 years [28]. Registry data from Dr. Roche, inventor of the device, reported an occlusion rate at 15 months of 93.2% for the great saphenous vein and of 86% for the small saphenous vein [29]. In 2024 a device similar to Varixio appeared under the name of Sclerofoam, offering the same stirring mechanism of action and both air and CO_2 capsules for mixing the sclerosing agent. The producer reports similar foam physical properties in the comparison with Varixio, yet we were not able to identify scientific publications related to the device.

In 2024, the latest evolution coming from the upgrade of the technology providing polidocanol 1% Cabrera microfoam was presented under the Mfoamer name. It is a fully automated device endowed with a monitor providing the possibility to choose from a wide range of gases percentages and drug concentrations, in a nitrogen-free context (from the lowest 0.1–3%, with several CO_2/O_2 percentages) [30].

Prospective multi-center studies on its clinical efficacy are ongoing.

It must be noted that, in the modern era, foam sclerotherapy by the above-mentioned devices almost always represents a conundrum in terms of legal responsibility. Indeed, no clinical governance document explicitly recommends their use, up to our search. Having the CE mark can provide some coverage in the European Union, yet no guidelines are officially endorsing their use. To the contrary, Varithena in the USA is an FDA-approved option supported by an American Vein Lymphatic Society position statement [31]. Yet, no major American guidelines can be found mentioning specifically the medical product of Varithena™. Despite that, a reimbursement code exists in its favor, witnessing the national recognition in US institutional health care.

In conclusion, it took 360 years of medical evolution to move from the empiricism to the evidence-based science that allows today safe and effective use of sclerotherapy.

The learning curve included the most disparate agents use, including mercurial preparations that poisoned the patients [7]. Other agents were acids of different nature, iron perchloride, iodine-tannin, 5% alcohol, mercury perchloride, carbolic acid, phenol, salvarsan, quinine, 50–60% glucose, luargol, sodium salicylate, sodium morrhuate, sodium bicarbonate, 20% sodium chloride, sodium citrate, grape sugar, chromate glycerin, ethanolamine oleate, and many more until polidocanol and sodium tetradecyl sulfate established their position as main sclerosing agents of the present era. Sodium tetradecyl sulfate was introduced in 1946 and used by Hobbs for his randomized trial. Polidocanol accessed the market 10 years before, but as anesthetic, indeed, then abandoned as it was causing clotting. Only in 1966, Otto Henschel, Scientific Director of Kreussler Pharma (Germany), provided it as a sclerosing agent [3]. Independently by the sclerosing agents, different injection strategies have been developed along the years. The two main visions were represented by the descending theory of Tournay and the ascending one from Sigg. Tournay advocated for the control of the reflux from the saphenofemoral junction down, in a sort of waterfall effect. To the contrary, Sigg campaigned for the ascending theory for which the treatment was performed from distal to proximal. Fegan followed the Sigg strategy, convinced of the main role of perforating vein incompetence [32]. Nowadays, practitioners are still divided in supporters of the ascending vs. descending theories, with no standardized recognized strategic protocols. This is very important to notice for the identification of the unmet needs to be fulfilled in the next near future. In fact, properly prepared foam, using the dedicated materials and methods, demonstrated high safety profiles and clinical efficacy, even by physician-compounded methods [19]. Yet, the variability in the used material, as well as in the preparation technique and in the eventual device, can lead to significant heterogeneity in the foam physical and related clinical features. Based on the above, sclerotherapy long-lasting history is clearly still dominant in today's practice, in which almost all patients are candidates for at least a tributary if not a saphenous trunk sclerotherapic treatment. Moreover, sclerotherapy is for sure here to stay in the future of phlebology, of course optimized in its performance in comparison with the current thermal tumescent radiofrequency and laser gold-standard. To do so, appropriate education of the practitioners for the correct material and methods use will be of paramount in order to minimize the human error. In this context, devices able to totally automatically provide the correct foam, made by the correct mix of drug and gas, will be of paramount importance, also in the context of the so much needed standardization for guidelines recognized by the clinical governance. Based on the empirical knowledge and the publications, proper sclerotherapy is not just a craftsman art for the many tips and tricks that can improve its performance, but also and first of all science that can and must be translated in the daily improvement of one of the most versatile and potentially effective tools at the disposal of the vein expert.

References

1. Janbon C, Laborde JC, Quere I. Aperçu historique du traitement des varices [History of the treatment of varices]. J Mal Vasc. 1994;19(3):210–5.
2. Millam D. The history of intravenous therapy. J Intraven Nurs. 1996 Jan-Feb;19(1):5–14.
3. Myers K. A history of injection treatments – II sclerotherapy. Phlebology. 2019;34:303–10.
4. Hodgson J. A treatise on the diseases of arteries and veins. London: J. Moyes; 1815.
5. Biegeleisen HI. Varicose veins, related diseases, and sclerotherapy: a guide for practitioners. USA: Eden Press; 1984.
6. Howard-Jones N. A critical study of the origins and early development of hypodermic medication. J Hist Med Allied Sci. 1947;2:201–49.
7. McLatchie JD. Treatment of varicose veins by intravenous injections. Annexe Thesis Digitisation Project 2019 Block 22;1928.
8. Orbach EJ, Petretti AK. The thrombogenic property of foam of a synthetic anionic detergent (sodium tetradecyl sulfate N.N.R.). Angiology. 1950;1:237–43.
9. McAusland S. The modern treatment of varicose veins. Med Press Cir. 1939;201:404–10.
10. Fluckiger P. Beitrag zur Technik der ambulanten Varizenbehandlung. Die Med Welt. 1963;12:617–21.
11. Gillesberger W. Die Ausrüstung des phlebologisch aktiven Dermatologen. Z Hautkrank. 1969;44:669–74.
12. Wollmann J-CGR. The history of sclerosing foams. Derm Surg. 2004;30:694–703.
13. Hobbs JT. Surgery and sclerotherapy in the treatment of varicose veins. A random trial. Arch Surg. 1974;109:793–6.
14. Hauer G. German patent DE 34 17 182 C2. Zwillings-Spritzen-Set, 9 May 1984.

15. Cabrera J, Cabrera J Jr, Garcia-Olmedo MA. New method of sclerosis in truncal varicose veins. Patol Vasc. 1995;4:35–7.
16. Monfreux A. Traitement sclérosant de grands troncs saphénes et collatéraux par la méthode MUS. Phlebologie. 1997;50:351–3.
17. Tessari L. Nouvelle technique pour l'obtention de scleromousse. Phlebologie. 1997;53:129.
18. Morrison N, Neuhardt DL, Rogers CR, McEown J, Morrison T, Johnson E, Salles-Cunha SX. Comparisons of side effects using air and carbon dioxide foam for endovenous chemical ablation. J Vasc Surg. 2008;47(4):830–6.
19. Gianesini S, Chi YW, Agüero C, et al. Fake-news-free evidence-based communication for proper vein-lymphatic disease management. Int Angiol. 2023;42(2):89–189.
20. Azmoun S, Liu Y, Tursun M, Liu S. Effect of catheter needle caliber on polidocanol foam stability in foam sclerotherapy. Front Neurol. 2024;15:1417788.
21. Lim SY, Tan JX, D'Cruz RT, Syn N, Chong TT, Tang TY. Catheter-directed foam sclerotherapy, an alternative to ultrasound-guided foam sclerotherapy for varicose vein treatment: a systematic review and meta-analysis. Phlebology. 2020;35(6):369–83.
22. Vähäaho S, Halmesmäki K, Mahmoud O, Albäck A, Noronen K, Venermo M. Three-year results of a randomized controlled trial comparing mechanochemical and thermal ablation in the treatment of insufficient great saphenous veins. J Vasc Surg Venous Lymphat Disord. 2021;9(3):652–9.
23. Bontinis V, Bontinis A, Koutsoumpelis A, et al. A network meta-analysis on the efficacy and safety of thermal and nonthermal endovenous ablation treatments. J Vasc Surg Venous Lymphat Disord. 2023;11(4):854–865.e5.
24. Leu AJ, Inderbitzi R. Balloon sclerotherapy: a new method for the treatment of truncal varicose veins. Vasa. 2008;37(2):165–73.
25. Carugo D, Ankrett DN, Zhao X, et al. Benefits of polido- canol endovenous microfoam (varithena.) compared with physician-compounded foam. Phlebology. 2016;31:283–95.
26. Kabnick LS, Jimenez JC, Coogan SM, et al. Comparative effectiveness of non-compounded polidocanol 1% endovenous microfoam (Varithena) ablation versus endovenous thermal ablation utilizing a systematic review and network meta-analysis. J Vasc Surg Venous Lymphat Disord. 2024;12(6):101896.
27. Roche E, Pons R, Roche O, et al. A new automated system for the preparation of sclerosing foam: a study of the physical characteristics produced and the device settings required. Phlebology. 2020;35(9):724–33.
28. Alongi G, Bissacco D, Cervi E. Three-year follow-up analysis of automated microfoam preparation system for great saphenous vein incompetence and varicose veins sclerotherapy treatment. Phlebology. 2024;39(7):471–6.
29. Roche E, Marqués C. First registry of patients treated with foam sclerotherapy using a new automated microfoam preparation device (2021–2022). Phlebology. 2025;40(4):235–42.
30. https://m-foamer.com.
31. Meissner MH, Di Iorio M, Davies A. 1% polidocanol endovenous microfoam (Varithena™) for the treatment of chronic venous disease: a position statement from the American Vein and Lymphatic Society. Phlebology. 2025;41(2):89–96. https://doi.org/10.1177/02683555251353150.
32. Fegan G. Varicose veins: compression sclerotherapy. Springfield: Charles Thomas; 1967.

Venous Patho-physiology Applied to the Sclerotherapy Act

2

Sergio Gianesini and Jospeh Dante Raffetto

1 Anatomy and Hemodynamics

The lower limb venous system can be divided into three compartments based on its location below, in between, or above the muscular fascia.

The deep system lies below the muscular fascia while the saphenous compartment resides in between the splitting of the muscular and saphenous fascia. The tributary system runs in the subcutaneous tissue [1, 2].

Below the muscular fascia, the pressure transmitted directly by the muscle contraction to the deep vein determines a higher velocity than the one exerted in the splitting of the fascia of the saphenous compartment. The generated pressure and the consequent velocity become even lower above the (muscular fascia?) fascia. This pressure gradient is translated into a velocity-increasing gradient from the surface toward the deepest compartments.

S. Gianesini (✉)
Department of Translational Medicine, University of Ferrara, Ferrara, Italy

Department of Surgery, Uniformed Services University of Health Sciences, Bethesda, MD, USA
e-mail: gnssrg@unife.it

J. D. Raffetto
Department of Surgery, Harvard Medical School, VA Boston Healthcare System, West Roxbury, MA, USA

Department of Surgery, Brigham and Women's Hospital, Boston, MA, USA
e-mail: joseph.raffetto@va.gov

The Venturi's effect states that the fluid will move from the slower toward the faster compartment in an aspiration (suction) effect resulting in the physiological drainage of the lower limb from the surface toward the deepest compartment [3].

Valvular incompetence leads to a subversion of this hierarchical order of venous emptying that is witnessed by a similar inversion of the related velocity gradient. In chronic venous disease, incompetent tributaries easily show higher velocities than the saphenous compartment, leading to increased turbulence and pathological wall stress with consequent inflammation [4].

The possible aspiration effect is of significant importance and consideration of the Venturi effect by the healthcare professional injecting sclerosants, particularly if in the foam formulation must be recognized because of the following principles:

1. The sclerosing agent can be inactivated by the blood flushing in the compartment by another venous region at different speeds based on the type of aspiration from one region to the other.
2. The contact time of the drug on the endothelium can be affected by the same flush speed described above (Fig. 2.1).

The communication among anatomical compartments can be realized by perforating veins connecting the deep system with the saphenous or the tributary of the saphenous system. Tributary veins can also originate and re-enter

S. Gianesini, Y. W. Chi (eds.), *Sclerotherapy*, https://doi.org/10.1007/978-3-032-32794-9_2

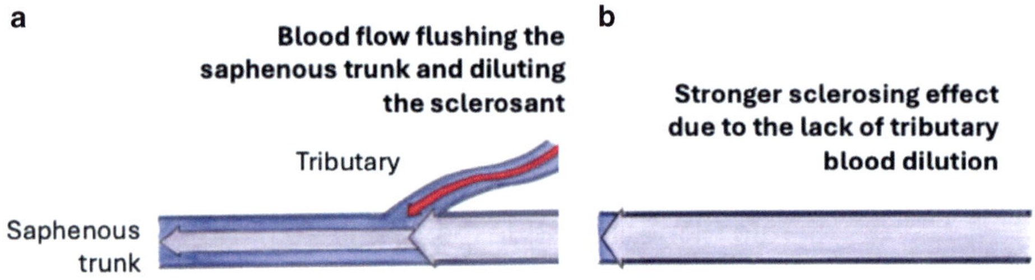

Fig. 2.1 (**a**) Sclerosant dilution/inactivation by the blood flushed in by a tributary along the targeted tract. (**b**) Sclerotherapy more intense action due to the lack of tributaries flushing along its tract. (Figure copyright: Dr. Celine Eggen (Centrum Oosterwal, Alkmaar (the Netherlands)))

in the same saphenous network. This aspect is of paramount importance in the context of a sclerotherapy injection as it can rapidly deviate the sclerosing agent delivered from the targeted compartment into another compartment/venous region.

The typical example is a very superficial tributary vein that is actually directly connected with the deep venous system, as frequently seen in muscular lower limbs of athletes. In this scenario, the healthcare professional must remember to carefully check the site and volume of the injection as it could quickly drain into the deep venous system [5].

It is important to understand the function of perforating veins as pressure equalizer between the different anatomical compartments [6].

The traditional definition of incompetence as an outward diastolic flow lasting more than 0.5 or 0.35 s should not confound the practitioner regarding the bi-directional flow of these communicating vessels [7, 8].

The multi-gate analysis of the perforating veins has demonstrated that only 84% of the outward diastolic flow lasting more than 500 ms presents a net outward diastolic flow in the thigh and decreases to 28.6% of the cases in the below knee region of the leg [9].

This hemodynamics aspect must be kept in mind whenever choosing the type of sclerosing agent and its concentration and volume as the net direction of the same drug drainage can change from case to case. This consideration applies both to the clinical scenarios dedicated to the sclerosis of the perforating veins and to the ones in which the target vein is another vessel but placed along a tract intersecting competent and/or incompetent perforators.

This concept also offers a reminder about the need of standardization and homogeneity in hemodynamics, particularly whenever dealing with scientific investigations on sclerotherapy performance.

As an example, when applying sclerotherapy along a saphenous trunk, it should be noted that the presence of multiple perforating veins along the tract, competent and/or incompetent, of small and/or large caliber, can alter the final concentration and volume that actually reaches the endothelium of the targeted vessel. For this reason, in everyday clinical practice, injecting foam in one single access for a long vein tract should be avoided in order to guarantee a homogeneous delivery of foam to act throughout the interested endothelium (Fig. 2.2).

The role of the hemodynamic load on the targeted vein segment must be considered on the targeted vein and the effect at the saphenofemoral junction, where the sclerosant agent blood-induced deactivation can significantly change based on the incompetence of the preterminal and/or terminal valve [10].

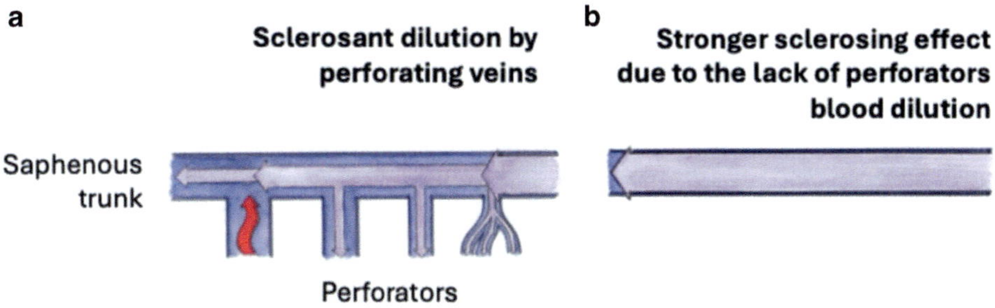

Fig. 2.2 (**a**) Presence of different perforating veins draining the sclerosant from the saphenous trunk into the deep venous system (white arrows) and/or diluting the same sclerosant by the deep venous blood reflux into the saphenous vein. (**b**) Foam sclerotherapy delivering a more powerful sclerosing process than in A due to the lack of drainage and/or dilution from the deep venous system in the depicted saphenous segment. (Figure copyright: Dr. Celine Eggen (Centrum Oosterwal, Alkmaar (the Netherlands)))

Even more, the incompetence of the ilio-femoral venous system, compared to the incompetence only of the terminal valve, can result in 5 times higher recurrence rate after sapheno-femoral ligation, highlighting the significant hemodynamic overload of sapheno-femoral junction reflux pattern delivers [11].

The choice of the correct volume, concentration, and injection site for a safe and effective sclerotherapy must include assessing the saphenous-femoral junctional reflux pattern; otherwise there is the risk of ineffective or even inadequate management.

The junctional evaluation challenge is also present in the small saphenous vein anatomic region.

A proper pre-procedural mapping is mandatory to determine the anatomical features of the sapheno-popliteal junction, including the presence of the popliteal fossa perforating veins.

The presence of popliteal fossa perforating veins has been reported in about 3% of patients. Incompetence in this segment can influence the indication toward sclerotherapy rather than surgery or endovenous thermal and non-thermal ablative procedures.

The proximity of perforating veins to the sapheno-popliteal junction in the popliteal fossa with nervous structures and/or its high flow reflux must be taken into consideration for the identification of the best therapeutic approach [12].

The sapheno-popliteal junction is an anatomic venous region of particular interest for the sclerotherapist as it is often constituted by a multi-channel network, which a sclerosing agent navigating in all these vessels can potentially provide a more complete occlusion of the whole anatomical structure compared to surgery and/or endovenous catheters.

Schweighofer et al. reported a total of 17% of specimens presenting a web-like connection at the popliteal fossa, while 6% had a duplicate junction [13].

It must also be remembered that up to 33% of sapheno-popliteal junctions are anatomically located over 12 cm from the popliteal skin crease [14].

The proper pre-operative mapping must identify the precise localization in order to guide the healthcare professional decision about the injection site, as well as the volume and concentration of the sclerosing agent (Fig. 2.3). Last but not least, the sapheno-popliteal junction represents an extremely delicate region for nerve-vessel interaction, for which the related anatomy must be known and recognized during ultrasound scanning. This

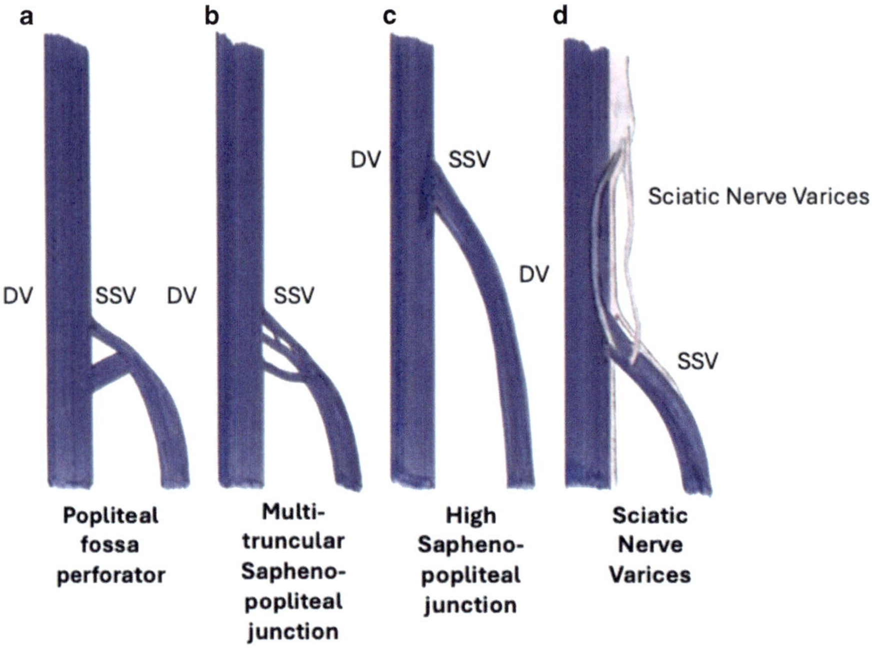

Fig. 2.3 (**a**) Popliteal Fossa perforating vein representing the main reflux source and therefore the therapeutic target, rather than the sapheno-popliteal junction. (**b**) Multi-truncular anatomy of the sapheno-popliteal junction requiring ablation of all its branches. (**c**) High sapheno-popliteal junction above the popliteal skin crease. (**d**) Sciatic nerve varices requiring special care in the vein treatment choice to avoid nerve injury favoring a sclerotherapy approach to other treatment options. DV: deep venous system. SSV: small saphenous vein. (Figure copyright: Dr. Celine Eggen (Centrum Oosterwal, Alkmaar (the Netherlands)))

includes the detection of eventual sciatic nerve varices that are not amenable to surgical or thermal procedures due to the high likelihood of nerve injury favoring a safer sclerotherapy option [15].

2 Histology

Understanding the histology of the targeted vessel is of paramount importance for proper sclerotherapy treatment. The typical example is noticed in Fig. 2.4, where the thin dilated tortuous tributary differs from the straight thicker wall saphenous trunk. Consequently, sclerosant agent selection and related concentrations and volumes must change based on the targeted vein features.

Before inducing a controlled damage of the vein wall with a sclerotherapy agent, a sclerotherapist must know the physiological histology and related changes that can occur after the sclerosing agent injection [16].

The features of the endothelium, of the media, and of the adventitia are fundamental for the sclerotherapy tailored to the targeted vein performance.

In this sense, the main target of the sclerosing agent is the endothelium.

It is formed by a mono-layer of flat cells attached to a basal lamina. These cells are metabolically active and express a cytoskeleton endowed of receptors that are fundamental for the biosignaling and the mechanotransduction of the physical forces of the venous flow into biochemical cellular messages. Laminar flows are translated into an anti-inflammatory and anti-thrombotic endothelial phenotype, turning pro-

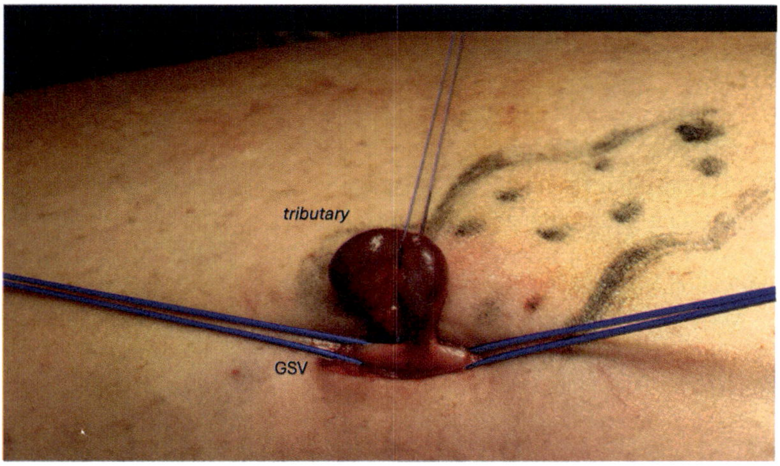

Fig. 2.4 Intraoperative picture clearly demonstrating the difference between the venous wall consistency of an incompetent tortuous tributary vein and the saphenous trunk. This aspect must be considered in the choice of the sclerosing agent and concentrations utilized. GSV: great saphenous vein

inflammatory and pro-thrombotic in case of turbulence [17–19].

Our research groups demonstrated how the suppression of the pathological reflux is able to normalize biomarkers of inflammation such as IP-10, RANTES, and PDGF [20].

Moreover, it was demonstrated the clear correlation between venous hemodynamics alteration, endothelial derangement, and release of inflammatory biomarkers [21].

The endothelial layer is kept together by different types of junctions (called tight junctions, adherens, and gap junctions).

Sclerotherapy intentionally destroys the endothelial layer and its junctions. While partial damage of these structures leads to recanalization, a properly performed sclerotherapy treatment provokes a total destruction resulting in a permanent fibrosis of the vessel [22–24].

A fundamental structure involved in this process is the glycocalyx. The glycocalyx is a carbohydrate-rich ciliary structure on the endothelium layer, composed of heparan sulfate, chondroitin sulfate, hyaluronic acid, syndecans, and glypicans.

Its main functions are to regulate the permeability of the endothelium as a sieve of various porosity, while also delivering protection to the same layer. It also regulates the coagulation balance and vessel contractility [25].

Sclerosants are able to rapidly solubilize, irritate, or damage the glycocalyx and the endothelium remaining structures, therefore exposing the endothelial membrane and initiating the cytolytic action and platelets' adhesion [26, 27].

Once the endothelium is exposed, subendothelial collagen and von Willebrand factor stimulate platelet adhesion and aggregation, leading to the creation of an initial thrombus scaffold that organizes into a fibrotic process in the following days [28–30].

Both the intrinsic and extrinsic pathways are involved. Tissue factor, expressed by the exposed subendothelial cells, binds to factor VIIa, leading to thrombin production and fibrin deposition. The initial platelets' aggregation is stabilized by this process, while fibroblasts infiltrate the coagulum. Neutrophils take 1–2 days to infiltrate the area, followed by macrophages involved in cellular debris elimination. The vascular remodeling is then mediated by cytokines such as IL-1, TNF, and VEGF.

The pillar of appropriate sclerotherapy is by achieving the perfect balance in the induction of a controlled inflammatory process. A mild inflammatory response leads to partial thrombosis, characterized by easy recanalization, while excessive wall damage can promote residual pigmentation and clinical discomfort to the patient [31, 32].

Histologically, recanalization often begins at segments where the endothelium survives sclerosant injury. Surviving endothelial cells can lead to the following events:

- Proliferate along the lumen.
- Reestablish junctions and barrier function.
- Initiate thrombolysis via fibrinolytic enzyme secretion.

Recanalization is facilitated when thrombus organization is incomplete. Histologic features include loose fibrin networks, sparse fibroblast infiltration, and inadequate collagen deposition.

MMP overactivity, insufficient TGF-β signaling, or compromised platelet aggregation can all contribute to thrombus instability [33].

Also, hemodynamic factors are involved in the possible recanalization of sclerotherapy-induced endothelial injury and thrombosis. In particular, high venous pressure can prevent thrombus compaction, hindering fibrosis, which is an aspect to take into consideration whenever injecting sclerosants near a tributary confluence.

Histological examination demonstrates persistent luminal channels lined by patchy endothelium when mechanical factors impede fibrosis [34].

Underneath the endothelium, a thin connective tissue matrix is made by collagen (type I and III), rare fibroblasts, elastic fibers, proteoglycans, and glycosaminoglycans.

Type 1 collagen is predominantly present in the adventitia and in the media, where it provides tensile strength.

Type 3 collagen is present mainly in the intima and subendothelial space, offering elasticity and reparative processes if needed.

After the endothelium is damaged by the sclerosing agent, exposed collagen mediates platelet adhesion, coagulation, and fibroblast activation [35–37].

Elastin fibers are more resistant to injury than collagen and they are relatively low in content in superficial veins compared to deep veins. High-concentration sclerosants and in particular foam sclerotherapy can fragment elastin fibers, leading to induration and long-term stiffness of the vessel [38, 39].

Fibronectin binds collagen and integrins on fibroblasts, producing a scaffold for the thrombus replacement with fibrotic tissue [40–42].

Fibroblasts are the main mediators of post-sclerotherapy vessel obliteration, and they are regulated by different cytokines and growth factors.

In particular, platelet-derived growth factor (PDGF) attracts fibroblasts to the induced thrombus. Transforming growth factor-beta (TGF-beta) differentiates fibroblasts into myofibroblasts. Vascular endothelial growth factor (VEGF) modulates angiogenesis in surrounding tissues. This process leads activated fibroblasts to migrate along fibronectin and collagen scaffolds, therefore organizing the thrombus. This migration is of paramount importance for the venous lumen obliteration, and its performance influences the recanalization risk after sclerosant injection [43–46].

Following endothelial injury, the intraluminal thrombus evolves in three stages:

(a) Acute Phase (Hours to 3 Days): Platelet-fibrin aggregation, neutrophils, and macrophages recruitment.
(b) Subacute Phase (3 Days to 2 Weeks): Fibroblast migration, initial collagen deposition, and thrombus contraction.
(c) Chronic Phase (Weeks to Months): Dense collagen deposition, vessel lumen collapse, and final fibrosis.

The evolution of endothelial injury and thrombus formation must be known by the sclerotherapist in order to plan proper follow-up and completion of any partially treated venous segments [33, 34, 47].

Fibroblasts interact with the extracellular matrix through integrins, enabling traction and contraction of collagen fibers. Myofibroblasts generate contractile forces collapsing the lumen and stabilizing the obliterated vessel [48, 49].

Matrix metalloproteinases degrade the extracellular matrix components to facilitate fibroblast migration and thrombus remodeling [50–54].

Histologic predictors of complete obliteration of sclerotherapy-treated vein include:

- Full circumferential endothelial injury.
- Adequate thrombus formation.
- Robust fibroblast recruitment and collagen deposition.
- Controlled inflammatory response.

From these aspects of endothelial injury and thrombus formation, it is important to understand why foam is more effective than liquid sclerotherapy. Foam sclerotherapy promotes complete endothelial contact with the sclerosing agent made possible by the foam ability to maximize its efficacy in the formation of a homogenous thrombus, making foam a valuable option for larger or thicker veins [55, 56].

A clear histological difference can be noted in the comparison between small superficial and deep veins. The larger vessels have an internal elastic lamina, even if often discontinuous. The presence of the internal elastic lamina provides resistance to the sclerosing agent's action, therefore requiring higher concentrations of sclerotherapy during treatment [57].

Following the dissection of the deeper layers of the vein wall, the smooth muscle and extracellular matrix component appear.

The venous tunica media is composed of circular smooth muscle cells, collagen fibers, rare elastic fibers, and interstitial matrix.

The vein decreases the amount of smooth muscle cells moving from the anatomical larger caliber veins toward the smaller superficial veins. In the most superficial layer of the skin, the media can be just a very thin strip of collagen, with very few or no muscular component.

Consequently, the more the superficial the veins are with only collagen composing the media, the more sclerotherapy injections will have to be performed at lower concentrations and at minimal injection pressures to prevent the higher risk of vessel rupture and extravasation.

Venous reflux leads to intraluminal venous hypertension that can alter the elastin and muscular components, favoring vessel dilation, with extracellular matrix expanding, leading to the instauration of a vicious cycle of histological damage and hemodynamic progressive impairment.

The progressive derangement of the endothelium layer, together with the above described muscular layer alteration induced by venous hypertension, facilitates the task of appropriate sclerotherapy in collapsing the vein and transforming it into a fibrotic chord.

This process directly involves the adventitia, which is physiologically composed of collagen, fibroblasts, mast cells, and rare elastic fibers. After the sclerotherapy injection, the adventitia produces collagen type I and III, contributing to the obliteration of the vein [30, 58].

Larger veins contain in their adventitia the vasa vasorum, which are microvessels supplying nutrients to the vein wall. The appropriate sclerosis is fundamental to avoid pain, induration, and recanalization.

The same concepts apply to the small sensory nerve fibers eventually spiraling around the target vessel. This also explains why some injections can lead to burning or stinging feelings, together with occasional paresthesia [59, 60].

Summing up in the context of venous sclerotherapy, telangiectasias are lacking smooth muscle cells and have a thin irregular basement membrane with minimal pericytic support.

Consequently, very low concentrations of sclerosant agent should be used when treating telangiectasias as they are more prone to pigmentation [31].

Reticular veins present a caliber of about 1–3 mm, have a thin yet recognizable smooth muscle layer, and when treated with sclerosing agents lead to a more consistent sclerotic/fibrotic process. Also, when treating reticular veins the concentration of the sclerosant agent must be kept at a minimal.

Another histological category can be identified in perforating veins and tributary/saphenous veins, characterized by the presence of adventitia layers and of a robust elastic lamina. In this context, foam rather than liquid sclerotherapy can be suggested to displace blood and maximize the surface contact with the endothelium.

The histological impact on clinical sclerotherapy must be taken into consideration when treating veins near the regions of venous valve levels. Valves present a specialized endothelial layer and a dense collagen and elastin structure to counteract the higher shear stress generated. This is translated in a higher resistance of the valves to the sclerotherapy action that can become evident in the form of segmental recanalization at their site. Proper sclerosing agent concentration choice must be done if a significant valvular structure is present along the targeted venous tract.

The same perivascular adipose tissue is to be looked as not a passive anatomical space, but rather as a reactive dynamic endocrine and paracrine organ releasing cytokines and venoactive substances that can influence venous tone and the inflammatory state of the treated vessel, which can include post-sclerotherapy induration phenomena [61, 62].

Consequently, special care must be used in avoiding sclerosing agent extravasation in order to avoid triggering reactions from the surrounding tissue with induration and possible fibrosis of the interstitial adipose space.

3 Sclerotherapy Complications in Histological Perspective

A partial recanalization occurs when the endothelial injury is discontinuous, the thrombus is unstable or incompletely organized, and the fibroblast migration is insufficient or when matrix metalloproteinases activity exceeds collagen deposition [33, 47, 54].

Another sclerotherapy treatment failure is represented by hyperpigmentation. Hyperpigmentation occurs when dermal macrophages phagocytose erythrocytes released during the thrombus organization. Hemosiderin deposition manifests as hyperpigmentation whose degree depends on the extent of the perivascular injury, the amount of thrombus breakdown, and the chronic inflammatory activity [56, 63–65].

Telangiectatic matting is a different process from residual hyperpigmentation and demonstrated by histology. Matting is a neoangiogenesis form occurring when angiogenic cytokines, especially VEGF, are secreted in response to incomplete thrombus organization or excessive inflammation. Telangiectatic matting occurs from an incomplete occluded leaking point and oftentimes requires a diagnostic revision of the case and a possible closure of the still persisting feeder vein.

Histologically, matting consists of thin-walled postcapillary venules, often with pericyte support [31, 66–68].

The sclerotherapy induration is associated with the excessive fibroblast activity and with the possible diffusion of sclerosant agent into the perivenous tissue. Histologically, specific inflammatory mediators are involved in the induration process of the following biological compounds:

- TGF-β upregulates collagen synthesis and myofibroblast differentiation.
- PDGF functions as a chemoattractant for fibroblasts.
- VEGF stimulates endothelial proliferation in neoangiogenesis.
- MMPs/TIMPs regulate extracellular matrix degradation and deposition.

Addressing the biological compounds involved in matting could lead to an improvement in the management of post-treatment sequelae for which they represent a possible treatment target for post-procedural venous active drugs.

Another histological complication of sclerotherapy injection is ulceration. Skin ulcerations occur when the sclerosant is too potent and/or in case of paravenous or intra-arterial injection [69].

Nerve injuries leading to paresthesia can occur following incorrect sclerotherapy injections. Superficial veins, particularly truncal veins, are closely associated with sensory nerves (saphenous, sural, lateral cutaneous branches). Nerve fibers course within the adventitia or immediately adjacent to the peri-adventitial space. An inflammatory process on the vein wall can be translated into activation of the nociceptors and exacerbated by perivascular edema compressing on the same nerve terminations. Perineural edema has been identified in related histologic sections. Minimizing nerve damage by avoiding too large a volume or too strong a concentration of sclerotherapy agent is of significant importance.

4 Sclerotherapy Agents Basic Science

A detailed description of the sclerosing agents is provided in the dedicated chapter, while herein their interaction with the vessel histology is reported.

Detergent sclerosants (polidocanol and sodium tetradecyl sulfate) solubilize the cell membranes by intercalating into the lipid bilayers. Detergents denature the cytoplasmic proteins, stimulate the cytoskeletal collapse, and cause detaching of the endothelial cells following disruption of the intercellular junctions and exposing the subendothelial collagen.

Few minutes following vein exposure to the detergent, histology shows vacuolization, nuclear condensation, and desquamation [22–24, 26, 27, 70].

Osmotic sclerosants (hypertonic dextrose or hypertonic saline) draw water from the endothelial cells by creating an osmotic gradient. The osmotic gradient leads to cell shrinkage and membrane destruction. The exposed basal lamina is associated with activation of platelet adherence. While the hyperosmolar option is effective in most superficial thin-walled veins, hyperosmolar agents are associated with a higher risk of perivascular tissue damage due to the less selective properties than the detergent agents [22, 23, 27].

Chemical irritants (chromated glycerin) induce protein denaturation and localized inflammation leading to endothelial necrosis and denudation resulting in subendothelial matrix exposure and thrombosis. The selectivity induced by chemical sclerosant damage is less than that obtained by detergents. However, controlling the depth and grade of the chemical sclerosing agent is difficult using irritants and is less commonly injected compared to the other types of sclerosants.

An important principle of sclerotherapy performance is the relation between the interaction of the sclerosing agent and the endothelial surface.

This is one of the features empowering foam formulations to increase the same endothelial lining denudation, to penetrate deeper in the vessel wall, while organizing a more structured initial thrombotic scaffold [55, 70].

It is well known that foam sclerotherapy compared to liquid sclerotherapy offers the advantage of displacing blood, hence avoiding dilution and inactivation of the sclerosing agent. Indeed, blood proteins are responsible for the rapid binding and neutralization of the sclerosing drug.

In a histologic comparison, it is evident how foam can produce a homogeneous endothelial derangement, even in large veins, while liquid sclerosants leave discontinuity in the injury pattern on the endothelial lining, with incomplete initial thrombus formation and a related higher risk of recanalization [55].

5 Integrating Histology and Clinical Decision-Making

The sclerosant choice and technique must bc adapted to the vein type:

(a) *Telangiectasias* (<1 mm) are thin-walled postcapillary venules, with minimal smooth muscle, highly responsive to low-concentration sclerosants. Histology predicts rapid endothelial destruction with minimal risk of deep tissue injury.
(b) *Reticular veins* (1–3 mm) are thin but with a continuous smooth muscle layer for which an increase in sclerosant concentration is required.
(c) *Perforator and truncal veins* (>3 mm) present a thicker media, a developed adventitia, and a partial elastic lamina. Foam formulations provide superior endothelial contact and uniform thrombus formation in this context.

In order to prevent complications from sclerotherapy, patient follow-up according to the histological changes is important:

- *Early Phase (1–2 Weeks)*: The time of thrombus organization and neutrophil/macrophage infiltration. In this phase, it is important to monitor for inflammation or matting.
- *Intermediate Phase (2–6 Weeks)*: This phase occurs when fibroblasts migrate, the extracellular matrix is altered, and the lumen begins to collapse. In this stage, optimizing fibrosis is fundamental. While evidence is lacking, keeping graduated compression in this phase is an empirical suggestion that has very limited risk and a potential benefit in favoring the sclerosis process.
- *Late Phase (2–6 Months)*: During this phase, a dense collagen structure is formed and the treated vessel is obliterated. Histology confirms the lumen closure or the eventual residual recanalization. In this stage, patient assessment including ultrasound scanning is recommended to confirm the result of the procedure.

In conclusion, the integration of histology into sclerotherapy is necessary for the healthcare professional interested in delivering an effective procedure with durable results and minimizing complications.

In particular, the practitioner must be familiar with the anatomy, hemodynamics, venous wall architecture, the endothelial biology, the extracellular matrix remodeling, and fibroblast activation. By understanding the principles of venous anatomy, venous structures, and composition, the pathophysiologic process of sclerotherapy interaction on the vessel lumen, and by selecting the proper sclerosing agent, concentration, and volume will enhance the clinician's efficacy and skill to perform safe and effective sclerotherapy.

References

1. Recek C. Pump activity influencing venous hemodynamics in the lower extremity. Int J Angiol. 2013;22:23–30.
2. Gianesini S, Occhionorelli S, Menegatti E, et al. CHIVA strategy in chronic venous disease treatment: instructions for users. Phlebology. 2015;30:157–71.
3. Gianesini S, Sisini F, Di Domenico G, et al. Lower limbs venous kinetics and consequent impact on drainage direction. Phlebology. 2018;33(2):107–14.
4. Gianesini S, Sisini F, Menegatti E, et al. Altered velocity gradient in lower limb chronic venous disease. Phlebology. 2019;34(1):17–24.
5. Davies CE, White AM, Whiteley MS. Varicose vein appearance caused by perforating vein incompetence detected after intense cycling. SAGE Open Med Case Rep. 2017;5:2050313X17747490.
6. Recek C. Competent and incompetent calf perforators in primary varicose veins: a resistant myth. Phlebology. 2016;31:532e40.
7. Sarin S, Scurr JH, Smith PD. Medial calf perforators in venous disease: the significance of outward flow. J Vasc Surg. 1992;16:40e6.
8. Labropoulos N, Mansour MA, Kang SS, Gloviczki P, Baker WH. New insights into perforator vein incompetence. Eur J Vasc Endovasc Surg. 1999;18:228e34.
9. Gianesini S, Menegatti E, Sisini F, et al. Comparison between duplex ultrasound and multigate quality doppler profile software in the assessment of lower limb perforating vein direction. Eur J Vasc Endovasc Surg. 2018;55(5):688–93.
10. Cappelli M, Molino Lova R, Ermini S, et al. Hemodynamics of the sapheno-femoral junction. Patterns of reflux and their clinical implications. Int Angiol. 2004;23(1):25–8.
11. Gianesini S, Occhionorelli S, Menegatti E, et al. Femoral vein valve incompetence as a risk factor for junctional recurrence. Phlebology. 2018;33(3):206–12.
12. Delis KT, Knaggs AL, Hobbs JT, Vandendriessche MA. The nonsaphenous vein of the popliteal fossa: prevalence, patterns of reflux, hemodynamic quantification, and clinical significance. J Vasc Surg. 2006;44(3):611–9.
13. Schweighofer G, Mühlberger D, Brenner E. The anatomy of the small saphenous vein: fascial and neural relations, saphenofemoral junction, and valves. J Vasc Surg. 2010;51(4):982–9.
14. Creton D. Saphenopopliteal junctions are significantly lower when incompetent. Embryological hypothesis and surgical implications. Phlebolymphology J. 2025;48:347–54.

15. Gianesini S, Menegatti E, Tacconi G, Scognamillo F, Liboni A, Zamboni P. Echo-guided foam sclerotherapy treatment of venous malformation involving the sciatic nerve. Phlebology. 2009;24(1):46–7.
16. Bergan JJ, Schmid-Schönbein GW, Smith PD, et al. Chronic venous disease. N Engl J Med. 2006;355:488–98.
17. Michel CC, Curry FE. Microvascular permeability. Physiol Rev. 1999;79(3):703–61.
18. Aird WC. Phenotypic heterogeneity of the endothelium: I. Structure, function, and mechanisms. Circ Res. 2007;100(2):158–73.
19. Curry FE, Adamson RH. Endothelial glycocalyx: permeability barrier and mechanosensor. Ann Biomed Eng. 2012;40(4):828–39.
20. Tisato V, Zauli G, Gianesini S, et al. Modulation of circulating cytokine-chemokine profile in patients affected by chronic venous insufficiency undergoing surgical hemodynamic correction. J Immunol Res. 2014;2014:473765.
21. Tisato V, Zauli G, Voltan R, et al. Endothelial cells obtained from patients affected by chronic venous disease exhibit a pro-inflammatory phenotype. PLoS One. 2012;7(6):e39543.
22. Hamel-Desnos CM, Desnos PR, Ferre B, Le Querrec A. In vivo biological effects of foam sclerotherapy. Eur J Vasc Endovasc Surg. 2011 Aug;42(2):238–45.
23. Weiss MA, Hsu JT, Neuhaus I, et al. Consensus for sclerotherapy. Dermatol Surg. 2014 Dec;40(12):1309–18.
24. Bai T, Jiang W, Chen Y, et al. Effect of Multiple Factors on Foam Stability in Foam Sclerotherapy. Sci Rep. 2018 Oct 24;8(1):15683.
25. Diaz JA, Gianesini S, Khalil RA. Glycocalyx disruption, endothelial dysfunction and vascular remodeling as underlying mechanisms and treatment targets of chronic venous disease. Int Angiol. 2024;43(6):563–90.
26. Chwała M, Szczeklik W, Szczeklik M, et al. Varicose veins of lower extremities, hemodynamics and treatment methods. Adv Clin Exp Med. 2015 Jan-Feb;24(1):5–14.
27. Guex JJ. Microsclerotherapy. Semin Dermatol. 1993 Jun;12(2):129–34.
28. Wakefield TW, Myers DD, Henke PK. Mechanisms of venous thrombosis and resolution. Arterioscler Thromb Vasc Biol. 2008;28(3):387–91.
29. Esmon CT. The interactions between inflammation and coagulation. Br J Haematol. 2005;131(4):417–30.
30. Evans CE, Iruela-Arispe ML, Zhao YY. Mechanisms of endothelial regeneration and vascular repair and their application to regenerative medicine. Am J Pathol. 2021;191(1):52–65.
31. Goldman MP, Sadick NS, Weiss RA. Cutaneous necrosis, telangiectatic matting, and hyperpigmentation following sclerotherapy. Etiology, prevention, and treatment. Dermatol Surg. 1995 Jan;21(1):19–29.
32. Taghinia AH, Upton J. Vascular Anomalies. J Hand Surg Am. 2018 Dec;43(12):1113–21.
33. Chabasse C, Siefert SA, Chaudry M, et al. Recanalization and flow regulate venous thrombus resolution and matrix metalloproteinase expression in vivo. J Vasc Surg Venous Lymphat Disord. 2015;3(1):64–74.
34. Mukhopadhyay S, Johnson TA, Duru N, et al. Fibrinolysis and inflammation in venous thrombus resolution. Front Immunol. 2019;10:1348.
35. Galley HF, Webster NR. Physiology of the endothelium. Br J Anaesth. 2004 Jul;93(1):105–13.
36. Ruggeri ZM. Adhesion mechanisms in platelet function. Circ Res. 2007;100(12):1673–85.
37. Farndale RW. The role of collagen in thrombosis and hemostasis. J Thromb Haemost. 2004;2(4):561–73.
38. Wali MA, al-Muzaini H, al-Sabti H. Changes of elastic and collagen fibers in varicose veins. Int Angiol. 2002;21(4):337–43.
39. Lim CS, Davies AH. Pathogenesis of primary varicose veins. Br J Surg. 2009 Nov;96(11):1231–42.
40. Singh P, Carraher C, Schwarzbauer JE. Assembly of fibronectin extracellular matrix. Annu Rev Cell Dev Biol. 2010;26:397–419.
41. Kanta J, Zavadakova A. Role of fibronectin in chronic venous diseases: A review. Vasc Med. 2020 Dec;25(6):588–97.
42. Patten J, Wang K. Fibronectin in development and wound healing. Adv Drug Deliv Rev. 2021 Mar;170:353–68.
43. Clark RA, Folkvord JM, Hart CE, et al. Platelet isoforms of platelet-derived growth factor stimulate fibroblasts to contract collagen matrices. J Clin Invest. 1989;84(4):1436–40.
44. Deng Z, Fan T, Xiao C, et al. TGF-β signaling in health, disease, and therapeutics. Signal Transduct Target Ther. 2024;9(1):61.
45. Chaudhary NI, et al. Inhibition of PDGF, VEGF and FGF signalling attenuates fibrosis. Eur Respir J. 2007;29(5):976–85.
46. Raffetto JD, Khalil RA. Mechanisms of lower extremity vein dysfunction in chronic venous disease. Int Angiol. 2021;40(4):370–8.
47. Savchenko AS, Martinod K, Seidman MA, et al. Neutrophil extracellular traps form predominantly during the organizing stage of human venous thromboembolism development. J Thromb Haemost. 2014;12(6):860–70.
48. Kattan WM, Alarfaj SF, Alnooh BM, et al. Myofibroblast-Mediated Contraction. J Coll Physicians Surg Pak. 2017 Jan;27(1):38–43.
49. Siadat SM, Ruberti JW. Mechanochemistry of collagen. Acta Biomater. 2023 Jun;163:50–62.
50. Mastenbroek TG, Feijge MA, Kremers RM, et al. Platelet-associated matrix metalloproteinases regulate thrombus formation and exert local collagenolytic activity. Arterioscler Thromb Vasc Biol. 2015;35(12):2554–61.
51. Nguyen KP, McGilvray KC, Puttlitz CM, et al. Matrix metalloproteinase-9 regulates vein wall biomechanics in murine thrombus resolution. PLoS One. 2015;10(9):e0139145.

52. Lu MJ, Zhang JQ, Nie ZY, et al. Monocyte/macrophage-mediated venous thrombus resolution. Front Immunol. 2024 Jul 19;15:1429523.
53. Deatrick KB, Obi A, Luke CE, et al. Matrix metalloproteinase-9 deletion is associated with decreased mid-term vein wall fibrosis in experimental stasis DVT. Thromb Res. 2013 Sep;132(3):360–6.
54. Kuzuya M, Iguchi A. Role of matrix metalloproteinases in vascular remodeling. J Atheroscler Thromb. 2003;10(5):275–82.
55. Hamel-Desnos C, Allaert FA. Liquid versus foam sclerotherapy: a systematic review. Phlebology. 2009;24(4):180–5.
56. Cabrera J, Fernández-García MD, García-Girón C, et al. Evaluation of the efficacy of polidocanol in the form of foam compared with liquid form in sclerotherapy of the greater saphenous vein: initial results. Dermatologic Surg. 2004;30(5):641–5.
57. Meissner MH. Lower extremity venous anatomy. Semin Intervent Radiol. 2005;22(3):147–56.
58. Raffetto JD, Mannello F. Pathophysiology of chronic venous disease. Int Angiol. 2014;33(3):212–21.
59. Price C. The anatomy of the saphenous nerve in the lower leg with particular reference to its relationship to the long saphenous vein. J Cardiovasc Surg (Torino). 1990 May-Jun;31(3):294–7.
60. Hwang J, Kim HJ. Superficial nerves of the leg: considerations for sclerotherapy and surgery. Anat Cell Biol. 2015;48(4):298–302.
61. Koenen M, Hill MA, Cohen P, et al. Obesity, Adipose Tissue and Vascular Dysfunction. Circ Res. 2021 Apr 2;128(7):951–68.
62. Stanek A, Brożyna-Tkaczyk K, Myśliński W. The Role of Obesity-Induced Perivascular Adipose Tissue (PVAT) Dysfunction in Vascular Homeostasis. Nutrients. 2021 Oct 28;13(11):3843.
63. Bossart S, Daneluzzi C, Cazzaniga S, et al. Skin hyperpigmentation after sclerotherapy with polidocanol: A systematic review. J Eur Acad Dermatol Venereol. 2023 Feb;37(2):274–83.
64. Aronniemi J, Castrén E, Lappalainen K, et al. Sclerotherapy complications of peripheral venous malformations. Phlebology. 2016 Dec;31(10):712–22.
65. Rabe E, Pannier F. Sclerotherapy of varicose veins with polidocanol based on the guidelines of the German Society of Phlebology. Dermatol Surg. 2010 Jun;36 Suppl 2:968–75.
66. Bertanha M, Jaldin RG, Moura R, et al. Sclerotherapy for Reticular Veins in the Lower Limbs: A Triple-Blind Randomized Clinical Trial. JAMA Dermatol. 2017 Dec 1;153(12):1249–55.
67. Ferrara N. Vascular endothelial growth factor: basic science and clinical progress. Endocr Rev. 2004;25(4):581–611.
68. Cabral G, Batagini N, Zerati A, et al. Telangiectatic Matting as a Complication After Aesthetic Procedures: A Case Report. Cureus. 2026 May 6;18(5):e108372.
69. Wong M, Parsi K, Myers K, et al. Sclerotherapy of lower limb veins: indications, contraindications and treatment strategies to prevent complications – a consensus document of the International Union of Phlebology-2023. Phlebology. 2023;38(4):205–58.
70. Joyce DP, De Freitas S, Woo EY, et al. Ultrasound-guided foam sclerotherapy as a therapeutic modality in venous ulceration. Surgeon. 2022 Oct;20(5):e206–13.

Sclerosing Agents

3

Sergio Gianesini, Makoto Mo, and Yung Wei Chi

1 Sclerosing Agents' Classification

The foundations of sclerotherapy date back to the seventeenth century, though early attempts were characterized by unacceptable complication rates. Successive refinements in chemical formulation marked distinct eras in sclerosant development. Early agents—including absolute alcohols, perchlorates, and iodine compounds—produced excessive tissue necrosis and systemic toxicity, limiting their viability. The advent of hypertonic saline in the mid-twentieth century represented an important shift toward safer osmotic agents, though injection pain and endothelial damage variability restricted widespread adoption [1]. The development of detergent sclerosants in the 1940s and 1950s laid the groundwork for modern practice. With the introduction of polidocanol (POL) in the 1960s and sodium tetradecyl sulfate (STS) in 1946, sclerotherapy acquired predictable pharmacologic behavior, improved tolerability, and broader international acceptance [2]. Subsequent decades expanded the role of these agents through investigations into foam sclerotherapy, which emerged in the 1990s and demonstrated superior efficacy for larger-diameter veins [3]. Today, POL and STS remain dominant, while osmotic agents retain niche roles. Their extensive clinical experience and regulatory approvals form much of the contemporary evidence base, enabling refined treatment algorithms for vein disease.

Sclerosants are broadly categorized into three categories:

1. Detergent sclerosants (e.g., polidocanol, sodium tetradecyl sulfate, ethanolamine oleate).
2. Osmotic sclerosants (e.g., hypertonic saline, hypertonic saline-dextrose combinations).
3. Chemical irritants (historical or specialized) (e.g., chromated glycerin, polyiodinated iodine solutions, absolute ethanol).

Each class exerts a distinct mechanism of endothelial damage, which in turn determines potency, safety profile, and optimal clinical use. Contemporary clinical practice relies primarily on POL and STS, as these agents combine high efficacy with low toxicity. Detergent (surfactant) agents act by disrupting lipid molecules within

S. Gianesini (✉)
Department of Translational Medicine, University of Ferrara, Ferrara, Italy

Department of Surgery, Uniformed Services University of Health Sciences, Bethesda, MD, USA
e-mail: gnssrg@unife.it

M. Mo
Department of Surgery, Yokohama City University, Yokohama, Japan

Japanese Society of Phlebology, Namiki Clinic, Yokohama, Japan

Y. W. Chi
Department of Cardiovascular Medicine, University of California, Davis Vascular Center, Sacramento, CA, USA

S. Gianesini, Y. W. Chi (eds.), *Sclerotherapy*, https://doi.org/10.1007/978-3-032-32794-9_3

the endothelial cell membrane. Their amphipathic structure allows them to insert into the lipid bilayer, causing rapid loss of membrane integrity, protein denaturation, cell lysis, exposure of subendothelial collagen, and initiation of thrombotic occlusion. They are potent even at low concentrations and allow formulation as foam, dramatically increasing surface contact and reducing dilution by blood [4]. Detergent sclerosants, including POL and STS, are amphiphilic molecules that disrupt endothelial cell membranes by altering lipid bilayer integrity. Their capacity for foam conversion provides enhanced potency and prolonged contact with the endothelium. These agents are the preferred choice for most leg vein applications [5]. Osmotic agents, such as sodium chloride (hypertonic saline) or sodium chloride combined with dextrose, rely on endothelial dehydration and protein denaturation. This results in endothelial shrinkage, intercellular junction breakdown, and subsequent thrombosis. Their efficacy is highly concentration-dependent, and they perform poorly when diluted by blood. They are less potent, require precise intraluminal placement, and cannot be foamed, making them primarily suitable for smaller, superficial telangiectasias. Chemical irritant agents, such as chromated glycerin, produce endothelial destruction through direct cellular toxicity. This leads to intense inflammatory reaction and high rates of irreversible fibrosis.

Although potent, they have limited availability and are used selectively due to greater risks of pigmentation and necrosis [6]. Independent of chemical class, all sclerosants aim to produce acute endothelial destruction leading to thrombotic occlusion, inflammation, and fibrotic remodeling of the treated vein. Sclerosis occurs in several stages: immediate endothelial cell death, subsequent platelet aggregation and thrombus formation, activation of inflammatory cascades, and progressive fibrosis with eventual obliteration of the lumen. The extent of destruction is influenced by concentration, volume, endothelial contact time, and the physical form (foam vs. liquid). Foam sclerotherapy enhances endothelial contact while displacing intravascular blood, increasing the efficiency of damage especially in larger veins [7]. Detergent sclerosants possess hydrophilic and hydrophobic domains that interact with endothelial cell membranes. Their mechanism involves the solubilization of membrane proteins and lipids, leading to morphological disruption and cell lysis. The effect is concentration-dependent and largely independent of blood pH or osmolarity. They retain efficacy even when diluted by blood, contributing to their predictable behavior under clinical conditions [8].

Osmotic agents induce endothelial damage through rapid osmotic shifts that desiccate and disrupt the cellular cytoplasm. Hypertonic saline creates intense osmotic gradients, drawing water out of endothelial cells, leading to dehydration, protein denaturation, and eventual cell death. However, efficacy is dependent on non-dilution by intravascular blood; even small volumes of blood mixing can significantly reduce potency. This requirement for precise intravascular placement limits their utility in tortuous or higher-diameter leg veins [9]. Chemical irritant sclerosants exert their effect through direct protein denaturation and cytotoxicity. Glycerin-based agents penetrate cells and denature intracellular proteins, culminating in rapid endothelial destruction. These agents may produce more intense pain and hyperpigmentation, necessitating cautious use.

2 Detergent Sclerosants

2.1 Polidocanol (Lauromacrogol 400)

Polidocanol is a non-ionic detergent sclerosant widely regarded for its safety and versatility. Derived from macrogol ethers (an alkyl polyglycol ether with amphiphilic properties), POL exhibits anesthetic properties that contribute to its favorable tolerability profile. Following injection, a portion of the agent binds plasma proteins immediately, while the remainder interacts with endothelial membranes.

It is approved for both liquid and foam formulations and is used for veins ranging from telangiectasias to saphenous trunks. POL acts by altering the surface tension of endothelial cell membranes, inducing reversible lipid layer expansion followed by irreversible membrane disruption. It is metabolized hepatically and renally, with a high therapeutic index and low systemic toxicity. Systemic levels after standard sclerotherapy doses remain far below toxic thresholds, even when treating extensive varicosities with foam. The elimination half-life is short—typically under 10 minutes—primarily because its detergent activity is neutralized almost instantly by plasma proteins. This rapid neutralization explains why systemic reactions are generally mild and transient and why POL is considered one of the safest sclerosants for repeated or high-volume injections [10]. When used in foam form, its potency increases several-fold due to improved endothelial contact [11].

Liquid POL is commonly employed for telangiectasias (0.25–0.5%), reticular veins (0.5–1.0%), and small varicosities. Foam POL (1–3%) is applied to larger tributary veins and incompetent saphenous trunks, often in outpatient settings. Numerous controlled trials have validated POL's efficacy in leg vein sclerotherapy, with occlusion rates exceeding 80–90% in appropriately selected veins [12].

POL demonstrates low rates of pain, pigmentation, and inflammatory responses compared with other agents [6]. Nevertheless, it can provoke transient visual disturbances, migraines, or chest tightness when used in foam form, likely due to microembolization phenomena; these events are typically self-limited [13]. A 2021 review highlighted the impossibility to report with strong certainty of evidence eventual differences in safety and occlusion rate performances among the different sclerosing agents, for which more appropriately collected and real-world scenario data are needed [14].

2.2 Sodium Tetradecyl Sulfate (STS)

STS is an anionic detergent sclerosant introduced in the mid-twentieth century. It remains a widely used and highly effective agent with robust clinical outcomes across a broad range of vein sizes.

STS is a derivative of sulfuric acid and acts by causing immediate denaturation of endothelial proteins, leading to cell death and subsequent fibrotic occlusion. Compared to POL, STS is generally considered more potent on a per-concentration basis. While also rapidly inactivated, it binds more aggressively to plasma proteins and has a higher potential for immunogenic interactions. Trace systemic levels have been measured for up to 30 minutes after large-volume injections, although concentrations remain low. Unlike POL, STS has documented cases of true IgE-mediated anaphylaxis, attributed partly to its protein-denaturation behavior that may generate antigenic complexes [15]. Liquid STS in lower concentrations (0.1–0.5%) is used for telangiectasias and small reticular veins, while higher concentrations (1–3%) are used for larger tributaries. Foam STS is commonly used for saphenous veins trunk as well as large residual varicosities, with multiple studies validating its effectiveness and durability [12]. Adverse effects include pigmentation, matting, localized pain, and urticaria. STS is associated with a higher incidence of anaphylactic reactions compared with POL due to its protein-denaturation mechanism [16]. Foam formulations may induce systemic symptoms similar to POL, though serious events remain rare. Table 3.1 sums up the suggested concentrations for the two main drugs used to perform both liquid and foam sclerotherapies. It must be noted that the herein reported table follows the empirical experience of the authors of this chapter and it does not represent a universally approved indication from the regulatory bodies of the different nations. Moreover, it must be highlighted how anatomical, histological, hemodynamics, clinical, and foam production methods can influence the final concentration and volume choice. For example, an immediately under-the-skin vein will lead to a decrease in the concentration to avoid eventual excessive inflammatory visible reactions that could lead to hyperpigmentation and/or induration.

Table 3.1 Empirically suggested concentration of POL and STS, in liquid and foam. The concentrations must be adjusted taking into consideration the specifics of each and every single case, based also on anatomical, histological, hemodynamic, clinical, and foam production aspects

Vein type	POL (%) liquid	POL (%) foam	STS (%) liquid	STS (%) foam
Teleangectasia	0.25–0.5	0.25	0.1–0.2	X
Reticular vein	0.5–1	0.25–0.5	0.2–0.5	0.2
Small varicosities (<4 mm)	1	0.5–1	0.5–1	0.5
Large varicosities (>4 mm)	2	1	1	0.5–1
Saphenous trunk	3	3	3	3
Perforator	3	3	3	3

A nearby venous confluence flushing blood at consistent speed and eventual turbulence will lead to an increase in the chosen concentration to counteract the same blood dilution effect. A saphenous trunk, because of its thicker and more endowed with muscular and connective tissue wall compared to a superficial tributary vein, will require a more aggressive sclerotherapy [17]. Last but not least, the foam production method can significantly influence the performance of the sclerosing act for which a "one concentration table fits all" format cannot be used. Indeed, the automated system producing 1% POL microfoam with nitrogen concentration <0.8% recently demonstrated competitiveness with both thermal tumescent and physician-compounded foam. A detailed analysis of this aspect is reported in the dedicated foam chapter of this textbook [18]. Further work is suggested to international scientific societies and clinical governance entities to produce detailed validated evidence-based concentration and volume tables that can guide the user in a therapeutic choice that must take into consideration far more variables than just the target vessel caliber.

Moreover, different countries follow different clinical governance approvals. The authors of this chapter recommend to follow the physician's own country regulatory indications.

2.3 Sodium Morrhuate

Sodium morrhuate is a mixture of sodium salts of unsaturated fatty acids, primarily oleic, palmitoleic, and linoleic acids. It functions as a surface-active detergent, disrupting lipid membranes and endothelial integrity upon intravascular injection [19]. Commercial preparations were historically available in concentrations ranging from 5% to 10%, typically supplied as sterile aqueous solutions buffered to physiologic pH. The detergent nature of sodium morrhuate results in nonselective cytotoxicity, accounting for both its efficacy and its propensity for adverse reactions [20]. In contemporary practice, its use is largely restricted due to safety concerns. It may still be encountered in resource-limited settings, patients intolerant to alternative agents, situations requiring strong sclerosant action in large-caliber veins. Documented adverse effects include severe pain during injection, skin necrosis following extravasation, ulceration and scarring, persistent hyperpigmentation. The risk of IgE-mediated hypersensitivity is notably higher with sodium morrhuate than with synthetic sclerosants [21, 22].

2.4 Ethanolamine Oleate

Ethanolamine oleate (EO) is a sclerosing agent with a long history of use in the treatment of varicose veins and other venous disorders such as esophageal varices or venous malformation. Chemically, EO is the oleic acid ester of ethanolamine and is classified among detergent sclerosants, sharing mechanistic features with sodium tetradecyl sulfate (STS) and polidocanol. Its amphipathic structure allows interaction with lipid membranes and plasma proteins, resulting in endothelial injury and subsequent venous obliteration. The primary mechanism of action of EO involves direct endothelial cytotoxicity through protein denaturation and disruption of cell membrane integrity. Contact between EO and the venous intima leads to endothelial desquamation, exposure of subendothelial collagen and activation of platelets and the coagulation cascade. This process results in intraluminal thrombosis, which subsequently undergoes organization and fibrotic transformation, ultimately producing permanent occlusion of the treated vein. Clinically, EO has been used primarily in liquid form for the treatment of reticular veins, varicose tributaries, and selected perforating veins. Reported concentrations range from 1% to 5%, with higher concentrations associated with increased endothelial destruction but also greater local inflammatory response and pain. Historically, EO was widely used in Europe and Asia before the broader adoption of polidocanol and STS, which offer improved tolerability profiles. Although EO can be prepared as a foam, its use in foam sclerotherapy is less common in contemporary practice due to limited standardization and a relative paucity of comparative safety data. Adverse effects associated with EO reflect its intermediate irritant potential. Common local reactions include injection pain, superficial thrombophlebitis, hyperpigmentation, and telangiectatic matting. Skin necrosis may occur following extravasation or inadvertent intra-arterial injection, though this remains uncommon with appropriate technique. Systemic complications are rare but hypersensitivity reactions have been reported. Compared with absolute ethanol, EO demonstrates a more controlled and localized injury pattern, with a lower incidence of severe tissue necrosis, albeit at the cost of reduced sclerosant potency. Histopathologic studies of veins treated with EO demonstrate complete endothelial loss, mural inflammation, and progressive replacement of thrombus by collagen-rich fibrous tissue. These changes are consistent with those observed following treatment with other detergent sclerosants, though EO may induce a more pronounced inflammatory infiltrate than polidocanol at equivalent concentrations [3]. In summary, while its role in modern phlebology has diminished in favor of agents with superior tolerability and a broader evidence base, EO remains a valid option for selected varicose veins when used by experienced practitioners with careful attention to technique and dosing [23].

3 Osmotic Sclerosants

3.1 Hypertonic Saline

Hypertonic saline (typically 20–23.4% sodium chloride) is a long-standing sclerosant known for its simplicity and purity but is associated with significant injection pain and localized irritation. Its mechanism relies solely on osmotic endothelial dehydration. Because efficacy is completely eliminated by dilution with blood, hypertonic saline requires precise intraluminal injection and is unsuitable for tortuous veins or veins larger than 1–2 mm in diameter. Owing to injection discomfort and limited potency, hypertonic saline is used primarily for very small telangiectasias, often in cosmetic practice. It cannot be used in foam form, significantly limiting its flexibility. Pain and burning sensations are common. Extravasation may cause ulceration or skin necrosis, and hypertonic saline may trigger vasovagal reactions. Pigmentation rates can be high if not properly managed. Hypertonic saline has no metabolic pathway; it is simply diluted in the bloodstream and contributes transiently to plasma osmolarity. When used in small volumes for telangiectasias, systemic osmotic effects are negligible [24]. Larger volumes, however, may cause discomfort, red cell crenation, or temporary fluid shifts if inadvertently injected in excessive quantities.

3.2 Hyperosmolar Saline-Dextrose Mixtures

Mixtures of sodium chloride and dextrose (e.g., 72% glycerin-based or NaCl–dextrose combinations) aim to reduce injection pain and enhance endothelial injury. Although less painful than pure hypertonic saline, these mixtures still require perfect intraluminal placement and cannot be used for larger veins. They may be employed for delicate telangiectasias where minimal inflammatory response is desired [25].

4 Chemical Irritant Sclerosants

4.1 Chromated Glycerin and Glycerin Solutions

Glycerin-based sclerosants (including 72% glycerin with chromated compounds in some regions) are both osmotic and irritant agents, as they exert also a potent endothelial toxicity, yet with minimal thrombosis formation. They are favored for extremely superficial or delicate telangiectasias in selected practices [26]. Their injection is associated with burning, and extravasation may produce pigmentation. Many countries have restricted availability due to concerns about contaminant toxicity and inconsistent formulations [27, 28]. Glycerin itself is metabolized through standard hepatic pathways, while chromated compounds carry toxicological considerations that have limited their availability [28].

4.2 Sodium Iodide and Polyiodide Solutions

These sclerosing agents are used mainly in older sclerotherapy protocols, now replaced by safer agents.

4.3 Sodium Salicylate

The use of salicylate compounds in venous sclerotherapy dates to the early- and mid-twentieth century, a period characterized by empirical exploration of injectable agents capable of producing controlled venous injury. Sodium salicylate was introduced as an alternative to more aggressive corrosive substances such as chromated glycerin or sodium morrhuate, offering a balance between endothelial toxicity and systemic tolerability [29]. Its adoption was particularly notable in Europe, where investigators sought sclerosants with predictable inflammatory responses and reduced risk of skin necrosis. Although sodium salicylate has largely fallen out of routine use with the advent of safer and more controllable detergent agents, it remains relevant from a historical, mechanistic, and comparative standpoint and continues to be referenced in specialized or resource-limited contexts. Sodium salicylate is the sodium salt of salicylic acid, with the chemical formula $C_7H_5NaO_3$. It is highly water-soluble and exhibits weak acidic properties in solution. Unlike detergent sclerosants, sodium salicylate does not disrupt lipid membranes through surfactant activity; rather, its sclerosing effect is mediated through direct chemical irritation and inflammation of the venous endothelium. Pharmacologically, salicylates are best known for their systemic anti-inflammatory, antipyretic, and analgesic effects. Paradoxically, when administered intravascularly at high local concentrations, sodium salicylate exerts a pronounced pro-inflammatory and cytotoxic effect on endothelial cells, leading to localized vascular injury without significant systemic absorption when used in appropriate doses. Early clinical series reported satisfactory obliteration rates for reticular veins and small varicosities using sodium salicylate, with success rates comparable to other sclerosants available at the time. However, efficacy in larger truncal veins was inconsistent, with higher recanalization rates compared to modern detergent agents. The relatively slow and inflammation-dependent mechanism of action may account for both its effectiveness in small-caliber veins and its limitations in larger venous segments, where blood flow rapidly dilutes the agent.

4.4 Absolute Ethanol

Absolute ethanol is an extremely potent sclerosant used mainly in interventional radiology for arteriovenous malformations. It causes complete endothelial and mural destruction, but with potential high rate of pain and complications. It is not used for routine venous insufficiency. It is usually indicated for extensive or infiltrative venous malformations, refractory lesions, and selected high-flow malformations with flow control. Ethanol is also used in mixed veno-lymphatic malformations. Extreme care must be applied in its use as complications include cardiopulmonary collapse, pulmonary hypertension, and nerve injury [30, 31].

4.5 Bleomycin

Bleomycin is an antineoplastic antibiotic with sclerosant properties mediated through DNA strand breaks and induction of endothelial apoptosis. Its effect is slower and less inflammatory than ethanol. It is indicated for lymphatic malformations, particularly macrocystic and mixed lesions, and selected venous malformations in anatomically sensitive areas such as the head and neck. To the contrary it shows lower efficacy in purely venous lesions compared with ethanol. Possible complications are fever, localized swelling, skin hyperpigmentation. Pulmonary toxicity is a possible concern, although rare at sclerotherapy doses [32, 33].

4.6 Doxycycline

Doxycycline acts as a sclerosant through inflammatory cytokine induction and inhibition of matrix metalloproteinases. It is widely used in lymphatic malformations. It can cause pain, fever, transient nerve irritation, and it brings a risk of tooth discoloration in young children [34].

5 Safety General Considerations

This chapter is focused on the two main detergent sclerosant agents (POL and STS) and on the dextrose solutions, as the most used worldwide. Specifics related to foam formulation and to malformations are to be found in the dedicated chapters. Both STS and POL are extremely safe if administered by expert physicians using appropriate technique and materials. They are both deactivated by plasma proteins, therefore quickly losing their action once they enter the bloodstream and with no direct effect in distal sites of the circulation [35–37]. Yet, complications can happen and they can become quickly major, moreover potentially in office-based settings where emergency action must be taken by the same doctor who performed the sclerotherapy act (Table 3.2).

A quite recent analysis from the World Health Organization Pharmacovigilance Databasc VigiBase reported that POL has been reported to be more associated with venous embolic/thrombotic events, ethanolamine with the higher pharmacovigilance disproportionality signal of cardiac arrhythmias and STS with more allergic reactions. It is of paramount importance that appropriate global registry data are collected in order to avoid erroneous conclusions on the real safety profiles in post-market surveillance. Also for this reason, all sclerotherapists should always report eventually encountered complications and participate as much as possible in real-world data collections [38].

Table 3.2 Sum-up table reporting the main sclerosing agents, their class/mechanism of action, the relative strength, the available concentrations, the indications, and safety profiles

Sclerosant	Mechanism of action	Potency	Common concentrations	Key indications	Clinical profile / notes
Polidocanol (Lauromacrogol 400)	Detergent (non-ionic surfactant)	Mild–Moderate	0.25%, 0.5%, 1%, 2%, 3%	Telangiectasias, reticular veins, varicose veins, foam sclerotherapy, low-flow venous malformations	Excellent; low pain, low necrosis risk, rare anaphylaxis
Sodium Tetradecyl Sulfate (STS)	Detergent (anionic surfactant)	Moderate–Strong	0.1%, 0.2%, 0.5%, 1%, 3%	Varicose veins, saphenous trunks, foam sclerotherapy, venous malformations	Good; higher pain and necrosis risk than polidocanol, rare anaphylaxis
Sodium Morrhuate	Detergent (fatty acid salt mixture)	Strong	5%, 10%	Large varicose veins (historical), limited use in venous malformations	Poor; high risk of pain, necrosis, hyperpigmentation, anaphylaxis
Ethanolamine Oleate	Detergent / chemical irritant	Moderate–Strong	2.5%, 5%	Esophageal varices, venous malformations	Moderate; hemolysis, renal toxicity
Hypertonic Saline (NaCl)	Osmotic agent	Mild	11.7%, 23.4%	Telangiectasias, very small veins	Fair; painful, high ulcer risk if extravasated
Chromated Glycerin	Osmotic + chemical irritant	Mild–Moderate	72%	Telangiectasias, reticular veins	Good; low necrosis risk, limited availability
Sodium Salicylate	Chemical irritant	Mild	10–20%	Small varices (historical)	Limited data; irritation common
Polyiodinated Iodine (Povidone-Iodine)	Chemical irritant	Mild	Variable	Rare/experimental use	Limited safety data
Ethanol (Absolute Alcohol)	Chemical toxin / protein denaturant	Very Strong	95–100%	Low-flow venous malformations, AVMs (specialist use)	Poor; high systemic toxicity, cardiopulmonary risk, nerve injury
Bleomycin	Cytotoxic antibiotic	Moderate	1 mg/mL (variable protocols)	Venous and lymphatic malformations (especially head & neck)	Good when low-dose; pulmonary toxicity risk at high cumulative doses
Doxycycline	Chemical irritant / antibiotic	Moderate–Strong	5–20 mg/mL	Venous and lymphatic malformations	Moderate; pain, inflammation, tissue injury possible

6 Regulatory Considerations

Sclerosing agents are regulated as medicinal products (drugs) when marketed as finished, labeled injectable products. They may also appear as medical devices in some contexts (e.g., delivery devices), but the active chemical sclerosant itself is treated as a drug in major jurisdictions [39]. A licensed marketing authorization (MA) or regulatory approval permits specific indications, concentrations, formulations, and routes of administration described on the product label. Off-label use refers to using an approved product outside its labeled indication, dose, or patient population and is common in sclerotherapy practice but carries medico-legal and regulatory implications for prescribers. Compounded formulations (locally prepared mixtures of active agents or concentrations not available as licensed products) are subject to distinct rules: In many countries, compounding is allowed under pharmacy/compounding statutes but brings heightened requirements for sterility, quality control, documentation, and, in some cases, manufacturer liability. In the USA, the Food and Drug Administration (FDA) regulates sclerosing agents as drugs when they are marketed as finished pharmaceutical products. Polidocanol (Asclera) and sodium tetradecyl sulfate (Sotradecol) have been the major products with FDA regulatory histories. STS has long-standing approvals for sclerotherapy indications, and polidocanol obtained approvals for specific vein types/doses following clinical trials and submission of safety data. In the EU, marketing authorization may be centralized (EMA) or national. However, many sclerosing agents are licensed at national level and clinical practice is commonly guided by European societies documents who are usually not lodged in the clinical governance institutions. National competent authorities set labeling and post-marketing obligations. For compounded/non-licensed use, member state laws and pharmacy regulations apply. Providers should follow local MA product labels and national guidance and document rationale when using off-label or compounded preparations; otherwise serious legal issues can arise. In the UK, Interventional Procedures guidance from NICE and MHRA (Medicines and Healthcare products Regulatory Agency) oversight shape practice and commissioning. MHRA applies drug regulation. Manufacturers and clinicians must comply with licensed indications, and they should always report adverse events. Regulatory agencies may require Risk Management Plans or post-marketing studies to further characterize safety. Post-marketing safety surveillance (spontaneous adverse event reporting, registries, post-authorization safety studies) is crucial because rare but serious events (neurological events, visual disturbances, pulmonary embolism) may only be detected after broader use considering their rarity. Foam sclerotherapy is widely used. Regulators consider both the active ingredient and the foam preparation method. When the foam preparation method is intrinsic to the product (e.g., a marketed microfoam kit), approval covers that method. Whenever foam is created by manual mixing (for example, physician-prepared three-way stopcock technique), the practice may be considered off-label for the product and raises questions about reproducibility, gas composition, and embolic risk. Therefore, using appropriate material and foam production methods is of paramount importance, particularly whenever opting for a physician-compounded foam. Regulatory and professional bodies commonly expect clinicians performing sclerotherapy to have documented training, competence in venous anatomy, hemodynamics and ultrasound if performing ultrasound-guided procedures, and access to resuscitation resources for rare allergic/anaphylactic reactions. Because sclerotherapy may be performed off-label, using compounded agents, or with small but non-negligible risks (e.g., transient visual symptoms, migraine, DVT), informed consent must explicitly state the product used (brand/generic), whether use is within the product label or off-label, known common and rare risks, expected benefits, alternatives (compression, endothermal ablation, surgery, etc.), and follow-up arrangements. Documentation of consent is important for medico-legal defensibility. Using a licensed product in accordance with its label generally reduces regulatory exposure. However, clinicians retain responsibility for safe patient selection, correct technique, dose limits, and post-procedure surveillance. Off-label use is permissible in many jurisdictions when supported by evidence and appropriate consent, but it increases legal risk if adverse events occur and standard of care is questioned. In the case of compounded or imported unlicensed products, liability may be shared among prescriber, dispensing pharmacy, and facility depending on local law. A sensitive topic is the one of sclerotherapy during pregnancy. The evidence about this clinical context is limited, so regulatory labels and professional guidelines should be consulted before treating these groups.

References

1. Myers K. A history of injection treatments—II sclerotherapy. Phlebology. 2019;34:303–10.
2. Weiss RA, Goldman MP. Advances in sclerotherapy. Dermatol Clin. 1995;13(2):431–45.
3. Wollmann JC. The history of sclerosing foams. Dermatol Surg. 2004;30(5):694–703; discussion 703. https://doi.org/10.1111/j.1524-4725.2004.30208.x. Erratum in: Dermatol Surg. 2005 Feb;31(2):249
4. Ma J, Chen Y, Zhang K, Yang T, Xie H, Yang X, Ding P. Study of vascular sclerosing agent based on the dual mechanism of vascular endothelial cell damage-plasmin system inhibition. Biochem Biophys Res Commun. 2023;680:135–40.
5. Rabe E, Pannier-Fischer F, Gerlach H, Breu FX, Guggenbichler S, Zabel M, German Society of Phlebology. Guidelines for sclerotherapy of varicose veins (ICD 10: I83.0, I83.1, I83.2, and I83.9). Dermatologic Surg. 2004;30(5):687–93. discussion 693
6. Duffy DM. Sclerosants: a comparative review. Dermatologic Surg. 2010;36(Suppl 2):1010–25.
7. Kern P. Sclerotherapy of varicose leg veins. Technique, indications and complications. Int Angiol. 2002;21(2 Suppl 1):40–5.
8. Parsi K. Interaction of detergent sclerosants with cell membranes. Phlebology. 2015;30(5):306–15.
9. Albanese G, Kondo KL. Pharmacology of sclerotherapy. Semin Intervent Radiol. 2010;27(4):391–9.
10. Alòs J, Carreño P, López JA, Estadella B, Serra-Prat M, Marinel-Lo J. Efficacy and safety of sclerotherapy using polidocanol foam: a controlled clinical trial. Eur J Vasc Endovasc Surg. 2006;31(1):101–7.
11. Hamel-Desnos C, Desnos P, Wollmann JC, Ouvry P, Mako S, Allaert FA. Evaluation of the efficacy of polidocanol in the form of foam compared with liquid form in sclerotherapy of the greater saphenous vein: initial results. Dermatologic Surg. 2003;29(12):1170–5. discussion 1175
12. Gianesini S, Obi A, Onida S, et al. Global guidelines trends and controversies in lower limb venous and lymphatic disease: narrative literature revision and experts' opinions following the vWINter international meeting in Phlebology, Lymphology & Aesthetics, 23–25 January 2019. Phlebology. 2019;34(1 Suppl):4–66.
13. Morrison N, Neuhardt DL, Rogers CR, McEown J, Morrison T, Johnson E, Salles-Cunha SX. Comparisons of side effects using air and carbon dioxide foam for endovenous chemical ablation. J Vasc Surg. 2008;47(4):830–6.
14. de Ávila Oliveira R, Riera R, Vasconcelos V, Baptista-Silva JC. Injection sclerotherapy for varicose veins. Cochrane Database Syst Rev. 2021;12(12):CD001732.
15. Jenkinson HA, Wilmas KM, Silapunt S. Sodium Tetradecyl sulfate: a review of clinical uses. Dermatologic Surg. 2017;43(11):1313–20.
16. Guex JJ. Complications and side-effects of foam sclerotherapy. Phlebology. 2009;24(6):270–4.
17. Birdina J, Pilmane M, Ligers A. The Morphofunctional Changes in the Wall of Varicose Veins. Ann Vasc Surg. 2017 Jul;42:274–84.
18. Kabnick LS, Jimenez JC, Coogan SM, et al. Comparative effectiveness of non-compounded polidocanol 1% endovenous microfoam (Varithena) ablation versus endovenous thermal ablation utilizing a systematic review and network meta-analysis. J Vasc Surg Venous Lymphat Disord. 2024;12(6):101896.
19. Tunick IS, Nach R. Sodium morrhuate as a sclerosing agent in the treatment of varicose veins. Ann Surg. 1932 May;95(5):734–7.
20. Imhoff E, Stemmer R. Classification et mécanisme d'action des sclérosants [Classification and mechanism of action of sclerosing agents]. Phlebologie. 1969;22(2):145–8.
21. Kang M, Yang A, Hannaford P, et al. Skin necrosis following sclerotherapy. Part 1: differential diagnosis based on classification of pathogenic mechanisms. Phlebology. 2022;37(6):409–24.
22. Kang M, Yang A, Hannaford P, Connor D, Parsi K. Skin necrosis following sclerotherapy. Part 2: risk minimisation and management strategies. Phlebology. 2022 Oct;37(9):628–43.
23. Ozaki M, Nomura T, Osuga K, et al. Effect and safety of ethanolamine oleate in sclerotherapy in patients with difficult-to-resect venous malformations: a multicenter, single-arm study. PLoS One. 2025;20(1):e0303130.
24. McCoy S, Evans A, Spurrier N. Sclerotherapy for leg telangiectasia–a blinded comparative trial of polidocanol and hypertonic saline. Dermatologic Surg. 1999;25(5):381–5. discussion 385–6
25. Zimmet SE. Sclerotherapy treatment of telangiectasias and varicose veins. Tech Vasc Interv Radiol. 2003;6(3):116–20.
26. Kern P, Ramelet AA, Wutschert R, et al. A double-blind, randomized study comparing pure chromated glycerin with chromated glycerin with 1% lidocaine and epinephrine for sclerotherapy of telangiectasias and reticular veins. Dermatologic Surg. 2011;37(11):1590–4.
27. Kern P, Ramelet AA, Wutschert R, et al. Single-blind, randomized study comparing chromated glycerin, polidocanol solution, and polidocanol foam for treatment of telangiectatic leg veins. Dermatologic Surg. 2004;30(3):367–72.
28. Georgiev M. Postsclerotherapy hyperpigmentations. Chromated glycerin as a screen for patients at risk (a retrospective study). J Dermatol Surg Oncol. 1993;19(7):649–52.
29. Sotiris D, Pallotta G, Nittari G, et al. An original approach for the treatment of varicose veins of the lower limbs. J Clin Aesthet Dermatol. 2020;13(8):E59–64.
30. Lai J, Xu Z, Chen H, et al. Comparison of bleomycin polidocanol foam versus absolute ethanol for sclero-

therapy of venous malformations. J Vasc Surg Venous Lymphat Disord. 2026 Mar;14(2):102352.
31. Lee BB, Laredo J, Kim YW, et al. Congenital vascular malformations: general treatment principles. Phlebology. 2007;22(6):258–63.
32. Alomari AI, Dubois J. Interventional management of vascular malformations. Tech Vasc Interv Radiol. 2011;14(1):22–31.
33. Okazaki T, Iwatani S, Yanai T, et al. Treatment of lymphangioma in children: our experience of 128 cases. J Pediatr Surg. 2007;42(2):386–9.
34. Burrows PE, Mitri RK, Alomari A, et al. Percutaneous sclerotherapy of lymphatic malformations with doxycycline. Radiology. 2008;246(3):123–31.
35. Parsi K, Exner T, Connor DE, et al. The lytic effects of detergent sclerosants on erythrocytes, platelets, endothelial cells and microparticles are attenuated by albumin and other plasma components in vitro. Eur J Vasc Endovasc Surg. 2008;36:216–23.
36. Connor DE, Cooley-Andrade O, Goh WX, et al. Detergent sclerosants are deactivated and consumed by circulating blood cells. Eur J Vasc Endovasc Surg. 2015;49:426–31.
37. Dabbs EB, Dos Santos SJ, Mainsiouw LE, et al. Implication of foam sclerosant inactivation by human whole blood in a laboratory setting. Phlebology. 2018;33:338–43.
38. Roselli A, Khouri C, Roustit M, et al. Safety profile of sclerosing agents: an analysis from the World Health Organization pharmacovigilance database VigiBase. Dermatologic Surg. 2019;45(12):1517–28.
39. Eckmann DM. Polidocanol for endovenous microfoam sclerosant therapy. Expert Opin Investig Drugs. 2009;18(12):1919–27.

Sclerotherapy Foam Production Techniques

4

Sergio Gianesini, Rodrigo Rial, and Yung Wei Chi

1 Evolution of Foam Sclerotherapy

Back in 1939, McAusland injected telangiectasia using froth obtained by shaking sodium morrhuate inside a rubber-capped bottle [1]. The origins of foam sclerotherapy can be traced to Orbach's "air-block" technique, introduced in the 1940s, which aimed to displace blood from the vein lumen prior to injection of a liquid sclerosant [2]. In 1953, Ree treated varicose using pure Etamolin foam generated by shaking a bottle containing the sclerosant and aspirating the bubbles into a syringe [3].

While conceptually sound, all these methods suffered from poor reproducibility, uncontrolled gas volumes, and inconsistent clinical outcomes. Prior to the 1990s, sclerotherapy was largely limited by the intrinsic drawbacks of liquid sclerosants: rapid dilution by intraluminal blood, poor contact with the venous endothelium, reduced efficacy in larger-caliber veins, unpredictable diffusion, and high recanalization rates. The need for a method that could displace blood, maintain stable endothelial contact, and enhance sclerosing potency led to experimental attempts at gas–liquid mixtures. While early reports of "froth" or air–liquid mixtures existed, these lacked reproducibility and standardization. It was Juan Cabrera Garrido who, in the early 1990s, systematically conceptualized and developed controlled sclerosant foam, establishing a reproducible method grounded in physical chemistry rather than empirical improvisation [4, 5]. The innovation was not merely technical but conceptual, redefining how sclerosants interact with venous blood and endothelium. Cabrera proposed foam not as a modified sclerosant, but as a delivery vehicle with distinct properties: blood displacement rather than dilution, increased surface area for endothelial contact, prolonged residence time within the target vein, homogeneous distribution along the venous lumen. Key physicochemical principles introduced by Cabrera included microbubble formation with controlled size distribution, surface tension stabilization to prevent premature coalescence, optimization of gas-to-liquid ratio to maximize foam stability while preserving injectability [6]. These principles distinguished Cabrera foam from earlier unstable froths and positioned foam as a pharmacomechanical tool rather than a simple formula-

S. Gianesini (✉)
Department of Translational Medicine, University of Ferrara, Ferrara, Italy

Department of Surgery, Uniformed Services University of Health Sciences, Bethesda, MD, USA
e-mail: gnssrg@unife.it

R. Rial
Vascular and Endovascular Department, University Hospital HM, Madrid, Spain

Y. W. Chi
Department of Cardiovascular Medicine, University of California, Davis Vascular Center, Sacramento, CA, USA
e-mail: ywchi@ucdavis.edu

S. Gianesini, Y. W. Chi (eds.), *Sclerotherapy*, https://doi.org/10.1007/978-3-032-32794-9_4

tion variant. Cabrera demonstrated that foam stability and structure were more critical determinants of efficacy than simply increasing sclerosant concentration [7]. Early clinical series published by Cabrera and contemporaries reported markedly improved occlusion rates in saphenous veins and major varicosities [6]. Moreover, these results challenged the prevailing view that sclerotherapy was unsuitable for truncal incompetence and paved the way for ultrasound-guided applications [6, 8]. The introduction of duplex ultrasound transformed foam sclerotherapy from a blind chemical procedure into a controlled, image-guided intervention. This evolution culminated in international consensus documents and guidelines formally recognizing ultrasound-guided foam sclerotherapy as a first-line or adjunctive treatment for varicose veins [9]. In 1998, Monfreux published about the MUS ("Méthode Ultra-Sonore," in English the Ultrasound Method) technique for saphenous trunks [10]. The MUS technique is based on targeted, segmental ultrasound-guided injection of sclerosant foam into the incompetent saphenous trunk, with controlled propagation and immediate hemodynamic interruption, rather than blind or diffuse sclerosant distribution. It was one of the first systematic truncal ultrasound-guided foam sclerotherapy techniques, preceding widespread standardization of foam preparation. The technique is characterized by duplex ultrasound mandatory use with real-time monitoring of the injection site, of the foam propagation, and of the junctions. The proposed concept is in favor of a controlled intraluminal filling, rather than a complete distal spread. The saphenous vein is treated in segments, not with a single large-volume injection, and the injection is typically performed below the saphenofemoral junction for the great saphenous vein and below the sapheno-popliteal junction for the small saphenous vein. Compression is applied proximally to prevent deep venous extension. Subsequently, the Tessari method introduced a two-syringe system connected by a three-way stopcock, allowing consistent bubble size and reproducibility [11]. While often credited as the origin of foam sclerotherapy, it represents a technical refinement of Cabrera's conceptual framework, not a conceptual departure [12]. Subsequent research explored alternative gases (CO_2, O_2, physiological gas mixtures) to reduce bubble persistence in systemic circulation and in particular neurological and visual side effects [13]. Later studies identified transient visual disturbances, migraine-like symptoms, and the role of right-to-left shunts such as patent foramen ovale [14]. Manual foam preparation remains subject to significant inter-operator variability. Factors influencing foam quality include syringe size and material, number and speed of pump exchanges, gas-to-liquid ratio, time elapsed between preparation and injection. These variables affect bubble size distribution, foam stability, and gas persistence, all of which influence clinical efficacy and safety [15]. The lack of standardization prompted the development of automated or semi-automated systems capable of delivering consistent, reproducible foam characteristics. Clinical development programs, including the pivotal VANISH-1 and VANISH-2 randomized controlled trials, were conducted in the early 2010s to evaluate the safety and efficacy of 1% polidocanol endovenous microfoam delivered by a high-tech canister for the treatment of incompetent saphenous veins and associated varicosities using a fully automated system called "Varithena" ® [16]. These trials demonstrated significant improvements in vein closure rates, symptom relief, and quality-of-life outcomes compared with placebo controls [17]. Varithena® became a regulated pharmaceutical product, characterized by a high-tech combination of biochemical mixing and internal circuit related rheological features, ensuring batch-to-batch consistency and compliance with Good Manufacturing Practice standards. The related microfoam demonstrated a median bubble diameter inferior to 100 micron and never greater than 500 micron. The O2/CO2 ratio is 65/35% in a 1/7 liquid/gas ratio [18, 19]. The instructions for users report to inject the foam not later than 75 s after it has been produced [20]. Varithena® transition marked a shift from operator-dependent foam creation to industry-controlled foam engineering, aligning foam sclerotherapy with modern pharmacological paradigms. For the first and

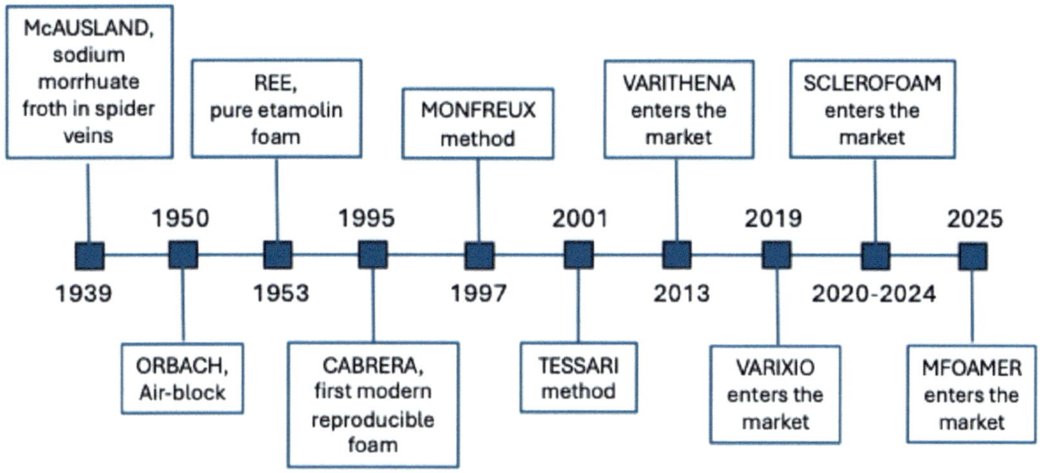

Fig. 4.1 Foam sclerotherapy historical milestones

only time in sclerotherapy history, foam was made totally operator-independent. Among the semi-automated systems, the most known in the global phlebology community is Varixio®. It uses a motor-driven system to mix sclerosant injected by the operator into a capsule containing gas under controlled conditions. This mechanization can potentially reduce variability and improve reproducibility across treatment sessions and centers, yet large solid data on the topic are missing in the scientific literature [21–23]. Recently, a similar device has been introduced in the market under the name of Sclerofoam® (not to be confounded with a sclerosing kit named in the same way and with trademark by Kreussler, https://www.aethoxysklerolinternational.com/wpcontent/uploads/2023/10/ScleroFoam_Flyer_Aktualisierung_KV_02.pdf), yet we were not able to identify any scientific reference about it. In general, large registries and randomized trials confirmed that, when performed within recommended parameters, foam sclerotherapy has a favorable safety profile comparable to other minimally invasive venous interventions. Research into nanobubble foams, automated delivery systems, and patient-specific foam rheology is now ongoing. The latest ongoing revolution in foam sclerotherapy is coming from the enhancement of the technology used for the Varithena® canister: A device called MFoamer™ has recently entered the market offering a full range of polidocanol concentration (from 0.1 to 3%) and gas mixtures (02/CO2 from 20/80 to 40/60, plus customizable percentages). Scientific literature production on the topic is ongoing and paving the way for a possible paradigm shift in fully automated sclerotherapy in all vein calibers [24]. Clearly, along the years appropriate foam sclerotherapy has moved from an art looking for its own science in a solid evidence-based potentially operator-independent valuable tool for chronic venous disease treatment (Fig. 4.1). At the same time, the need of education on its fundamentals and best practice has increased, making its use suitable only for the practitioners truly committed in the related practice training.

2 Foam Hemodynamics and Clinical Features

The superiority of foam over liquid sclerosant in many clinical scenarios can be explained by fundamental hemodynamic and pharmacologic principles. In liquid sclerotherapy, the injected sclerosant mixes immediately with intraluminal blood, leading to rapid dilution and a reduction in effective concentration at the endothelial surface. In contrast, foam acts as a space-occupying medium that displaces blood from the vein lumen, replacing it with a sclerosant-rich interface that directly contacts the endothelium [15].

From a hemodynamic perspective, foam behaves as a viscoelastic plug rather than a freely flowing liquid. When injected under ultrasound guidance, foam advances along the vein as a coherent column, pushing blood ahead of it and minimizing turbulent mixing [25]. This "plug flow" phenomenon increases residence time within the target vein and reduces washout into the deep venous system when appropriate compression and positioning are applied [26]. Experimental vein models have demonstrated that foam achieves more complete blood displacement than liquid injections, even at lower sclerosant doses [27]. Pharmacologically, the increased efficiency of foam allows clinicians to achieve equivalent or superior endothelial injury with lower absolute amounts of active drug. This dose-sparing effect is particularly relevant in extensive treatments or in patients requiring multiple sessions, as it may reduce systemic exposure and toxicity. Moreover, the gas–liquid interface of foam increases the effective surface area of the sclerosant, enhancing interaction with endothelial cell membranes and facilitating detergent-induced cell lysis. Foam also enables better control of sclerosant distribution under ultrasound visualization. The echogenicity of foam allows real-time monitoring of its propagation within superficial veins, perforators, and junctional regions [8]. This visualization capability represents a major advance over liquid sclerotherapy, where the injected solution is often invisible once diluted in blood. Ultrasound-guided foam sclerotherapy thus combines mechanical blood displacement, enhanced pharmacologic action, and image-guided precision in a single technique. While the theoretical advantages of foam are compelling, clinical experience has clearly demonstrated that not all foams are equivalent. Foam quality, encompassing bubble size, homogeneity, stability, drainage behavior, and resistance to coalescence has direct implications for both efficacy and safety [27]. Poorly prepared foam may collapse rapidly, behave like a liquid, or fragment into large bubbles that migrate unpredictably, and undermining the very advantages foam is intended to provide [28]. Bubble size distribution is a key determinant of foam behavior within veins. Smaller, more uniform bubbles tend to produce cohesive foams with predictable flow characteristics, whereas highly polydisperse foams are prone to rapid coalescence and uneven endothelial contact. Stability, often expressed as foam half-life or drainage time, determines the usable working window between foam production and injection, as well as the persistence of foam within the treated vein. Excessively unstable foam may lose its structure before effective sclerosis occurs, while overly stable foam may increase the risk of unintended migration if not carefully controlled. Clinical studies and consensus documents emphasized that foam production techniques must be standardized within each practice to ensure reproducible results [29]. Variability in syringe size, connector type, mixing intensity, and gas composition can lead to significant interoperator and inter-session differences in foam quality, complicating outcome assessment and increasing the risk of complications. For vascular experts, understanding and controlling foam production is therefore integral to optimizing treatment outcomes, particularly in truncal vein sclerotherapy and complex venous disease. Beyond efficacy, foam quality also intersects with safety considerations. Transient neurologic symptoms, visual disturbances, and migraine-like phenomena have been reported after foam sclerotherapy, and while these events are uncommon, their occurrence has prompted careful examination of foam characteristics and injection techniques [14]. Although the pathophysiology is multifactorial, inappropriate foam volume, rapid injection, and uncontrolled proximal spread are more consistently implicated than foam production alone [30]. Producing foam with predictable, reproducible properties is a foundational step in minimizing risk and maintaining high standards of care in advanced venous practice. In summary, the transition from liquid to foam sclerotherapy represents a major evolution in the treatment of varicose veins, driven by improved hemodynamic efficiency, enhanced pharmacologic action, and superior imaging control. These benefits, however, are inseparable from the quality of the foam itself. A thorough understanding of the principles underlying foam production is essential for vascular experts seeking to fully exploit the potential of foam sclerotherapy while maintaining safety and reproducibility.

3 Fundamental Concepts in Foam Sclerotherapy Production

The clinical success of foam sclerotherapy is inseparably linked to the physical behavior of sclerosing foams. While the pharmacologic action of detergent sclerosants such as polidocanol and sodium tetradecyl sulfate is well established, their therapeutic effectiveness in foam form is profoundly influenced by the laws of soft matter physics governing gas–liquid dispersions. For vascular experts, an understanding of foam physics is not an academic exercise but a practical necessity, as subtle variations in foam structure can translate into significant differences in intravascular behavior, endothelial injury, efficacy, and safety. Sclerosing foams are complex, metastable systems that evolve continuously from the moment of their creation. Their behavior is governed by interfacial phenomena, fluid dynamics, and time-dependent structural changes such as drainage, coalescence, and gas diffusion. Unlike industrial foams designed for long-term stability, medical sclerosing foams must strike a balance between sufficient persistence to achieve endothelial destruction and timely breakdown to minimize systemic dissemination, while navigating in the tortuous venous network. This balance is achieved or lost through the interaction of physical parameters that are directly influenced by foam production techniques. A sclerosing foam is a gas-in-liquid dispersion in which the continuous phase is a liquid sclerosant solution and the dispersed phase consists of gas bubbles separated by thin liquid films known as lamellae. From a physicochemical standpoint, sclerosing foam belongs to the broader class of aqueous foams, sharing properties with foams used in food science, detergents, and materials engineering, while exhibiting distinct features related to its medical application. Unlike emulsions, where two immiscible liquids are dispersed, foams are inherently unstable systems because gas has a strong thermodynamic tendency to escape from the liquid phase. The persistence of a foam therefore depends on the ability of surface-active molecules, in this case detergent sclerosants, to stabilize the gas–liquid interface and slow the processes that lead to foam collapse. Polidocanol and sodium tetradecyl sulfate act not only as endothelial toxins but also as surfactants, lowering surface tension and enabling foam formation. Clinically used sclerosing foams are typically polydisperse, meaning that bubble sizes vary within the foam, although the degree of polydispersity depends heavily on the production method. Foam generated manually at the bedside is metastable by design: it is intended to persist for seconds to minutes, rather than hours, reflecting the need for a limited but effective intravascular residence time. From a functional perspective, sclerosing foam can be conceptualized as a drug delivery vehicle that temporarily replaces intravascular blood with a sclerosant-rich interface. This conceptual shift, from liquid injection to space-occupying foam delivery, has profound implications for how sclerosant dose, distribution, and contact time are understood and controlled in clinical practice. At the core of foam physics lies the gas–liquid interface. Each bubble in a sclerosing foam is enveloped by a thin liquid film stabilized by surfactant molecules that align at the interface, with their hydrophobic tails oriented toward the gas phase and hydrophilic heads toward the liquid phase. This arrangement reduces interfacial tension, allowing bubbles to form and persist long enough for clinical use. Interfacial tension is a critical parameter because it governs bubble formation, stability, and resistance to coalescence. High interfacial tension favors rapid bubble collapse, whereas excessively low interfacial tension may promote uncontrolled foam expansion and altered flow behavior. Detergent sclerosants achieve an optimal intermediate reduction in surface tension, enabling foam formation while maintaining sufficient lamellar strength. The choice of gas has a direct influence on interfacial dynamics. Room air, composed largely of nitrogen and oxygen, produces foams with relatively low gas solubility in blood, resulting in slower bubble dissolution and greater foam persistence. In contrast, carbon dioxide is highly soluble in blood and aqueous solutions, leading to more rapid gas diffusion out of bubbles and faster foam decay [31]. These physicochemical differences explain many of the observed clinical distinctions between air-based and CO_2-based foams. Under shear stress during injection or intravascular flow, the interfacial layer must deform without rupturing. Excessive shear can disrupt lamellae, converting foam into a liquid-like dispersion before effective sclerosis occurs. This phenomenon underscores the importance of injection technique, needle diameter, and catheter selection in preserving foam integrity. Bubble size and spatial arrangement define the architecture of a sclerosing foam and are among the most important determinants of its intravascular behavior. Based on the bubble diameter, the foam can be classified as micro (<250 micron), mini (250–200 micron) or macro (>500 micron). Laboratory data show that the lower the polidocanol concentration is, the smaller the bubble size becomes. Moreover, the wetter (higher than ¼ liquid/ratio) the foam is the smaller the bubble is, both for polidocanol and sodium tetradecyl sulfate. At the same time, the wetter the foam is the slower the coarsening becomes [32]. In general, smaller bubbles increase total surface area, enhancing contact between the sclerosant and the endothelium, while larger bubbles may promote faster gas escape and uneven distribution. Manually produced foams are typically polydisperse, containing a wide range of bubble diameters, often spanning one order of magnitude. Excessive variability can lead to heterogeneous behavior, with smaller bubbles stabilizing the foam while larger bubbles dominate flow dynamics and coalescence. In experimental vein models, highly polydisperse foams have been shown to fragment unpredictably, leading to incomplete blood displacement and patchy endothelial exposure [25]. Foam architecture evolves as bubbles pack together, forming polyhedral structures separated by thin liquid films. In dense foams, bubbles adopt polygonal shapes to minimize surface energy, while in wetter foams they remain more spherical. The transition between these states is influenced by liquid content, bubble size distribution, and gravity-driven drainage. From a clinical perspective, foam architecture influences cohesiveness, the ability of foam to advance as a unified column rather than dispersing into individual bubbles. Cohesive foams are associated with more predictable propagation under ultrasound and more effective blood displacement in truncal veins. Production techniques that generate excessively coarse or excessively wet foams tend to compromise this cohesiveness, reducing therapeutic efficiency. Foam decay is an inevitable, time-dependent process governed by three principal mechanisms: drainage, coalescence, and gas diffusion (Ostwald ripening). Understanding these mechanisms is essential for appreciating why foam must be used promptly after production and why its properties change continuously during handling and injection. Drainage refers to the gravitational flow of liquid out of the foam lamellae toward dependent regions. As liquid drains, films become thinner and more susceptible to rupture. Drainage rate depends on liquid viscosity, bubble size, and the thickness of lamellae, all of which are influenced by sclerosant concentration and foam production method. Clinically, excessive drainage results in "wet foam" converting toward a liquid state before effective sclerosis occurs. Coalescence occurs when adjacent bubbles merge following rupture of the intervening lamella, producing larger bubbles with reduced surface area. Coalescence accelerates foam breakdown and increases heterogeneity within the foam structure. Factors promoting coalescence include high polydispersity, excessive mechanical stress, and delayed injection. Gas diffusion, also known as Ostwald ripening, involves the transfer of gas from smaller bubbles (with higher internal pressure because of the smaller radius) to larger bubbles (with lower internal pressure). This process leads to progressive growth of large bubbles at the expense of smaller ones, contributing to foam coarsening over time. Gas solubility plays a major role in this mechanism, explaining the faster decay of CO_2-based foams compared with air-based foams. Collectively, these processes define the usable lifetime of a sclerosing foam. From a clinical standpoint, foam should be injected during the early phase of its evolution, when bubble size distribution, stability, and cohesiveness are optimal. Delayed injection increases variability and undermines reproducibility, emphasizing the need for streamlined workflows and standardized production protocols.

4 Foam Quality Determinants

Foam quality is a central determinant of both the efficacy and safety of foam sclerotherapy. Unlike liquid sclerosants, which are relatively stable and predictable after preparation, sclerosing foam is a metastable physicochemical system whose properties evolve continuously from the moment of its production. Its clinical performance depends on a complex interaction between chemical composition, physical structure, and time-dependent degradation processes. For vascular experts, foam quality should be regarded as a modifiable therapeutic variable, comparable in importance to sclerosant concentration, injected volume, or ultrasound guidance. Suboptimal foam may behave essentially as a diluted liquid, whereas optimized foam can function as an efficient intravascular drug delivery system capable of achieving consistent endothelial injury with reduced drug dose. The two detergent sclerosants most widely used for foam sclerotherapy polidocanol and sodium tetradecyl sulfate. Both agents act as surfactants, lowering surface tension at the gas–liquid interface and enabling foam formation, while simultaneously exerting cytotoxic effects on the venous endothelium. Despite these shared properties, important differences exist in their physicochemical behavior and clinical profiles, which influence foam quality. Polidocanol is a non-ionic surfactant characterized by relatively low surface tension and good foamability across a range of concentrations [33]. It tends to produce foams with moderate stability and a favorable safety profile, which has contributed to its widespread use in Europe and in controlled microfoam formulations. Sodium tetradecyl sulfate, an anionic surfactant, is more potent in terms of endothelial injury but may generate foams with different stability characteristics depending on concentration and gas composition. Sclerosant concentration plays a dual role. Pharmacologically, higher concentrations increase the extent and depth of endothelial damage. Physically, concentration affects interfacial rheology, lamellar thickness, and resistance to drainage and coalescence. Experimental studies have shown that very low sclerosant concentrations may produce unstable, "wet" foams that collapse rapidly, while excessively high concentrations may paradoxically reduce foam quality by increasing viscosity and impairing homogeneous bubble formation [34]. Clinically, foam sclerotherapy allows the use of lower sclerosant concentrations compared with liquid sclerotherapy for the same target vein diameter, due to improved blood displacement and prolonged endothelial contact time. This dose-sparing effect is one of the key advantages of foam but is contingent upon producing foam with appropriate physical properties. Consequently, sclerosant concentration should always be selected in conjunction with foam production parameters rather than in isolation. The liquid-to-gas (L:G) ratio is one of the most critical determinants of foam structure and behavior. It defines the relative volume of sclerosant solution to gas within the foam and directly influences bubble size, liquid content, stability, and injectability. In clinical practice, most manually produced foams use L:G ratios ranging from 1:3 to 1:4, which have been identified as a practical compromise between stability and ease of injection. Lower gas fractions (e.g., 1:1 or 1:2) result in wetter foams with higher liquid content, which may behave more like liquids and provide inferior blood displacement. Conversely, very high gas fractions (e.g., ≥1:6) produce drier foams that may be initially voluminous but are often fragile, prone to rapid coalescence, and difficult to inject smoothly. From a physical perspective, increasing the gas fraction reduces lamellar thickness and increases susceptibility to rupture and drainage. From a clinical standpoint, excessively dry foam may fragment during injection or within the vein, leading to unpredictable distribution and reduced endothelial contact. Thus, the optimal L:G ratio is not simply the one that produces the most visible foam, but the one that yields cohesive, injectable foam with sufficient intravascular persistence.

Standardization of the L:G ratio is essential for reproducibility. Variations in syringe size, connector dead space, and gas compressibility can lead to unintentional deviations from the intended ratio. For this reason, expert practice emphasizes the use of consistent equipment and validated protocols for foam preparation. The type of gas used to generate sclerosing foam has a profound impact on foam stability, bubble persistence, and intravascular behavior. The most commonly used gases include room air, carbon dioxide (CO_2), and mixtures of CO_2 and oxygen. Room air-based foams are generally more stable because nitrogen, which constitutes the majority of air, has low solubility in blood and aqueous solutions. This results in slower gas diffusion out of the bubbles and prolonged foam persistence. Such stability can be advantageous when longer working times are required or when treating long venous segments. CO_2-based foams, by contrast, are less stable due to the high solubility of carbon dioxide in blood. Bubbles dissolve more rapidly, leading to faster foam decay and a shorter effective lifespan. This reduced stability requires rapid injection and streamlined workflows but may limit the duration of bubble persistence in the circulation. CO_2/O_2 mixtures exhibit intermediate behavior, combining reduced nitrogen content with manageable handling characteristics. Gas solubility also influences foam-aging mechanisms, particularly Ostwald ripening, whereby gas diffuses from smaller bubbles to larger ones. Highly soluble gases accelerate this process, promoting faster foam coarsening and collapse. Temperature is an often under-appreciated determinant of foam quality. It influences gas solubility, liquid viscosity, interfacial tension, and drainage dynamics. In general, higher temperatures increase gas solubility and reduce liquid viscosity, accelerating foam decay [35]. Even modest temperature differences, such as those between a cool procedure room and body temperature, can significantly alter foam behavior once injected. From a practical perspective, foam is usually produced at room temperature and injected into veins at near-body temperature, where accelerated degradation occurs. This temperature shift reinforces the importance of prompt injection after foam preparation. For experts seeking maximal reproducibility, maintaining consistent environmental conditions and minimizing delays between production and injection are essential components of quality control. Time is an intrinsic determinant of foam quality. From the moment of production, sclerosing foam undergoes continuous structural evolution driven by drainage, coalescence, and gas diffusion. These processes collectively define foam aging, which progressively alters bubble size distribution, stability, and cohesiveness. Early-phase foam, immediately after production, typically exhibits optimal characteristics for sclerotherapy: relatively uniform bubble size, adequate stability, and good injectability. As time passes, liquid drains from lamellae, bubbles coalesce, and larger bubbles grow at the expense of smaller ones. Clinically, this manifests as increased injection resistance or, conversely, sudden loss of foam structure resulting in liquid-like behavior. Numerous experimental and clinical studies emphasize that time-to-injection is a critical variable in foam sclerotherapy. Delayed injection increases variability and reduces reproducibility, even when all other production parameters are standardized. For this reason, expert protocols typically specify maximum acceptable intervals between foam preparation and injection, particularly when using less stable gas compositions. In summary, foam quality is the product of multiple interdependent determinants. Mastery of these variables allows vascular experts to tailor foam characteristics to specific clinical scenarios, maximizing efficacy while maintaining safety. Understanding and controlling sclerosant type and concentration, liquid-to-gas ratio, gas composition, temperature, and time-dependent aging are fundamental prerequisites for high-level foam sclerotherapy practice.

5 Manual Foam Production Techniques

Manual foam production remains the most widely used approach for generating sclerosing foam in daily clinical practice. Despite the development of controlled, proprietary microfoam systems, physician-compounded foam continues to play a central role due to its flexibility, low cost, adaptability to different clinical scenarios, and immediate availability. However, manual foam production is intrinsically operator-dependent and subject to significant variability, which can directly affect foam quality, intravascular behavior, efficacy, and safety. For vascular experts, manual foam production should be understood not as a simple preparatory maneuver but as a technical procedure governed by physical principles. The choice of mixing system, syringes, connectors, number of passes, and handling time all contribute to the final foam characteristics. In 1997, Monfreaux introduced its method for physician-compounded foam: a glass syringe containing liquid sclerosant and with an outlet sealed by a cap. The piston is pulled back so to generate a sub-atmospheric pressure, sucking air into the syringe. A quite liquid foam with large bubbles is generated. A significant variability can be found following the different pressure that can be applied to aspirate air [10]. In 2001, the Tessari method was described, and it reported two syringes connected by a three-way stopcock, allowing repeated transfer of sclerosant solution and gas between the syringes to generate foam through turbulent mixing [11]. In its classic configuration, one syringe contains the liquid sclerosant and the other contains gas, typically room air. A commonly used liquid-to-gas ratio ranges from 1:3 to 1:4, although variations exist depending on operator preference and clinical indication. The syringes are connected via a three-way stopcock, and the mixture is passed rapidly back and forth for a defined number of cycles, usually between 10 and 20 passes (Fig. 4.2). Caution must be applied in the variability associated with the number of times and the pressure on the plunger as these two aspects can impact the physical properties of the generated foam. Apart from this operator-dependent aspect, variability can also be generated by the amount of stopcock dead space. Possible advantages of this production method can be found in its simplicity and low cost, with no need of specialized equipment. At the same time, this last aspect can be considered as a limit, in light of the significant variation in foam production happening even just changing the type of syringe.

A technical variant is to rotate the three-way stopcock by 45% so to increase the turbulence and the density of the sclerosing foam. It must be noted that this is an empirical consideration still lacking evidence-based published support and can exacerbate the lack of standardization and reproducibility of the Tessari method.

The double syringe system (DSS) (Fig. 4.3) is a manual foam production technique conceptually similar to the Tessari method but typically using a straight female-to-female Luer connector instead of a three-way stopcock [33]. This modification alters the flow path and shear profile during mixing, leading to differences in foam characteristics.

Two syringes, one containing sclerosant and the other gas, are connected directly via a Luer connector. Foam is generated by rapidly transferring the contents back and forth between the syringes for a predefined number of passes, commonly between 10 and 30 strokes. The absence of a stopcock may reduce unintended gas trapping and ratio distortion. DSS-generated foam may exhibit a slightly more uniform bubble size distri-

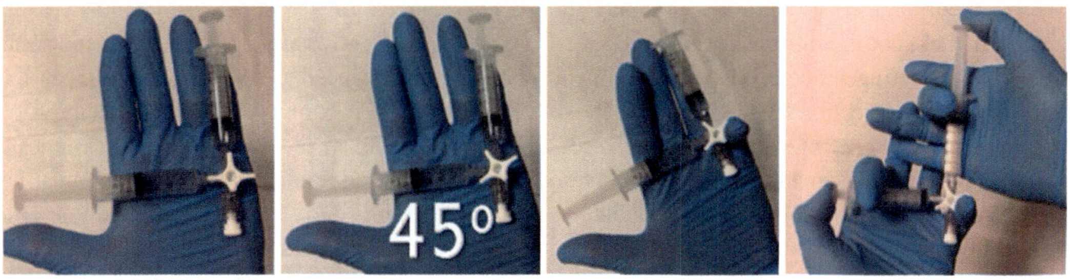

Fig. 4.2 *Tessari method:* two syringes connected by a three-way stopcock

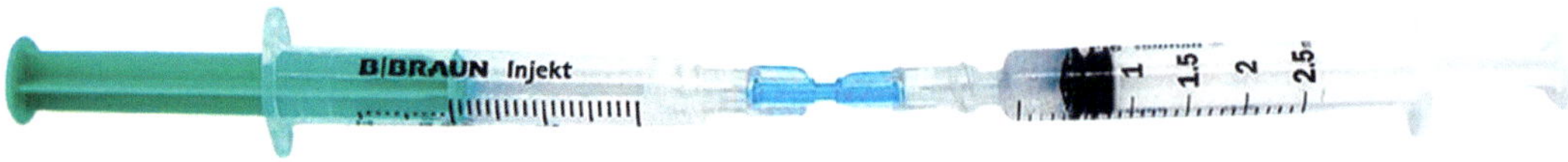

Fig. 4.3 Double syringe system female-to-female Luer connector, involving two syringes containing gas and liquid, respectively. The angle of the bending of the connector can alter the generated turbulence and related foam features. Picture copyright: Dr. Serge Mako, Kreussler Pharma (France)

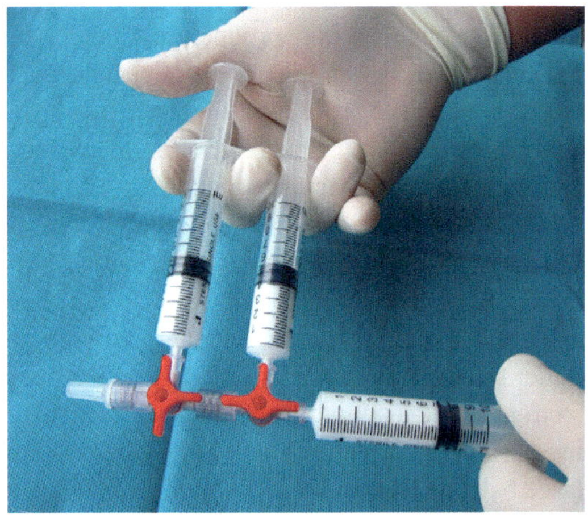

Fig. 4.4 Multi-syringe system, from the open access publication Xu J, Wang YF, Chen AW, Wang T, Liu SH. A modified Tessari method for producing more foam. SpringerPlus. 2016 Feb. 19;5:129

bution than classic Tessari foam, although both systems remain polydisperse [36]. A recent retrospective publication showcased the DSS method competitiveness in a retrospective evaluation of great and small saphenous vein treatment by sodium tetradecyl sulfate sclerotherapy [37]. Despite these advantages, DSS remains operator-dependent and sensitive to syringe diameter, connector internal diameter, and mixing technique, underscoring the need for strict protocol standardization. Recognizing the variability inherent in the classic Tessari method, several modified Tessari techniques have been proposed to improve foam consistency, injectability, and handling characteristics. Using smaller-diameter syringes can increase shear forces during mixing, resulting in smaller average bubble size and improved foam homogeneity. However, excessive shear may also accelerate foam degradation if overmixed. Different stopcock designs and orientations influence turbulence and dead space volume. High-quality, low-dead-space stopcocks can reduce unintended dilution and improve reproducibility. Standardizing the number and speed of syringe passes is one of the most effective ways to reduce inter-operator variability. Foam properties change significantly beyond a certain number of mixing cycles, for which there is a need for predefined protocols [38]. Multi-syringe systems extend the basic Tessari principle by incorporating a third syringe into the circuit. In these configurations, foam is generated between two syringes and then collected into a third syringe for injection (Fig. 4.4).

A variant is represented by a specific three-syringe technique designed to improve injection smoothness [39]. By collecting foam into a "clean" syringe that has not undergone repeated plunger movements, this method reduces plunger friction and allows more controlled injection, particularly through small-gauge needles. Multi-syringe and tourbillon systems do not fundamentally alter foam physics but improve ergonomics and delivery precision. They are particularly useful in delicate applications, such as perforator veins or small-caliber tributaries, where injection control is paramount. Of course this comes with the cost of an increased complexity, of a greater risk of ratio drift if not carefully managed. Additional connections also increase potential for air leakage. Summing up, several are the technical sources of variability in manual foam, which is inherently variable. Operator-Dependent factors are the speed and force of syringe passes, the number of mixing cycles, as well as the subjective assessment of "acceptable" foam appearance. To this, equipment-related factors must be added, taking into consideration the syringe diameter, volume, and lubrication, the connector type and internal geometry, the dead space and gas compressibility. Last but not least, process-related factors must be taken into consideration as well, such as liquid-to-gas ratio inaccuracies, time delay between production and injection, temperature and environmental conditions (anatomy and hemodynamics in the surroundings of the injection site). Uncontrolled variability can lead to inconsistent endothelial contact, unpredictable foam migration, and difficulty comparing outcomes between sessions or operators.

6 Considerations on Material and Equipment

In foam sclerotherapy, materials and equipment should be regarded as active determinants of therapeutic performance, not neutral accessories. At an advanced level of practice, foam quality is no longer conceptualized as a binary outcome ("good" versus "poor" foam), but rather as the result of controlled interactions between device geometry, surface chemistry, and operator-applied energy. Even when sclerosant concentration, gas composition, and liquid-to-gas ratio are rigorously standardized, subtle differences in syringes, connectors, and mixing mechanics can produce clinically relevant changes in foam microstructure and intravascular behavior. From a physics standpoint, manual foam production is a turbulent multiphase dispersion process in which gas fragmentation, lamella formation, and early foam aging occur simultaneously. The devices used during this process define the shear field, flow regime, and boundary conditions under which bubbles are created and stabilized. For expert operators treating truncal veins, perforators, or recurrent disease, mastery of equipment-related variables is essential for achieving reproducible closure rates while minimizing adverse events. Syringe volume is frequently discussed in terms of convenience, yet its internal diameter is the parameter of primary physical importance. For a given plunger velocity, smaller-diameter syringes generate higher shear rates, promoting more efficient gas fragmentation and smaller initial bubble diameters. Bench studies demonstrate a direct inverse relationship between syringe internal diameter and mean bubble size when other variables are held constant [34]. In contrast, larger-volume syringes generate lower shear forces and tend to produce coarser, more polydisperse foams, particularly when combined with low-turbulence connectors. While such foams may be acceptable for large superficial varices, they are less suitable for truncal veins or perforators where cohesive, plug-like flow is desired [26]. Syringe selection should therefore be target-specific rather than generic. Small-diameter syringes are preferable when precision, homogeneity, and predictability are prioritized, whereas larger syringes may be justified only when foam volume requirements outweigh microstructural considerations. Plunger lubrication, typically achieved using silicone oil, introduces an often under-appreciated variable into foam production. Silicone reduces friction and improves smoothness of plunger motion, but it also modifies operator feedback and mixing regularity. Excessively lubricated plungers may glide unevenly, leading to irregular shear application and inconsistent bubble formation. Furthermore, variability in silicone coating thickness between syringe manufacturers and even between production lots can alter injection resistance and mixing dynamics, together with the same foam tensioactive properties [41]. For high-volume or research-oriented centers, this variability represents a significant confounder when attempting to standardize foam production protocols. Top-level practice therefore favors strict equipment consistency, often including a single syringe manufacturer, a fixed syringe volume, a lot tracking whenever possible. The appropriate sclerotherapy culture must approach the matter mirroring the quality control principles used in pharmaceutical compounding and interventional device trials. Three-way stopcocks, classically used in the Tessari method, introduce nonlinear flow paths with abrupt directional changes. These geometric features increase turbulence intensity and promote gas fragmentation. However, they also introduce significant internal volume (dead space) and multiple zones of flow stagnation. From a foam physics perspective, stopcock geometry creates heterogeneous shear fields, resulting in broader bubble size distributions compared with linear connectors. While this may enhance initial foam formation, it also accelerates early coalescence and foam aging if mixing is excessive. At an expert level, stopcocks should be viewed as high-energy mixing devices whose benefits must be balanced against their intrinsic variability. Selection of low-dead-space, high-precision stopcocks is therefore essential for reproducibility. Straight female-to-female Luer connectors, commonly used in DSS, create a more axially symmetric flow path with reduced turbulence and lower internal volume. This geometry favors more uniform shear distribution and often produces foam with narrower bubble size. However, reduced turbulence means that adequate foam quality requires intentional compensation through increased mixing passes or higher plunger velocities. Failure to adjust technique accordingly may result in under-mixed, unstable foam. For expert operators, straight connectors offer superior process control, particularly when foam production protocols are rigorously standardized and reproducibility is prioritized over maximal turbulence. Dead space represents one of the most insidious sources of error in manual foam production. Defined as the internal volume not directly governed by plunger displacement, dead space can systematically distort the intended liquid-to-gas ratio. Because gas is compressible and liquid is not, dead space preferentially traps gas during mixing, effectively increasing the gas fraction beyond the nominal ratio. This phenomenon becomes increasingly significant as total foam volume decreases, making it particularly relevant in expert-level treatments of perforators and small truncal segments. Additionally, repeated cycling of foam through dead space accelerates lamellar thinning and bubble coalescence, contributing to premature foam aging. Expert protocols therefore emphasize minimization of connector volume, elimination of unnecessary junctions, and consistent priming techniques. Mixing energy is determined by the integrated shear applied over time, incorporating plunger velocity, stroke length, syringe diameter, and connector geometry. Insufficient energy results in incomplete gas dispersion and unstable foam, whereas excessive energy disrupts lamellae and accelerates foam decay. Importantly, optimal mixing energy is system-specific. The same number of passes may produce fundamentally different foam characteristics depending on syringe size and connector design. This explains why protocols cannot be universally transferred between institutions without recalibration. For expert users, mixing energy should be conceptualized as a controlled variable, not an intuitive action. The number of mixing passes is a practical surrogate for total energy input and one of the few parameters easily standardized across operators. A nonlinear relationship between number of passes and foam quality is present: initial passes reduce bubble size, an optimal plateau is reached, and further passes promote coalescence and instability [18]. Most expert protocols converge on 10–20 passes for Tessari-based systems, with adjustments based on syringe diameter and connector geometry. Exceeding this range does not improve foam quality and may degrade it. Defining and enforcing a standardized number of passes remains one of the most effective strategies for reducing inter-operator variability in high-volume expert centers.

Materials and equipment selection represents a strategic component of foam sclerotherapy, not a logistical afterthought. Syringe geometry, lubrication, connector design, dead space, and mixing mechanics collectively define the shear environment in which foam is created and aged. Mastery of these variables enables predictable foam behavior, reproducible outcomes, and safe expansion of foam sclerotherapy into complex venous territories (Table 4.1). Laboratory data suggest that polidocanol 3% produces a more stable foam than sodium tetradecyl sulfate 3%, yet endothelial and media damage is greater following sodium tetradecyl sulfate action. These data must be confirmed ex vivo and in the different foam production conditions before generalizing them in relation to the several different concentrations and gas combinations [41]. Gas selection is one of the most debated and clinically consequential aspects of foam sclerotherapy. Unlike other determinants of foam quality, which primarily influence local intravascular behavior, gas composition directly links foam physics with sys-

Table 4.1 Main factors influencing foam production performance

Main factors influencing foam production performance
A) Foam production technique
1. Manual (Monfreaux, Double Syringe System, Tessari, etc)
2. Semi-automated (Varixio™, Sclerofoam™)
3. Fully automated (Varithena™, MFoamer™)
B) Materials & equipment
1. Syringe and needles geometry
2. Lubrication
3. Connector design
4. Dead space
5. Mixing mechanic
6. Sclerosing drug
C) Gas componenT
1. Nitrogen, Oxygen, Carbon Dioxide, Mixtures
2. Liquid / Gas (wet vs dry)
3. Temperature

temic biological effects. The choice of gas affects bubble stability, foam persistence, embolic potential, endothelial contact time, and ultimately both efficacy and safety. For the vascular expert, gas selection should not be guided by dogma or tradition, but by a nuanced understanding of gas solubility, diffusion kinetics, foam-aging mechanisms, and procedural workflow. Room air is the most commonly used gas in physician-compounded foam sclerotherapy worldwide. Its widespread adoption is largely due to availability, ease of use, and favorable foam stability characteristics. Air consists primarily of nitrogen (≈78%) and oxygen (≈21%), with nitrogen being poorly soluble in blood and aqueous solutions. The low solubility of nitrogen confers prolonged bubble persistence, resulting in foams with longer half-life and greater structural stability. However, prolonged bubble persistence also implies slower biological clearance. Echocardiographic studies have demonstrated transient right-heart echogenic signals following air-based foam injections, reflecting the passage of gas bubbles through the venous circulation [42]. While clinically significant neurologic events are rare, their association with paradoxical embolism via right-to-left shunts has been documented [30]. Carbon dioxide has been proposed as an alternative gas for foam sclerotherapy because of its high solubility in blood and rapid diffusion across biological membranes. CO_2-based foams dissolve significantly faster than air-based foams, resulting in shorter bubble persistence and more rapid systemic clearance. From a foam physics perspective, CO_2 produces less stable foams with shorter half-life and accelerated drainage and coarsening. This reduced stability necessitates rapid injection following foam production and meticulous procedural coordination. Delays that would be inconsequential with air-based foam may render CO_2 foam ineffective by the time of injection. Clinically, CO_2 foam may reduce the duration of intravascular gas persistence and has been associated with a lower incidence of transient visual disturbances and migraine-like symptoms in some series. However, its reduced stability may compromise efficacy in larger veins or longer segments unless technique is adapted accordingly. Thus, CO_2 foam is best suited for short-segment treatments, small-caliber veins, or scenarios where rapid gas clearance is prioritized over maximal foam persistence. Mixtures of carbon dioxide and oxygen have been developed to achieve a balance between foam stability and biological clearance. By reducing nitrogen content while retaining manageable handling characteristics, CO_2/O_2 mixtures aim to combine the safety advantages of CO_2 with improved foam performance compared with pure CO_2. Clinically, this translates into a shorter working window than air foam but greater robustness than CO_2 alone. A randomized clinical study comparing air-based foam with CO_2/O_2-based foam reported a modest improvement in truncal vein occlusion rates and reduced hyperpigmentation in the CO_2/O_2 group, although neurologic events were too infrequent to draw definitive conclusions [31]. The fundamental trade-off in gas selection lies between foam stability and biological clearance. Stable foams provide prolonged endothelial contact and predictable intravascular behavior, whereas rapidly clearing foams reduce the duration of gas persistence in the circulation. From a mechanistic standpoint, stability enhances therapeutic efficacy by increasing residence time and minimizing dilution, while rapid clearance may reduce the theoretical risk of systemic gas embolization. However, clinical evidence suggests that procedural factors such as injected foam volume, injection speed, patient positioning, and venous anatomy play a more decisive role in adverse events than gas choice alone. The goal is not maximal stability or maximal clearance per se, but appropriate matching of foam properties to the clinical context. In advanced practice, gas selection should be individualized based on target vein characteristics, treatment extent, patient risk profile, and operator workflow. CO_2/O_2-based foam may be preferred in patients with known right-to-left shunts, migraine history, or heightened sensitivity to transient neurologic symptoms, provided that technique is adapted to compensate for reduced stability. CO_2/O_2 mixtures offer a compromise solution in centers equipped to support their use. Importantly, no gas choice can substitute for meticulous technique. Limiting total foam volume, avoiding forceful injection, and maintaining ultrasound control of foam propagation remain the most effective safety measures regardless of gas composition. Gas selection is therefore best understood as one component of an integrated, physics-informed treatment strategy, rather than as an isolated determinant of outcome.

7 Proprietary Microfoam Systems

The emergence of controlled and proprietary microfoam systems represents a conceptual and technological inflection point in the evolution of foam sclerotherapy. Traditional physician-compounded foam, while effective in expert hands, remains intrinsically dependent on operator technique, equipment variability, and time-sensitive handling. These sources of variability directly affect bubble size distribution, stability, intravascular flow behavior, and ultimately clinical outcomes. Controlled microfoam systems aim to transform foam sclerotherapy from a craft-based procedure into a standardized endovenous therapy, aligning it with contemporary expectations for reproducibility, regulatory oversight, and evidence-based adoption. For vascular experts, these systems do not replace technical knowledge; rather, they shift the locus of control from bedside foam generation to engineered foam specification and delivery strategy. While manual foam production techniques can achieve excellent outcomes in experienced hands, several limitations become evident at scale:

- Inter-operator variability, even within expert centers.
- Inter-session variability for the same operator.
- Dependence on syringe geometry, stopcock design, and gas source.
- Difficulty standardizing foam dose and microstructure across studies.

Even minor variations in mixing energy, timing, or connector dead space produce measurable differences in foam behavior. These differences are magnified in multicenter trials, where reproducibility is essential for regulatory approval and guideline endorsement. Controlled microfoam systems were developed to meet specific engineering and clinical objectives:

- Fixed gas composition, typically low-nitrogen (according to FDA requirements it must be under 0.8% Nitrogen) [45].
- Narrow bubble size distribution, reducing polydispersity.
- Predictable foam decay kinetics, minimizing operator timing dependence.
- Reproducible injectability, including catheter compatibility.

From a regulatory perspective, it must be stress-out that how the regulatory approval of a device does not necessarily mean it is also approved by the clinical governance and by the institutions in charge of the official national guidelines. Up to our knowledge, the only automatic foam production device approved by the regulatory body and by the clinical governance is Varithena® and only for United States and Canada. Varithena® is a commercially manufactured polidocanol endovenous microfoam using a proprietary canister-based system. It combines polidocanol (1%) with an extremely low-nitrogen gas mixture, producing microbubbles with a highly controlled size distribution, typically smaller and more uniform than physician-compounded foams. From a physical standpoint, Varithena® demonstrates reduced Ostwald ripening, increased resistance to coalescence, stable plug-like propagation under physiologic flow conditions [18]. These characteristics result in predictable intravascular displacement of blood, reduced fragmentation, and consistent endothelial exposure along the treated segment [43]. Varithena® represents the first foam sclerosant to undergo large-scale randomized, placebo-controlled trials leading to regulatory approval for truncal vein treatment. This repositioned foam sclerotherapy as a primary endovenous modality, comparable in scope to thermal ablation in selected patients [44]. Clinical trials demonstrate significant improvements in Venous Clinical Severity Score (VCSS), symptom burden, cosmetic appearance, Duplex-confirmed vein closure [43]. Durability studies confirm persistence of benefit at 1 year and beyond, reinforcing Varithena® as a therapeutic option [45]. Unlike Varithena®, which standardizes the foam itself, semi-automated foam generators aim to standardize the process of foam creation, while preserving freedom in sclerosant type, concentration, and gas selection. The typical example is a device named Varixio® which is an electromagnetic driven foam generator designed to deliver precise control over liquid-to-gas ratio, mixing energy, and foam density. It eliminates variables such as plunger speed and number of passes. Its rotor can speed up to 4000 rpm. Bench evaluations show that Varixio® can produce foam at concentrations as low as Polidocanol 0.25% or sodium tetradecyl sulfate 0.2%, bubble diameter less than 250 μm (from 84 ± 14 to 119 ± 6. average 100 μm), with a mean half-life of up to 5.2 min and a liquid:gas ratio between 1:5 and 1:7 [21]. In 2024, a monocentric retrospective study, reported a total occlusion of the great saphenous vein in all treated cases at 1 year follow up, dropping to a partial recanalization rate of 26.8% after 36 months, with a complete one in 6.1% of cases [46]. The following year a retrospective publication highlighted occlusion rate at 15 months of 93.2% (41/43) for the great saphenous vein and 86% (13/15) for the small saphenous vein. Complications were reported in 3.1% of sessions, ranging in between mild and moderate [22].

Meanwhile, a similar device named Sclerofoam entered the market, offering a similar semi-automated foam production method, based on the use of gas capsules and an electromagnetic rotor (max 5000 rpm). Up to our knowledge, no scientific data have been published using this device, for which further evidence is needed in support of the producer website claims ("<120 micron bubble diameter," "up to 5–6 min durability"). Current evidence suggests that foam produced by semi-automated methods presents intermediate characteristics between physician-compounded foam and fully automated microfoam production, making it a process-control adjunct rather than a replacement for Varithena®. Up to our knowledge, the only currently available alternative to Varithena® for a fully automated foam production is MFoamer®, a high-tech device operating by means of an electro-mechanical closed circuit, combining several possible combinations of O_2 and CO_2 gas mixtures, with Polidocanol or Sodium tetradecyl sulfate ranging from 0.1% all the way to 3% (Fig 4.5).

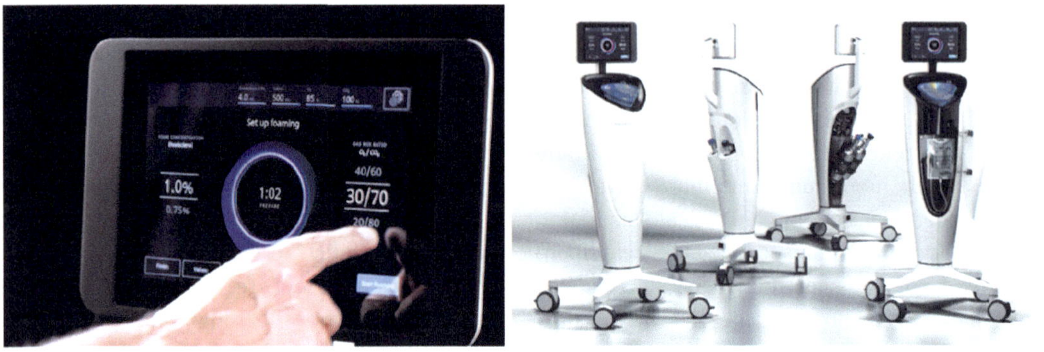

Fig. 4.5 MFoamer® device. Picture available here https://m-foamer.com

8 Integration of Foam Production with Delivery Technique

Foam sclerotherapy must be conceptualized as a continuous system rather than a sequence of discrete steps. Foam generation, delivery, intravascular propagation, and endothelial interaction are mechanically and temporally inseparable processes. Any disruption or mismatch between foam properties and delivery technique can negate the advantages of even the most sophisticated foam formulation. For advanced practitioners, the key question is not *whether* a foam is stable in vitro, but whether it remains functionally intact during injection, transit, and intravascular deployment under physiologic conditions. Needle gauge defines the initial shear environment encountered by foam at the moment of injection. As internal diameter decreases, wall shear rate increases nonlinearly, exposing foam to intense mechanical stress over very short time scales. Even brief exposure to such stress can alter bubble size distribution, disrupt lamellae, and accelerate foam aging. Experimental studies demonstrate that injection through fine-gauge needles ($\geq$27G) increases bubble fragmentation, broadens polydispersity, shortens effective foam half-life in vivo [47]. These effects are not inherently undesirable but must be aligned with clinical intent. In superficial telangiectasias or reticular veins, rapid dispersion and limited persistence may be advantageous. In contrast, truncal and perforator treatments demand cohesive, plug-like foam propagation, which is compromised by excessive needle-induced shear. Injection speed is a second-order but highly influential variable. Rapid plunger depression generates transient pressure spikes and turbulent flow, amplifying shear beyond that predicted by needle diameter alone. Slow, controlled injection minimizes turbulence, preserves foam microstructure, and improves ultrasound-visible predictability of propagation. Needle gauge and injection velocity should be selected as a coupled system, tailored to target vein diameter, foam stability profile, and desired extent of intravascular propagation. Catheter-directed foam sclerotherapy was developed to overcome the limitations of point injection in long or large-diameter veins. By positioning the delivery point within the target segment, catheter-based techniques allow spatial decoupling of access and treatment zones, enabling controlled retrograde or segmental foam deployment. This approach is particularly relevant for large truncal veins, recurrent or neovascularized segments, tortuous anatomy unsuitable for thermal ablation [48]. Catheters impose unique mechanical stresses on foam in the form of the prolonged wall shear during transit, the potential jetting effects at the catheter tip and a sensitivity to lumen diameter, length, and surface finish. Manual foam may undergo significant degradation when delivered through long, narrow-lumen catheters; therefore, controlled microfoam and mechanically standardized foams might represent a better choice as they exhibit greater resistance to catheter-induced breakdown. Expert catheter-based strategies often employ controlled withdrawal techniques, injecting foam incrementally as the catheter is retracted. This allows uniform treatment of long segments while limiting uncontrolled proximal migration. However, the technique demands precise coordination. A detailed description of catheters for sclerotherapy delivery is reported in Chap. 10. Independently by the delivery method, shear stress is the dominant physical force linking foam production, injection, and intravascular behavior. Foam lamellae are thin liquid films stabilized by surfactants: when exposed to shear beyond a critical threshold, these films thin and rupture. Shear arises from needle or catheter transit, injection velocity, interaction with blood flow, changes in vein caliber and curvature. Foam degradation under shear is nonlinear. Moderate shear may refine bubble size and improve homogeneity, whereas excessive or sustained shear accelerates drainage, coalescence, and loss of cohesive structure. Shear should be conceptualized as a dose-dependent modifier of foam quality, analogous to energy input during mixing. The objective is not to eliminate shear, but to apply it deliberately and within tolerable limits. Another aspect that can modify the final foam feature is the perivenous tumescence that can be used to reduce the vessel caliber, rather than for anesthetic purposes. Indeed, it can exert profound mechanical and hemodynamic effects by reducing the vein diameter, displacing intraluminal blood, and dampening local venous flow. These effects enhance foam-wall contact and reduce dilution, allowing lower foam volumes to achieve effective endothelial injury. By decreasing vein caliber and flow velocity, tumescence reduces shear forces acting on foam, promoting cohesive intraluminal propagation and prolonging effective contact time. In catheter-directed and controlled microfoam applications, tumescence acts synergistically to improve predictability and safety [49].

9 Foam Volume, Distribution, and Migration Control

Among all adjustable variables in foam sclerotherapy, foam volume and spatial distribution represent the most powerful and potentially hazardous determinants of outcome. Unlike thermal ablation, where energy deposition is largely confined to the treated segment, foam introduces a mobile, compressible, and buoyant multiphase system whose behavior is dictated by venous anatomy, hemodynamics, and operator technique. Success in foam sclerotherapy depends less on "how much foam" is injected and more on where, how fast, and under what boundary conditions it is allowed to propagate. In foam sclerotherapy, "dose" is a multidimensional construct. The biologically effective dose depends on the sclerosant concentration, the foam volume, the gas fraction and solubility, the bubble size distribution and stability, the endothelial contact time and the degree of blood displacement. Increasing any single component (e.g., volume) without controlling the others does not linearly increase efficacy and may disproportionately increase systemic exposure. This explains why excessive foam volumes may fail to improve closure rates while increasing neurologic or cardiopulmonary signals. Endothelial injury induced by detergent sclerosants demonstrates threshold and saturation behavior. Once the endothelium is adequately exposed and denuded, additional foam confers diminishing therapeutic benefit but continues to contribute gas and sclerosant to the circulation. Maximal foam volume is rarely optimal foam volume. The goal is to reach the biological injury threshold uniformly along the target segment, not to exceed it. Consensus documents and expert guidelines consistently recommend limiting physician-compounded foam volumes per session, typically to ≤10 mL, emphasizing staged treatment when necessary [9]. In contrast, controlled microfoam trials demonstrate that standardized dosing, rather than larger volumes, achieves durable symptom and appearance improvements [43]. Truncal veins and tributary veins represent fundamentally different hemodynamic environments. Truncal veins are high-capacitance conduits with axial flow, reflux pathways, and direct connections to the deep venous system. Tributaries and reticular veins, by contrast, are lower-flow, more compartmentalized structures. In truncal treatment, the objective is segmental, uniform endothelial exposure without uncontrolled proximal migration. Excess foam volume in a truncal vein increases the probability of junctional spillover, deep venous entry, systemic bubble load. Controlled microfoam systems offer advantages here by reducing variability in propagation and fragmentation. For tributary and reticular veins, the goal shifts toward distributed micro-dosing through multiple access points. Smaller foam volumes injected at multiple sites reduce the driving pressure for migration while achieving adequate local injury. Foam migration into the deep venous system is governed by pressure gradients generated during injection, reflux channels and perforators, buoyancy and patient positioning, excessive injected volume or velocity. Migration control is achieved through stacked safeguards, such as proximal manual or ultrasound-guided compression at junctions, limb elevation or reverse Trendelenburg positioning, segmental injection rather than bolus delivery, slow injection velocity, immediate post-injection compression, selection of rapidly soluble gases in high-risk patients. Ultrasound is not merely confirmatory but interventional. Echogenic foam allows real-time visualization of direction and velocity of propagation, segmental filling patterns, entry into perforators or deep veins. This transforms foam sclerotherapy into a closed-loop system, where injection parameters are continuously adjusted based on observed behavior. Experienced practitioners actively modulate delivery by pausing injection when foam approaches junctions, adjusting compression or limb position dynamically, terminating injection upon adequate segmental coverage, using ultrasound to confirm foam dissipation before further injection. Ultrasound serves as the primary risk-mitigation interface, analogous to fluoroscopy in complex endovascular procedures.

10 Safety Considerations Related to Foam Production

Safety in foam sclerotherapy is inseparable from the physics of foam generation and degradation, the physiology of venous and cardiopulmonary circulation, and the operator's capacity to modulate these variables in real time. Unlike thermal or mechanical ablation modalities, foam sclerotherapy deliberately introduces a compressible gas phase into the venous system, transforming a localized intervention into a potentially systemic physiologic perturbation. Adverse phenomena should not be conceptualized as unpredictable "complications," but rather as expected outcomes when defined physical thresholds are exceeded. Neurologic manifestations following foam sclerotherapy form a continuum ranging from benign, transient sensory phenomena to rare ischemic injury. These include visual disturbances (scintillating scotoma, blurred vision, hemianopic phenomena), migraine-like aura with or without headache, transient ischemic attack, ischemic stroke (exceptionally rare) [50]. Critically, the temporal clustering of symptoms, typically within minutes of injection, strongly implicates a gas-mediated mechanism rather than thrombotic embolization [13]. Resolution within minutes to hours further supports a functional, reversible process in most cases. Experimental models demonstrate that foam bubbles entering the cerebral circulation can cause transient microvascular obstruction, endothelial mechanotransduction and irritation, disruption of neurovascular coupling. Importantly, these effects may occur without permanent infarction, explaining why neuroimaging is often normal in symptomatic patients. The pathophysiology closely resembles decompression sickness and contrast microbubble phenomena observed in echocardiography. This mechanistic understanding is essential: gas embolism and thromboembolism are biologically distinct entities, requiring different prevention strategies. Patent foramen ovale (PFO) is present in approximately 25–30% of adults, with variable shunt magnitude and dynamic behavior [51]. In most individuals, the shunt is functionally silent, however, foam sclerotherapy introduces conditions that can transiently unmask shunt patency. Factors facilitating paradoxical embolism include acute increases in right atrial pressure, Valsalva maneuvers during or after injection, postural changes, large or rapidly injected foam volumes. However, PFO presence alone is not sufficient to cause neurologic events. The interaction between shunt anatomy, foam characteristics, and procedural technique ultimately determines risk. Routine screening for PFO is not universally recommended, but selective screening may be appropriate in patients with migraine with aura, prior unexplained neurologic events, planned high-volume treatment. The goal is risk stratification, not risk elimination, allowing informed selection of foam volume, gas composition, and delivery strategy. Gas solubility is a dominant determinant of bubble persistence. Nitrogen, the major component of room air, exhibits low blood solubility and slow diffusion, resulting in prolonged intravascular residence. Clinical comparisons between air-based foam and CO_2 or CO_2/O_2 foams suggest a reduction in transient neurologic symptoms with more soluble gases, particularly in patients prone to migraine-like phenomena [31]. However, differences in major neurologic outcomes remain difficult to demonstrate due to low event rates. Importantly, highly soluble gases produce less stable foam, necessitating compensatory adjustments in technique to maintain efficacy. Safety begins at foam production. Fundamental principles include using the lowest effective foam volume, avoiding excessive gas fractions, favoring standardized or controlled microfoam when large segments are treated. Foam aging should be minimized, as coalescence and Ostwald ripening increase bubble size and unpredictability. Injection-related risk mitigation includes slow, steady injection to avoid pressure spikes, segmental dosing rather than bolus delivery, proximal compression at junctions, patient positioning to counteract buoyancy-driven migration. Expert safety governance included the pre-procedural identification of neurologic risk factors, the informed consent addressing transient neurologic symptoms, the post-procedural observation in high-risk patients. In expert hands, these strategies convert foam sclerotherapy into a predictable and controllable intervention, rather than a probabilistic one. In contemporary expert practice, foam sclerotherapy must be understood not merely as a procedural skill, but as a complex, operator-mediated manufacturing and delivery process. The "product" administered to the patient is a time-dependent, metastable dispersion, whose characteristics are influenced by human behavior, device geometry, environmental conditions, and workflow timing. As foam sclerotherapy has moved from individual expert practice into high-volume centers, multicenter trials, and regulated therapeutic pathways, variability has emerged as a dominant threat to safety, efficacy, and scientific credibility. At the highest level of practice, excellence is therefore defined not by isolated technical brilliance, but by the ability to design, implement, and maintain systems that reliably reproduce optimal foam characteristics across operators, patients, and time. Foam production in expert practice must be conceptualized as a controlled process, analogous to pharmaceutical compounding or contrast preparation in interventional radiology. Without formal constraints, foam properties vary continuously as a function of mixing energy and timing, gas compressibility, syringe and connector type and geometry, operator motor patterns, environmental temperature, and delays. This intrinsic instability mandates explicit procedural boundaries. At a minimum, the following must be standardized:

1. Liquid-to-gas ratio(s).
2. Gas composition (air, CO_2, CO_2/O_2).
3. Syringe volume and manufacturer.
4. Connector type and dead space.
5. Mixing technique (manual vs. mechanical).
6. Number and cadence of mixing passes.
7. Maximum allowable time from foam generation to injection.

Critically, acceptable tolerances (e.g., ±1 pass, ±10 s) should be defined, in order to possess a quality control instrument. Guidelines and recommendations in general should take into consideration the sclerosing drug concentration adjustment based on all the above-mentioned foam features as the power of the sclerotherapy act is clearly not dependent only by one parameter. Intra-operator and inter-operator variability can persist even among senior clinicians, particularly in manual foam production. This reflects fundamental human factors' limitations rather than lack of expertise. Mechanical and controlled microfoam systems reduce, but do not abolish, operator dependence. While foam generation becomes standardized, delivery, volume selection, and migration control remain operator-governed, reinforcing the need for comprehensive training. Documentation is not administrative overhead but a scientific data capture system. Without granular documentation, correlations between foam variables and outcomes cannot be established. An expert documentation framework should systematically capture:

- Sclerosant type and concentration.
- Foam type (manual, mechanical).
- Gas composition.
- Total foam volume and segmental allocation.
- Injection sites and technique.
- Ultrasound findings (pre-, intra-, post-procedure).
- Immediate and delayed adverse events.

This dataset enables root–cause analysis when outcomes deviate from expectations. Participation in registries further allows benchmarking against peer institutions and contributes to the external validity of foam sclerotherapy as a modality. Currently a global real-world data collector has been made available for free and in more than ten languages from all continents (https://v-registry.com). It must also be noted that visual inspection remains the fastest quality check but correlates only imperfectly with objective foam parameters such as bubble size distribution and stability. "Creamy" appearance does not guarantee optimal in vivo performance. Nevertheless, expert visual assessment should systematically evaluate homogeneity, absence of macroscopic bubbles, drainage rate, temporal stability over defined intervals.

11 Failures Identification and Related Solution

In expert foam sclerotherapy practice, failure is rarely accidental. Instead, it reflects predictable breakdowns at the interface between foam physics, delivery mechanics, and venous physiology. High-level mastery is therefore defined not by the absence of failure, but by the ability to recognize early warning signals, identify root causes, and intervene decisively before clinical consequences emerge. Unlike device-based ablation, foam sclerotherapy lacks a single failure point. Errors may originate during foam generation, storage (even seconds matter), injection, or intravascular propagation. Troubleshooting must therefore be anticipatory, structured, and grounded in failure-mode analysis, rather than reactive improvisation. Wet or unstable foam represents one of the most common and most underestimated failure modes in expert practice. It is characterized by high liquid fraction, rapid gravitational drainage, lamellar thinning and rupture, loss of plug-like intravascular behavior. On ultrasound, unstable foam manifests as diffuse echogenic haze, rapid disappearance, and poor segmental filling. Clinically, this translates into inadequate endothelial injury despite apparently correct sclerosant concentration. At expert level, wet foam should be analyzed across four domains:

1. *Formulation Variables*
   - Low gas-to-liquid ratio.
   - Inappropriate sclerosant concentration for foam stabilization.
2. *Process Variables*
   - Insufficient mixing energy.
   - Inconsistent mixing cadence.
   - Delay between production and injection.
3. *Environmental Variables*
   - Elevated ambient or syringe temperature.
   - Heat transfer from operator's hands.

4. *Delivery Variables*
   - Excessive blood dilution due to inadequate compression or high flow hemodynamics from nearby confluences.

These factors are often additive, meaning that marginal deviations in several domains can collectively precipitate failure. Preventively, expert centers should enforce strict time-to-injection limits, control environmental temperature, use ultrasound as a functional stability assay. Another aspect to consider is the excessive bubble size which is not merely a cosmetic imperfection: it directly alters buoyancy, embolic potential, and migration dynamics. Large bubbles fragment unpredictably under shear, resist pulmonary filtration, increase the probability of paradoxical embolization. Thus, bubble size must be considered a safety-critical parameter, not just an efficacy determinant. Excessive bubble size reflects insufficient shear during foam generation or post-generation coalescence. Key determinants include large-diameter syringes producing low shear, minimal connector turbulence, low number of mixing passes, foam aging with Ostwald ripening, nitrogen-rich gas compositions. Notably, attempting to correct large bubbles by forceful injection is counterproductive, as it introduces uncontrolled shear and pressure spikes. Coarse foam should never be injected to avoid waste, while foam exceeding visual or ultrasound size thresholds is to be discarded. On the other side, injection resistance is a sentinel sign of system mismatch. It indicates discordance between foam rheology, delivery device geometry, intravascular opposing conditions. Ignoring resistance and increasing force is a critical expert error, as it converts mechanical impedance into pressure-driven risk. Injection resistance may arise from overly stable or viscous foam, narrow-gauge needles or long catheters, catheter kinking or malposition, partial thrombosis or venous spasm, foam dehydration within the delivery system, access mispositioning. Flow irregularities, such as jerking, jetting, or sudden release, create localized pressure spikes, promoting foam fragmentation and proximal migration. In this scenario, it is important to cease the injection immediately, to proceed with an ultrasound verification of the intravascular conditions, evaluation of the available tools (such as needle/catheter size and patency), to reformulate foam, eventually changing access site. At the highest level of practice, excellence is defined by early recognition of failure signatures, decisive interruption of unsafe processes, structured correction and prevention, continuous learning from deviations. In this framework, failure becomes a source of refinement, and foam sclerotherapy evolves into a mature, highly controlled endovenous therapy based on science and ethics.

12 Emerging Research and Future Directions

Foam sclerotherapy is transitioning from a predominantly empirical technique to a physics-informed, quantitatively governed therapeutic modality. While early development focused on demonstrating feasibility and clinical efficacy, contemporary research is increasingly directed toward understanding causality—that is, how measurable foam properties translate into predictable biological and clinical outcomes. Traditional descriptors of foam quality such as "dense," "creamy," and "stable" are inherently subjective and operator-dependent. While they remain useful heuristics, they lack the precision required for reproducibility, cross-study comparison, or regulatory science. Emerging research seeks to replace qualitative judgment with formal metrology, defining foam in terms of quantifiable parameters such as mean bubble diameter and distribution width, polydispersity indices, gas volume fraction, drainage half-life, coalescence and Ostwald ripening rates, viscosity and yield stress under shear. These parameters allow foam to be treated as a characterizable formulation, analogous to a drug suspension or emulsion. State-of-the-art characterization techniques include high-speed optical and confocal microscopy, automated image analysis with machine-learning-based segmentation, laser diffraction and light scattering, electrical impedance spectroscopy, microfluidic flow visualization platforms. However, a central challenge persists: most measurements are performed under static or simplified conditions, whereas clinical foam experiences dynamic shear, blood interaction, and temperature gradients. Bridging this gap remains a major research priority. This is particularly evident in the need of using gasses that can significantly differ in their solubility in the bloodstream. A fundamental advancement is indeed the need to lower the nitrogen concentration almost to zero, while guaranteeing the necessary foam stability. The critical insight is that quantitative characterization must be context-specific, reflecting not only foam formulation but also delivery and hemodynamic conditions. Early bench models were instrumental in elucidating basic foam behavior, but they lack wall compliance and viscoelasticity, realistic venous geometry and bifurcations, pulsatile flow and reflux dynamics, blood–foam biochemical interactions. As a result, their predictive value for clinical performance is limited, particularly for truncal veins and junctional regions. Recent advances have produced high-fidelity vein model systems incorporating compliant silicone or polymeric walls mimicking venous elasticity, patient-derived or anatomically accurate geometries, controlled flow/reflux and pressure gradients, blood analogs or whole blood to simulate dilution and protein effects [25]. Advanced vein models are increasingly viewed as preclinical validation tools, enabling comparison of foam generation systems, gas compositions, and delivery strategies prior to human studies. For expert readers, this suggests a future in which bench performance becomes a prerequisite for clinical adoption, analogous to device testing in endovascular interventions. Temperature influences virtually every physical property relevant to foam performance, including gas solubility and diffusion, liquid viscosity, drainage rate, coalescence kinetics. Despite this, environmental temperature and thermal handling are rarely controlled or documented in clinical practice. Experimental studies demonstrate that modest temperature variations (±5–10 °C) alter foam half-life, shift bubble size distributions, modify resistance to shear-induced degradation [40]. These findings imply that ambient room conditions, warming of syringes by hand, delays between preparation and injection may introduce systematic but unrecognized variability. Emerging concepts include temperature-regulated foam generators and insulated or actively controlled syringes. Despite extensive work on foam physics, direct linkage between physical foam parameters and clinical endpoints remains limited. Most trials report foam type and volume but omit quantitative descriptors such as bubble size or stability. This disconnection hampers mechanistic interpretation of outcomes, cross-study comparison, rational optimization of foam characteristics for specific vein phenotypes. Current research should aim to establish correlations between bubble size distribution and neurologic risk, foam stability and occlusion durability, gas solubility and systemic exposure, rheologic behavior and catheter deliverability. Such correlations would enable predictive modeling, allowing clinicians to select foam characteristics tailored to vein diameter, anatomy, and patient risk profile. Future clinical trials are likely to mandate standardized foam characterization, stratify outcomes and indications by physical foam parameters, support regulatory frameworks treating foam as a defined formulation rather than a generic technique. In conclusion, the whole chapter signals a paradigm shift: foam physics becomes a clinical variable, subject to optimization and governance rather than tacit assumption.

References

1. McAusland S. The modern treatment of varicose veins. Med Press Circular. 1939;201:404–10.
2. Orbach EJ. Contributions to the therapy of the varicose complex. J Int Coll Surg. 1950;13(6):765–71.
3. Ree A. Etamolin foam in the treatment of varicose veins. A new method. Acta Dermatovenerol. 1953;33:435–6.
4. Cabrera J. New sclerotherapy method for truncular varices. Patología Vascular. 1995;10(4):55–71.
5. Tisi PV, Beverley C, Rees A. Injection sclerotherapy for varicose veins. Cochrane Database Syst Rev. 2006;4:CD001732.

6. Cabrera J, Cabrera J Jr, Garcia-Olmedo MA. Treatment of varicose long saphenous veins with sclerosant in microfoam form: long-term outcomes. Phlebology. 2000;15:19–23.
7. Kern P, Ramelet AA, Wutschert R, et al. Single-blind randomized study comparing polidocanol foam and liquid in sclerotherapy. Dermatologic Surg. 2004;30:718–22.
8. Smith PC. Chronic venous disease treated by ultrasound guided foam sclerotherapy. Eur J Vasc Endovasc Surg. 2006;32(5):577–83.
9. Gianesini S, Obi A, Onida S, et al. Global guidelines trends and controversies in lower limb venous and lymphatic disease: narrative literature revision and experts' opinions following the vWINter international meeting in phlebology, Lymphology & Aesthetics, 23–25 January 2019. Phlebology. 2019;34(1 Suppl):4–66.
10. Monfreux A. Traitement sclérosant des troncs saphéniens et de leurs collatérales de gros calibre par la méthode MUS. Phlebologie. 1997;50:351–3.
11. Tessari L, Cavezzi A, Frullini A. Preliminary experience with a new sclerosing foam in the treatment of varicose veins. Dermatologic Surg. 2001;27:58–60.
12. Cavezzi A, Tessari L. Foam sclerotherapy techniques: different gases and methods. Phlebology. 2009;24:247–51.
13. Morrison N, Neuhardt DL. Foam sclerotherapy: cardiac and cerebral monitoring. Phlebology. 2009;24(6):252–9.
14. Gillet JL. Neurological complications of foam sclerotherapy: fears and reality. Phlebology. 2011;26(7):277–9.
15. Eckmann DM, Kobayashi S, Li M. Microvascular embolization following polidocanol microfoam sclerosant administration. Dermatologic Surg. 2005;31(6):636–43.
16. King JT, O'Byrne M, Vasquez M, VANISH-1 Investigator Group, et al. Treatment of truncal incompetence and varicose veins with a single Administration of a new polidocanol endovenous microfoam preparation improves symptoms and appearance. Eur J Vasc Endovasc Surg. 2015;50(6):784–93.
17. Todd KL 3rd, Wright DI, VANISH-2 Investigator Group. The VANISH-2 study: a randomized, blinded, multicenter study to evaluate the efficacy and safety of polidocanol endovenous microfoam 0.5% and 1.0% compared with placebo for the treatment of saphenofemoral junction incompetence. Phlebology. 2014;29(9):608–18.
18. Carugo D, Ankrett DN, Zhao X, et al. Benefits of polidocanol endovenous microfoam (Varithena®) compared with physician-compounded foams. Phlebology. 2016;31(4):283–95.
19. U.S. Food and Drug Administration. Summary basis of approval: Varithena® (polidocanol injectable microfoam). FDA; 2013.
20. https://www.bostonscientific.com/content/dam/varithena/hcp/Varithena_Instructions_for_Use.pdf
21. Roche E, Pons R, Roche O, et al. A new automated system for the preparation of sclerosant foam: a study of the physical characteristics produced and the device settings required. Phlebology. 2020;35(9):724–33.
22. Roche E, Marqués C. First registry of patients treated with foam sclerotherapy using a new automated microfoam preparation device (2021–2022). Phlebology. 2025;40(4):235–42.
23. Gianesini S, Chi YW, Agüero C, et al. Fake-news-free evidence-based communication for proper vein-lymphatic disease management. Int Angiol. 2023;42(2):89–189.
24. Kabnick LS, Jimenez JC, Coogan SM, Gache L, Frame D, Gunnarsson C, Ozsvath K. Comparative effectiveness of non-compounded polidocanol 1% endovenous microfoam (Varithena) ablation versus endovenous thermal ablation utilizing a systematic review and network meta-analysis. J Vasc Surg Venous Lymphat Disord. 2024;12(6):101896.
25. Bottaro E, Paterson J, Zhang X, et al. Physical vein models to quantify the flow performance of sclerosing foams. Front Bioeng Biotechnol. 2019;7:109.
26. Hill D, Hamilton R, Fung T. Assessment of techniques to reduce sclerosant foam migration during ultrasound-guided sclerotherapy of the great saphenous vein. J Vasc Surg. 2008;48(4):934–9.
27. Meghdadi A, Jones SA, Patel VA, et al. Foam-in-vein: a review of rheological properties and characterization methods for optimization of sclerosing foams. J Biomed Mater Res B Appl Biomater. 2021;109(1):69–91.
28. Peterson JD, Goldman MP. An investigation into the influence of various gases and concentrations of sclerosants on foam stability. Dermatologic Surg. 2011;37(1):12–7.
29. Breu FX, Guggenbichler S. European consensus meeting on foam Sclerotherapy, April, 4–6, 2003, Tegernsee, Germany. Dermatol Surg. 2004;30(5):709–17.
30. Parsi K. Paradoxical embolism and foam sclerotherapy. Phlebology. 2012;27:147–67.
31. Beckitt T, et al. Air versus physiological gas for foam sclerotherapy. Eur J Vasc Endovasc Surg. 2011;42:115–21.
32. Cameron E, Chen T, Connor DE, et al. Sclerosant foam structure and stability is strongly influenced by liquid air fraction. Eur J Vasc Endovasc Surg. 2013;46(4):488–94.
33. Hamel-Desnos C, Desnos P, Wollmann JC, et al. Evaluation of the efficacy of polidocanol in the form of foam compared with liquid form in sclerotherapy of the greater saphenous vein: initial results. Dermatologic Surg. 2003;29(12):1170–5.
34. Carugo D, Ankrett DN, O'Byrne V, et al. The role of clinically-relevant parameters on the cohesiveness of sclerosing foams in a biomimetic vein model. J Mater Sci Mater Med. 2015;26(11):258.
35. Buonsante GF, Marques MA, Barros BCS, et al. Impact of temperature on the production of 1% poli-

docanol foam: comparison between the Tessari and double-syringe techniques in an experimental study. J Vasc Bras. 2025;24:e20250010.
36. Ouvry P, Allaert FA, Desnos P, et al. Efficacy of polidocanol foam versus liquid in sclerotherapy of the great saphenous vein: a multicentre randomised controlled trial with a 2-year follow-up. Eur J Vasc Endovasc Surg. 2008;36(3):366–70.
37. Mariani F, Carbone L, Sozio G, et al. Ultrasound-guided foam sclerotherapy of the saphenous trunks is associated with a low 5-year recurrence rate and improved quality of life in patients with chronic venous disease: a multicenter study. J Vasc Surg Venous Lymphat Disord. 2025;13(4):102212.
38. Xu J, Wang YF, Chen AW, et al. A modified Tessari method for producing more foam. Springerplus. 2016;5:129.
39. Whiteley MS, Patel SB. Modified Tessari tourbillon technique for making foam sclerotherapy with silicone-free syringes. Phlebology. 2015;30(9):614–7.
40. Bai T, Jiang W, Chen Y, et al. Effect of multiple factors on foam stability in foam Sclerotherapy. Sci Rep. 2018;8(1):15683.
41. McAree B, Ikponmwosa A, Brockbank K, et al. Comparative stability of sodium tetradecyl sulphate (STD) and polidocanol foam: impact on vein damage in an in-vitro model. Eur J Vasc Endovasc Surg. 2012;43(6):721–5.
42. Bush RG, Derrick M, Manjoney D. Major neurological events following foam sclerotherapy. Phlebology. 2008;23(4):189–92.
43. Gibson K, Kabnick L, Varithena® 013 Investigator Group. A multicenter, randomized, placebo-controlled study to evaluate the efficacy and safety of Varithena® (polidocanol endovenous microfoam 1%) for symptomatic, visible varicose veins with saphenofemoral junction incompetence. Phlebology. 2017;32(3):185–93.
44. Vasquez M, Gasparis AP, Varithena® 017 Investigator Group. A multicenter, randomized, placebo-controlled trial of endovenous thermal ablation with or without polidocanol endovenous microfoam treatment in patients with great saphenous vein incompetence and visible varicosities. Phlebology. 2017;32(4):272–81.
45. Todd KL 3rd, Wright DI, VANISH-2 Investigator Group. Durability of treatment effect with polidocanol endovenous microfoam on varicose vein symptoms and appearance (VANISH-2). J Vasc Surg Venous Lymphat Disord. 2015;3(3):258–64.
46. Alongi G, Bissacco D, Cervi E. Three-year follow-up analysis of automated microfoam preparation system for great saphenous vein incompetence and varicose veins sclerotherapy treatment. Phlebology. 2024;39(7):471–6.
47. Skuła M, Hobot J, Czaja J, et al. The effect of the calibre and length of needle on the stability of sclerosing foam. Phlebology. 2021;36(4):322–8.
48. Parsi K. Catheter-directed sclerotherapy. Phlebology. 2009;24(3):98–107.
49. Dos Santos JB, Júnior WC, Porta RM, Puggina J, da Silva DF, Puech-Leão P, de Luccia N, da Silva ES. Catheter-directed foam sclerotherapy with tumescence of the great saphenous vein versus ultrasound-guided foam sclerotherapy: a randomized controlled trial. Phlebology. 2020;35(2):84–91.
50. Wong M, Parsi K, Myers K, et al. Sclerotherapy of lower limb veins: indications, contraindications and treatment strategies to prevent complications—a consensus document of the International Union of Phlebology-2023. Phlebology. 2023;38(4):205–58.
51. Hagen PT, Scholz DG, Edwards WD. Incidence and size of patent foramen ovale during the first 10 decades of life: an autopsy study of 965 normal hearts. Mayo Clin Proc. 1984;59(1):17–20.

5 Sclerosant Bubbles' Physics, Biochemistry, and Translational Medicine Properties

Juan Cabrera García Olmedo and Sergio Gianesini

The endothelium is the goal. Blood is only the obstacle.

—Juan Cabrera García-Olmedo

1 Introduction

1.1 Foundational Safety Principles of Pharmaceutical Microfoam

When physicians first encounter injectable sclerosing microfoam, a small set of recurrent questions almost invariably arises. These questions are not naïve: they are the natural expression of clinical prudence when a therapy introduces gas into the vascular system. Historically, such concerns were amplified by early experiences with manually prepared, air-based foams. Addressing these questions explicitly and calmly is therefore a necessary starting point.

J. C. García Olmedo
Pharmacology Unit, International Institute of Phlebology, Granada, Spain
e-mail: juancabrera@cabrera.health

S. Gianesini (✉)
Department of Translational Medicine, University of Ferrara, Ferrara, Italy

Department of Surgery, Uniformed Services University of Health Sciences, Bethesda, MD, USA
e-mail: gnssrg@unife.it

At the origin of pharmaceutical Cabrera microfoam, in 1993, the central safety challenge was framed in very simple terms: what happens to the microbubbles once they are injected?

Understanding this question required following what may be called *the therapeutic journey of injectable sclerosing microbubbles*, from their moment of injection, through their site of action, and finally to their physiological resolution.

"Do the Bubbles Remain Active Once They Leave the Treated Vein?"

In the target vein, microfoam is deliberately structured to be highly active: it displaces blood, occupies the lumen, and places the sclerosant in direct contact with the endothelium. However, this activity is strictly local. Once the foam exits the treated segment and mixes with circulating blood, in general, the sclerosing action ends. Amphipathic molecules such as polidocanol are rapidly stripped from the bubble surface by plasma proteins and erythrocyte membranes, leading to immediate pharmacological neutralization. Beyond the site of action, bubbles no longer carry sclerosing capacity.

S. Gianesini, Y. W. Chi (eds.), *Sclerotherapy*, https://doi.org/10.1007/978-3-032-32794-9_5

"If Bubbles Reach the Heart or Lungs, Can They Carry the Sclerosant and Cause Damage?"

As microfoam leaves the treated venous segment and enters progressively wider vessels, the structured foam column disperses. Individual bubbles detach from one another and the thin sclerosant film that initially coated each bubble is rapidly washed away by the surrounding blood. What remains is no longer a drug-carrying structure, but a transient gaseous "ghost."

From a pharmacological safety perspective, the nature of this residual gas then becomes the only relevant factor. Pharmaceutical microfoam is generated using physiological gases—carbon dioxide and oxygen—with minimal nitrogen content. These gases are highly soluble in blood and readily diffuse across the pulmonary membrane. Consequently, residual microbubbles dissolve and are eliminated through normal respiration within seconds to minutes, without obstructing the pulmonary microcirculation or delivering active drug to distant organs.

"What About the Brain, Especially in Patients with Right-To-Left Shunts?"

This question was one of the most critical ones during early safety evaluations. Preclinical and clinical studies specifically addressed this scenario, demonstrating that microbubbles composed of physiological gases and controlled size traverse capillary beds without producing occlusion or ischemic injury, even when transiently present in the arterial circulation. This behavior contrasts sharply with nitrogen-rich air bubbles, which are poorly soluble and persist intravascularly.

"Why Doesn't this Treatment Sclerose the Deep Venous System?"

The answer lies in control and visibility. Pharmaceutical microfoam is echogenic and injected under ultrasound guidance, allowing the operator to monitor its progression in real time. More importantly, its therapeutic action is self-limited: once diluted by blood and removed from the confined environment of the target vein, its activity ceases. The deep venous system is therefore not exposed to an active sclerosant under correct technique.

"Does the Induced Thrombosis Pose a Risk of Embolization?"

The thrombotic process following microfoam sclerotherapy is mural and adherent by design. Endothelial injury exposes subendothelial collagen, promoting platelet aggregation directly along the vessel wall. The resulting thrombus grows as a continuous, wall-attached structure that evolves into fibrosis, rather than as a free-floating clot prone to embolization.

"Does this Apply to Any Type of Foam?"

No. The safety principles described here apply exclusively to pharmaceutical-grade microfoam. They cannot be extrapolated to manually prepared or air-based foams. Home-made foams typically contain high nitrogen levels, larger and heterogeneous bubbles, and lack internal structural coherence, leading to slower dissolution and unpredictable intravascular behavior. By contrast, pharmaceutical microfoam is defined by controlled micronization, minimal nitrogen content, and rapid physiological neutralization once its local action is complete.

This understanding of the *therapeutic journey of injectable microbubbles* is central to the original development of the technique and remains its ethical foundation. By design, pharmaceutical microfoam respects the most classical principle of medicine: *primum non nocere*. With these foundations established, the mechanistic and pharmacological concepts developed in the following sections can be approached without residual concern.

In this context, microfoam must be understood as a pharmaceutical form in its own right, where dose, distribution, and duration are encoded by structure.

1.2 The Concept of Action and Sclerosis

Human interaction with individual physiology remains extremely limited, even today. Our physical and intellectual constraints restrict both our perception and manipulation of the human body. We cannot perceive biological detail without sophisticated instruments. We rarely understand it fully and again we rely on complex tools whenever we attempt to intervene, if we are confident that such intervention will not cause harm.

Within this context, we define *action* as the final voluntary act upon the patient, the last deliberate event before the clinician loses direct control over the ensuing biological cascade. The administration of a drug, the mechanical stripping of a vein or the chemical injury of an endothelium are all examples of *action* in this sense. What follows these acts, the tissue reaction, the inflammation, and the repair, unfold according to biological laws that the physician can only partially anticipate.

Sclerosis, therefore, represents a unique category of therapeutic action: an intentional, localized, and irreversible transformation of living tissue. It is the deliberate induction of a controlled injury that leads to fibrosis and vessel closure. Unlike most pharmacological interventions, which aim to restore normal function, sclerotherapy seeks to destroy a pathological structure by triggering its biological self-destruction.

This concept of "controlled therapeutic injury" stands as a distinct pharmacological principle, one that merges the physical, chemical, and biological domains into a single act of action.

The use of sclerosing agents in foam form is not a recent innovation. Historical accounts document the therapeutic use of foamed sclerosants as early as 1939, when agitation-based techniques were employed to enhance endothelial contact in the treatment of varicose veins [1].

Subsequent work in the 1940s and 1950s, particularly by Orbach, further explored the clinical potential of foam sclerotherapy, establishing foundational concepts that would later be revisited and refined [2].

In 1993, Cabrera and collaborators introduced a profound evolution of this idea, later consolidated in U.S. Patent 5,676,962, describing injectable microfoam composed of a sclerosing agent, very small microbubbles and physiologic gases. The innovation transformed sclerotherapy from a technique suited only for small-caliber veins (<8 mm) into one capable of treating large-caliber varicose veins (≥8 mm) safely and effectively.

In early theoretical formulations (1993), a simplified yet powerful definition of sclerosing action was proposed as the product of two fundamental variables: the concentration of the sclerosant at the endothelial surface and the duration of its contact. There is little more a sclerotherapist can aspire to achieve than to place the sclerosant precisely at its site of action and ensure it remains there long enough to produce the desired endothelial injury. This concept, intuitive in theory but challenging in practice, has guided more than three decades of pharmaceutical and technological refinement, still evolving today and enabling new therapeutic frontiers. This dual dependency forms the foundational equation of *action* in sclerotherapy:

$$\text{Sclerosing Action} = \text{Sclerosant Concentration} \times \text{Endothelial Contact Time}$$

Ultimately, every act of sclerotherapy reduces to the clinician's ability to optimize these two variables. The *action* may be appropriate for the therapeutic objective, insufficient to achieve sclerosis or excessive—leading to undesired damage. Mastering this balance defines both the science and the art of sclerotherapy.

However, the observable *sclerosing effect*, the stable histological outcome, does not follow identically in all patients. To account for biological variability, a proportionality constant k is introduced, still undetermined experimentally, which links the physical–chemical action to its biological consequence:

$$\text{Sclerosing Effect} = k \times (\text{Sclerosant Concentration} \times \text{Endothelial Contact Time})$$

When $k \approx 1$, the local action translates efficiently into effect;

When $k < 1$, the tissue exhibits lower susceptibility (e.g., thicker glycocalyx, faster plasma neutralization), and when $k > 1$, the endothelium is more vulnerable (e.g., fragile membranes, reduced protein buffering).

This expression serves as a clinical rule of thumb: to enhance the therapeutic effect within safe limits, one may adjust either the effective concentration at the interface or the exclusive laminar contact time. The proportionality constant k encapsulates interindividual biological variability and awaits future experimental determination.

2 Pharmaceutical Concepts

2.1 Specific and Nonspecific Drugs

The surface of a cell resembles a complex forest far more than a barren desert. The cellular membrane is populated by receptors, transport channels, signaling molecules and countless other structures essential to cellular function. Inside the cell, the number of macromolecules and specialized organelles is even greater, forming an extraordinarily complex and dynamic environment.

In pharmacology, these active cellular structures are typically the targets of drugs, which act by increasing, decreasing, or blocking their activity. The interaction between a drug and its receptor, known as the *drug–receptor interaction*, is generally highly specific. This principle of molecular recognition defines the precision of most modern pharmacological therapies.

However, this concept of *specificity* does not apply to sclerosing agents. Sclerosants belong to the class of nonspecific drugs, agents whose action is governed not by receptor binding but by physicochemical interactions with biological structures. Instead of targeting a particular molecular site, they act on the cellular membrane as a whole, dissolving and disrupting its organization. The result is a loss of membrane integrity, cell lysis, and, ultimately, irreversible sclerosis of the treated tissue.

Among this group, detergent-based sclerosants such as polidocanol and sodium tetradecyl sulfate (STS) stand out. These compounds are amphiphilic: each molecule contains both hydrophilic and lipophilic segments, allowing them to insert spontaneously into lipid bilayers. The outcome is the destabilization of membrane structure, the loss of selective permeability, and eventual endothelial cell destruction.

Polidocanol, the principal sclerosant used in microfoam formulations, is a nonionic amphipathic alcohol with the molecular formula $C_{30}H_{62}O_{10}$. It belongs to the class of fatty alcohol ethoxylates, characterized by a hydrophobic alkyl chain and a hydrophilic polyoxyethylene segment. Its physicochemical properties—surface tension of approximately 31.8 mN/m and density near 0.97 g/cm^3—explain its ability to integrate into lipid membranes and modify interfacial forces.

This nonspecific mode of action situates sclerotherapy at the crossroads between pharmacology and physical chemistry. Its predictability arises not from molecular selectivity but from controlled exposure, a balance between concentration, contact time, and mechanical delivery that determines whether the result will be gentle endothelial irritation or complete sclerosis.

For nonspecific drugs such as sclerosants, therapeutic outcome cannot be inferred from molecular identity alone; it emerges from how exposure is structured in space and time.

2.2 Amphipathic Substances: Developing Clinical Intuition

Matter is generally neutral, yet at the molecular scale small fluctuations in electric charge can be detected. Some atoms strongly attract neighboring electrons and create an uneven distribution of charge across the molecule. This property, called polarity, is typical of molecules containing electronegative atoms (electron-hungry atoms) such as oxygen, nitrogen, or fluorine. Water is the best-known polar molecule and many of its remarkable physical properties arise from this polarity.

Other molecules are strongly nonpolar, with atoms that show little attraction for neighboring electrons. As a result, they form electrically uniform and completely neutral surfaces. This is the case for substances like fats and oils.

But what happens when a single molecule contains both a polar and a nonpolar part? These are amphipathic molecules. This chimeric configuration truly exists in nature and is, in fact, one of the most fundamental features underlying the origin and maintenance of life itself, as it drives the formation and stability of every known biological membrane. Amphipathic molecules spontaneously orient themselves in solution: the nonpolar segment seeks other nonpolar environments, while the polar region aligns toward water when it is present. They behave like molecular compasses, spontaneously rotating until they adopt a configuration in which their fatty tails cluster together, hidden from water, while their polar heads form a continuous shell in contact with the surrounding aqueous environment. This self-organizing behavior is both spontaneous and emergent, and it underlies one of the fundamental processes in the formation and stabilization of cell membranes.

To develop a useful intuition about amphipathic substances, imagine a molecule acting as a bilingual interpreter, fluent in both the language of water and the language of fat. One end, the hydrophilic head, seeks the company of water molecules; the other end, the hydrophobic tail, avoids water and prefers lipids. When such a molecule meets a cell membrane it naturally aligns: one side facing water, the other embedded in fat.

This dual personality allows amphipathic molecules to align at interfaces and reduce surface tension. At sufficient concentrations, they organize into micelles, where the hydrophobic tails hide inside while the hydrophilic heads face the surrounding water. When they encounter a biological membrane, they insert into its lipid layer, disturbing its architecture. If enough of them insert, the membrane weakens, loses its barrier properties, and eventually ruptures.

In sclerotherapy, this property explains why agents like polidocanol and sodium tetradecyl sulfate (STS) can damage endothelial cells. Their amphipathic structure allows them to insert into the lipid bilayer of the endothelium, destabilizing it until the cell ruptures. When the sclerosant is presented as a microfoam, the amphipathic molecules concentrate at the gas–liquid surface of each bubble, creating millions of microinterfaces where molecular interactions occur simultaneously.

Understanding amphipathic substances, therefore, is not about mastering chemistry but about developing intuition for how microfoam behaves in real tissue. Their capacity to align, penetrate, and destabilize cell membranes is what gives them their clinical efficacy. This concept naturally leads to the next section, where we explore in greater depth how these molecules interact directly with the endothelial membrane.

2.3 Sclerosant–Endothelium Interaction: Endothelial Disruption Driven by Amphipathic Properties

The interaction between sclerosants and the venous endothelium is a fundamental event in sclerotherapy. Molecules such as polidocanol and sodium tetradecyl sulfate (STS) exploit this principle: the hydrophobic tail of each molecule penetrates the membrane's lipid core, while the hydrophilic head remains exposed to the aqueous plasma environment. This asymmetric arrangement destabilizes the bilayer, leading to localized defects that merge into macroscopic lesions. What begins as a molecular rearrangement becomes a macroscopic event with endothelial denudation and vessel sclerosis.

The mechanism of action of polidocanol and sodium tetradecyl sulfate (STS) is concentration dependent. At concentrations above 0.2%, polidocanol induces endothelial disruption and cell lysis. When its *action* is properly managed, this leads to predictable sclerosis with an excellent safety profile. When the molecule integrates into the endothelial lipid bilayer, it reduces membrane surface tension, leading to osmotic imbalance, calcium influx, and ultimately apoptosis or necrosis of the endothelial cells. Once the endothelial lining is destroyed, exposure of the subendothelial collagen triggers adherent thrombosis and, subsequently, fibrosis, resulting in permanent occlusion of the treated vein.

Unlike drugs with a specific target, sclerosants are nonspecific pharmacologic agents whose outcome depends on the physical state and distribution of the agent at the site of action. *Every accessible portion of the cell membrane can serve as a target for sclerosing agents*. The development of pharmaceutical-grade microfoam, as implemented in validated formulations characterized by controlled micronization and physiological gas mixtures, provides unprecedented control over these conditions. The foam architecture markedly increases the effective interfacial contact area between polidocanol molecules and the venous endothelium by several orders of magnitude compared to liquid sclerosants. This enhanced interface stabilizes the agent long enough to produce controlled endothelial destruction before it is rapidly inactivated by plasma proteins and erythrocyte membranes [3, 4].

Clinically, this means that understanding the amphipathic behavior of these molecules is essential for optimizing foam preparation and predicting their interaction with the endothelium. In practice, the sclerosant's potency depends on how easily these molecules can reach and align at the membrane surface. When delivered as microfoam, they concentrate at the gas–liquid interface, exponentially increasing their available surface area and enhancing the probability of interaction. This is why the microfoam form is not merely a delivery system: it is a pharmacological amplifier of amphipathic behavior.

This nonspecific but highly controllable mechanism situates sclerotherapy at the intersection of pharmacology, biophysics, and engineering. The sclerosant's potency is governed not by molecular affinity but by exposure dynamics, the combination of concentration, contact time, and mechanical delivery. Understanding these parameters transforms what was once an empirical technique into a reproducible pharmacological process, bridging the molecular structure of polidocanol with the macroscopic vascular outcomes observed in clinical practice.

For the practicing phlebologist, understanding amphipathic molecules is less about memorizing chemistry and more about visualizing this dynamic interplay between water, lipids, and interface. The sclerosant works precisely because it can exist comfortably in all three environments and, in doing so, destabilizes the delicate balance that maintains vascular wall integrity. This conceptual foundation naturally leads to the next topic: how to maximize the interaction between polidocanol and the endothelial membrane, where these amphipathic principles manifest in clinical reality. What ultimately governs this interaction is not only concentration, but the extent and organization of the interface through which contact occurs.

2.4 Pharmaceutical Concept of Active Surface

The concept of active surface is central to understanding how microfoam technology transforms a liquid sclerosant into a three-dimensional pharmaceutical system. In classical pharmacology, the notion of active surface rarely appears, since most drugs act by binding to specific molecular receptors. However, for sclerosing agents such as polidocanol, efficacy depends not on receptor affinity but on how much of the agent can physically contact the target tissue, the vascular endothelium, at any given time [5, 6].

The *active surface* can be defined as the total interfacial area where the sclerosant molecules are available to interact with the endothelial membrane. The larger this area, the greater the probability of molecular exchange and membrane disruption.

In the liquid form of sclerosant, the contact surface is limited to the narrow film between the injected solution and the blood. In contrast, when the sclerosant is converted into microfoam with controlled micronization and a high gas–liquid interface density, the gas–liquid surface of each microbubble becomes a new pharmacologically active surface. Pharmaceutical implementations typically operate within micrometric bubble size ranges and employ physiological gas mixtures to ensure both efficacy and safety [3].

This surface magnification ensures that billions of microbubbles can interact simultaneously with the endothelium, multiplying the opportunities for membrane disruption and accelerating the onset of sclerosis.

From a biophysical standpoint, this concept unites geometry and pharmacology. The effective active surface determines both the rate and intensity of endothelial injury, just as receptor density determines drug potency in classic pharmacology. Smaller bubbles and a uniform size distribution produce a higher total surface area and greater pharmacologic efficiency, a relationship expressed mathematically as $A \propto n^{1/3}$ at constant gas volume.

Clinically, understanding the active surface concept helps explain why pharmaceutical-grade microfoam achieves superior outcomes compared with hand-made foams: greater homogeneity, longer half-life, and predictable endothelial interaction. The microfoam therefore acts not merely as a vehicle but as a surface amplifier, translating the molecular amphipathic behavior of polidocanol into a macroscopic pharmacologic advantage that bridges chemistry, geometry, and clinical efficacy.

Thus, in sclerotherapy, the concept of active surface is not merely theoretical: it is a measurable determinant of efficacy. Understanding and controlling it is essential for designing foams with predictable performance, balancing potency with safety. However, increasing active surface alone is insufficient. The therapeutic behavior of microfoam depends critically on how that surface is structurally organized.

The concept of active surface area introduced here can be further formalized and explored quantitatively. For readers interested in a geometric and energetic treatment of surface scaling in microfoam, a complementary analysis is provided in Appendix A.

2.5 Design Principles of Therapeutic Pharmaceutical Microfoam

Representative microstructural configurations illustrates distinct geometric regimes of foams commonly encountered in experimental and clinical contexts.

Polyhedric foam (top left) exhibits rigid lamellar junctions and polyhedral deformation, resulting in mechanical brittleness, rupture under shear, and suboptimal post-action disaggregation.

Borderline foam (top right) represents an unstable transitional regime with limited reproducibility and unpredictable behavior.

Tangent-Bubble Kugelschaum (TBK) (bottom left) is defined by micrometric spherical bubbles in tangential contact, providing elastic cohesion, piston-like intravascular behavior, effective endothelial contact, and controlled post-action metabolization. Kugelschaum dispersed in liquid (bottom right) consists of isolated bubbles lacking connectivity, unable to generate mechanical displacement or sustained therapeutic action and functionally behaving as a turbid liquid.

This figure delineates the structural space of injectable foams and highlights that only the TBK regime supports reproducible efficacy and systemic safety in large-volume sclerotherapy.

The term *foam* is widely used in sclerotherapy, yet it encompasses materials with profoundly different physical organizations and, consequently, radically different biological

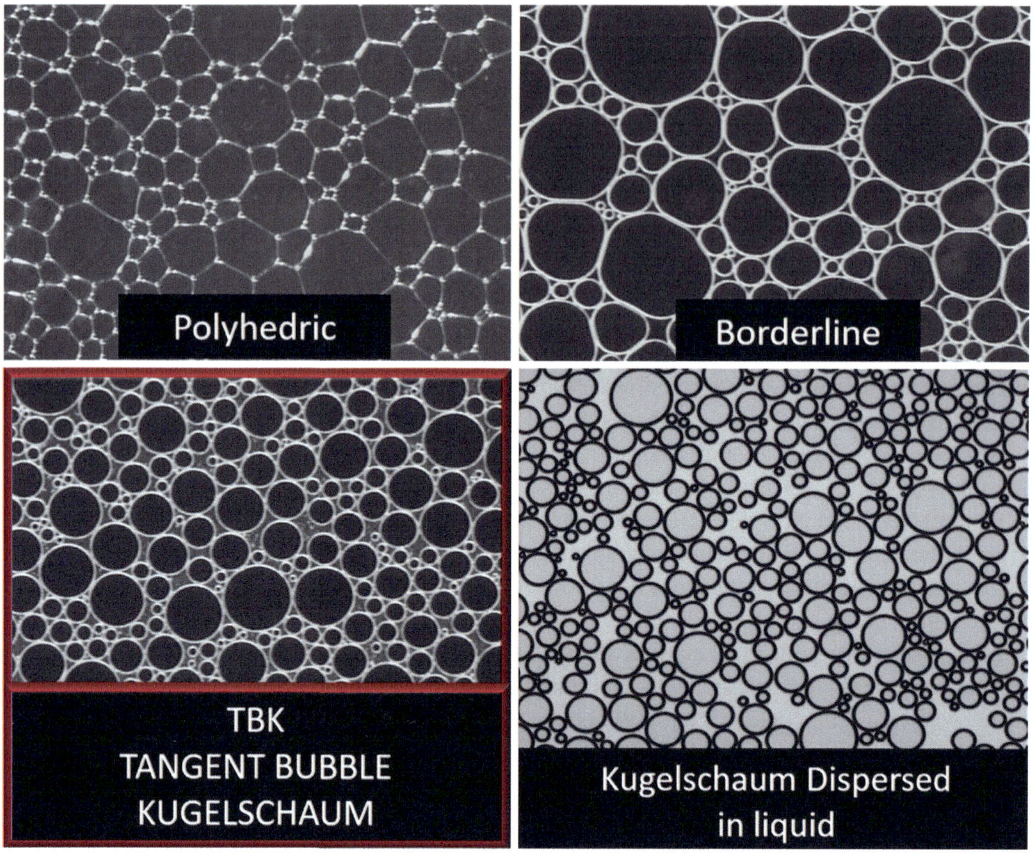

Fig. 5.1 Structural regimes of foams and their functional relevance in sclerotherapy

behaviors. Visual similarity or shared chemical composition does not imply functional equivalence. What determines whether a foam can act as a therapeutic system, particularly at large injected volumes, is not its appearance, but its structural regime.

Figure 5.1 provides a structural map of foams commonly encountered in clinical and experimental settings. Rather than depicting a continuum of quality, it delineates distinct geometric regimes, each associated with characteristic mechanical behavior, intravascular performance, and metabolic fate. These regimes are not interchangeable.

This distinction is essential: therapeutic microfoam occupies only a narrow region of this structural space and provides the conceptual foundation for the design principles discussed below.

As illustrated in Fig. 5.1, four archetypal configurations can be identified.

Polyhedric foams are characterized by rigid lamellar junctions and polyhedral deformation of bubbles. This geometry confers apparent stability at rest but proves mechanically fragile. Under shear, such as during passage through needles or catheters, these foams fracture abruptly. Fragmentation not only compromises coherent lumen occupation, but also generates poorly controlled gas–liquid fragments that disaggregate inefficiently and are suboptimal for predictable metabolization.

Borderline foams occupy an unstable transitional regime between polyhedric and spherical configurations. Their behavior is inherently variable: minor perturbations in shear, temperature, or composition may shift them toward premature collapse or excessive rigidity. From a therapeutic standpoint, this regime lacks reproducibility and cannot be relied upon for controlled large-volume treatment.

Kugelschaum dispersed in liquid consists of isolated spherical bubbles suspended in a continuous liquid phase. Although bubbles may be small, their lack of mutual contact prevents collective mechanical behavior. These systems do not act as foams in the therapeutic sense: they fail to displace blood, do not sustain endothelial contact, and behave functionally as turbid liquids rather than as intravascular tools.

Only one regime fulfills the simultaneous requirements of cohesion, adaptability, action, and safe disappearance: the tangent-bubble Kugelschaum (TBK).

In a TBK, bubbles are approximately spherical, micrometric in size, and connected through point-to-point (tangential) contact. This geometry avoids rigid lamellar constraints while preserving connectivity. The result is a foam that is neither brittle nor dispersed, but elastically coherent.

Mechanically, TBK foams can deform, roll, and rearrange locally without losing collective integrity. This enables them to pass through needles without catastrophic rupture and to advance intravascularly as a cohesive, piston-like column capable of displacing blood and uniformly contacting the endothelium, even in large-caliber veins.

Pharmacologically, the TBK regime provides the optimal balance between active surface availability and temporal stability. Amphipathic sclerosant molecules remain concentrated at gas–liquid interfaces, long enough to exert controlled endothelial injury, yet the structure does not trap the system in a persistent, non-dissociable state.

Critically, the same tangential organization that supports action also enables orderly post-action disassembly. Once structural confinement is lost beyond the target vein, bubbles detach individually and are rapidly stripped of sclerosant by blood components, dissolving according to the high solubility of physiological gases. Action, neutralization, and metabolization therefore form a continuous and self-limiting sequence.

Within this framework, a pharmaceutical microfoam can be defined structurally rather than procedurally:

A pharmaceutical microfoam is a tangent-bubble Kugelschaum (TBK) with bubble radium in the micrometric range, in which bubbles have tangential neighbors and are filled with physiological gases such as carbon dioxide and/or oxygen with nitrogen content below 0.8%.

This definition intentionally excludes foams that fall outside the TBK regime, regardless of how they are prepared or how similar they may appear macroscopically. It also clarifies why not all "foams" are therapeutically equivalent, and why large-volume sclerotherapy cannot be reliably performed outside this structural window.

The structural map presented in Fig. 5.1 makes explicit a central principle of pharmaceutical microfoam:

Structure does not modulate function: it enables it.

Outside the TBK regime, therapeutic action and safe metabolization decouple. Foams either lose coherence before acting or persist beyond their useful window. Within the TBK regime, by contrast, geometry encodes function: mechanical displacement, endothelial contact, and physiological clearance emerge naturally from structure.

For this reason, TBK should be regarded not as an idealized or optional configuration, but as the minimal structural condition under which injectable microfoam becomes a reproducible, scalable, and safe pharmaceutical tool.

Table 5.1 Structural determinants of pharmaceutical microfoam and their pharmacological implications

Structural parameter	Physical meaning	Pharmacological implication	Clinical relevance
Bubble size distribution	Partitioning of gas volume across bubbles	Determines total endothelial contact surface	Homogeneous lumen occupation
Interfacial surface area	Gas–liquid–endothelium interface	Site of sclerosing action	Effective endothelial exposure
Structural coherence	Degree of bubble connectivity	Sustains piston-like behavior	Controlled displacement of blood
Gas composition	CO_2/O_2 vs N_2 content	Solubility and elimination rate	Systemic safety
Temporal stability	Persistence of structure over time	Duration of effective contact	Predictable therapeutic window
Echogenicity	Acoustic reflectivity	Real-time visualization	Ultrasound-guided control

2.6 Bubble Micronization: Increasing the Active Surface and Enhancing Sclerosing Capacity

Sclerosants act through their amphipathic nature, embedding themselves in cell membranes and producing direct endothelial damage. As nonspecific agents, their efficacy depends primarily on the extent and duration of contact between the active substance and the endothelial surface. Micronization of bubbles markedly increases the total active surface area available for interaction, thereby maximizing contact between the sclerosant and the venous endothelium and enhancing the transfer of active molecules to the target tissue.

From a pharmaceutical perspective, bubble micronization represents one of the key engineering and pharmacological advances that distinguishes pharmaceutical microfoam from manually prepared foams. As described in Cabrera's 1993 patent and supported by subsequent analyses, microfoams with controlled bubble size distributions, typically in the 20–100 μm range, produced with defined gas–liquid ratios and physiological CO_2/O_2 mixtures with minimal nitrogen content, achieve a favorable balance between stability, safety, and sclerosing efficiency [3, 6]. These parameters represent one validated pharmaceutical implementation of the broader principle that bubble micronization amplifies active surface availability and prolongs effective endothelial contact. In this way, a simple liquid solution is transformed into a dynamic delivery system with amplified local potency. Recalling the fundamental relationship governing sclerosing action, Sclerosing Action = Sclerosant Concentration × Contact Time, bubble micronization enhances both terms simultaneously. By increasing the available interfacial surface, micronized foam limits immediate dilution by blood flow and maintains close proximity between the sclerosant and the endothelium, thereby extending effective contact time and facilitating molecular transfer. Empirical observations support this principle. Pharmaceutical-grade microfoam prepared under controlled conditions exhibits a substantially prolonged intravascular dwell time relative to air-based and manually prepared foams, reflecting its homogeneous bubble size distribution and resistance to coalescence [3]. These properties reduce drainage, prolong endothelial contact, and improve mechanical blood displacement, while also mitigating Ostwald ripening and preserving structural stability across injections. Clinically, pharmaceutical-grade microfoam enables the treatment of large-caliber veins (≥8 mm) using higher injection volumes while maintaining complete lumen occupation and uniform endothelial denudation without systemic toxicity. From a clinical standpoint, increased bubble uniformity directly translates into greater active surface availability and improved therapeutic efficiency. Bubble size uniformity is therefore not merely an engineering achievement but a pharmacological requirement, defining the boundary between empirical sclerotherapy and a fully realized pharmaceutical technology, one in which physics, chemistry, and vascular physiology converge to optimize both efficacy and safety. In pharmaceuti-

The Priming Effect

In the early 1990s, foam sclerotherapy was regarded as suitable only for small and medium veins, while large truncal veins were treated surgically or with thermal ablation.

In February 1993, Juan Cabrera (Jr.) explored the idea that a small, strategically placed priming injection of microfoam could provoke a reflex vasospasm in a large horizontal vein. This initial spasm would narrow the lumen, expel intraluminal blood, and transform the vein, momentarily, into a smaller, more manageable target for complete foam occupation and sclerosis. The goal was ambitious: to extend the reach of sclerotherapy beyond its traditional limits and to conceive a unified therapeutic technology for veins of all calibers.

This physiological mechanical sequence, *priming dose → progressive vein contraction → full foam occupation → sclerosis*, was later confirmed and formalized within the Cabrera group and validated both experimentally and clinically [5, 7]. The same procedural logic is now reflected in modern Varithena® practice: clinicians inject ≤5 mL of pharmaceutical-grade microfoam, confirm vasoconstriction by duplex ultrasound, and, if necessary, add small aliquots until full occupation is achieved.

As *Coleridge Smith* noted, "*The first injection produces spasm of the treated vein and facilitates the passage of foam to more proximal veins with the subsequent injections.*" [8]

Similarly, Bradbury et al. [9] advised injecting slowly, waiting for spasm to occur and resuming only after the foam clears, again mirroring the priming-and-fill strategy.

Together, these observations confirm that this priming effect is not an abstract notion but a reproducible physiological event that has become standard practice in modern foam sclerotherapy. Its first formulation in 1993 marked one of the earliest deliberate attempts to bridge small-vein sclerotherapy with the treatment of large truncal veins, thus expanding the therapeutic horizon of venous disease.

A modest experimental insight matured into a fundamental principle: a minimal initial dose invites the vein to contract and the subsequent foam injection and occupation complete the closure.

cal microfoam, geometry does not modulate dose: it defines it. The key structural features governing the pharmacological behavior of pharmaceutical microfoam are summarized in Table 5.1.

3 Microfoam in the Site of Action

The following sections invite the reader to dive deeper into a field still unfamiliar to many physicians—where pharmaceutical microfoam demonstrates that even the largest venous trunks can be treated safely, effectively, and reproducibly, provided that the right structure and formulation are in hand, as achieved in validated pharmaceutical implementations capable of safely delivering volumes ≥20 mL.

3.1 Large Vein Sclerosis: From Historical Limitations to Structure-Driven Solutions

Endovenous management of large-caliber truncal veins (typically ≥8 mm) has long been dominated by surgery and thermal ablation techniques, including endovenous laser ablation (EVLA) and radiofrequency (RF) closure. While effective, these approaches are inherently invasive, resource-intensive, and frequently require tumescent anesthesia and a semi-surgical environment.

More recently, the availability of pharmaceutical-grade, FDA-approved microfoam (Varithena™) has expanded the therapeutic landscape, offering a non-thermal, non-tumescent alternative capable of achieving comparable or superior occlusion rates in large truncal veins with reduced procedural burden and improved patient tolerance.

Traditionally, sclerotherapy was considered most suitable for smaller varicosities, with limited evidence supporting its use for larger trunks due to concerns about inconsistent sclerosant behavior and efficacy in high-flow, large-diameter veins [10].

Early attempts to extend sclerotherapy to larger veins relied on increasing sclerosant concentration or injection volume or on the use of manually produced foams generated by agitation techniques. Although conceptually appealing, these approaches resulted in foams with highly variable bubble size and stability, leading to inconsistent intravascular behavior and unpredictable clinical outcomes [11].

Extending the scope of sclerosants from small to large veins therefore represented a major clinical challenge—and, at the time, only a bold supposition.

In February 1993, a simple physiological hypothesis was explored: that a small, strategically delivered priming dose of microfoam could provoke a defensive vasospasm in a large horizontal vein.

By allowing the foam to rise and contact the superior endothelial surface, this initial stimulus was observed to induce progressive venous contraction, expelling intraluminal blood and transiently reducing the vessel diameter. A vein previously considered "surgical-sized" could thus be transformed into a temporarily smaller and more manageable target for complete foam occupation and sclerosis.

This sequence, priming dose → progressive contraction → full foam occupation → sclerosis, provided a physiological and mechanical solution to the long-standing challenge of treating large-caliber veins using a single, sclerotherapy-based technology and laid the conceptual foundation for what would later become modern pharmaceutical microfoam therapy. This sequence becomes mechanically possible only when microfoam behaves as a coherent intravascular system, rather than as a fragmented dispersion.

In essence, a minimal priming dose invites the vein to contract and subsequent microfoam delivery completes closure within a temporarily reduced lumen: an approach that extends sclerotherapy beyond its traditional limits and toward a unified therapeutic framework applicable to veins of all sizes.

The validity of this concept was subsequently confirmed in clinical studies. Trials employing polidocanol 1% microfoam formulated with physiological CO_2/O_2 gas mixtures demonstrated high and reproducible occlusion rates in the great saphenous vein, with outcomes comparable to thermal ablation techniques and improved predictability relative to manually prepared foams [7].

From a mechanistic standpoint, the priming effect can be understood as a sequence of coupled physical, chemical, and physiological interactions: (i) a priming phase in which a small amount of microfoam contacts the superior venous wall and induces localized irritation and vasospasm; (ii) a contraction phase during which muscular constriction progressively reduces venous diameter; (iii) an occupation phase in which the lumen becomes sufficiently small to allow complete foam filling; and (iv) a sclerosis phase characterized by uniform endothelial injury leading to fibrosis and permanent closure.

The buoyancy of microfoam ensures preferential action at the endothelial surface, while the amphipathic nature of polidocanol guarantees effective membrane disruption upon contact. Simultaneously, the use of physiological gas mixtures ensures rapid absorption and elimination of excess bubbles, maintaining safety even in patients with patent foramen ovale [12].

Clinically, the priming effect enables a staged, ultrasound-guided closure of large veins without catheters, thermal injury, or surgical trauma. By integrating physics, pharmacology, and vascular

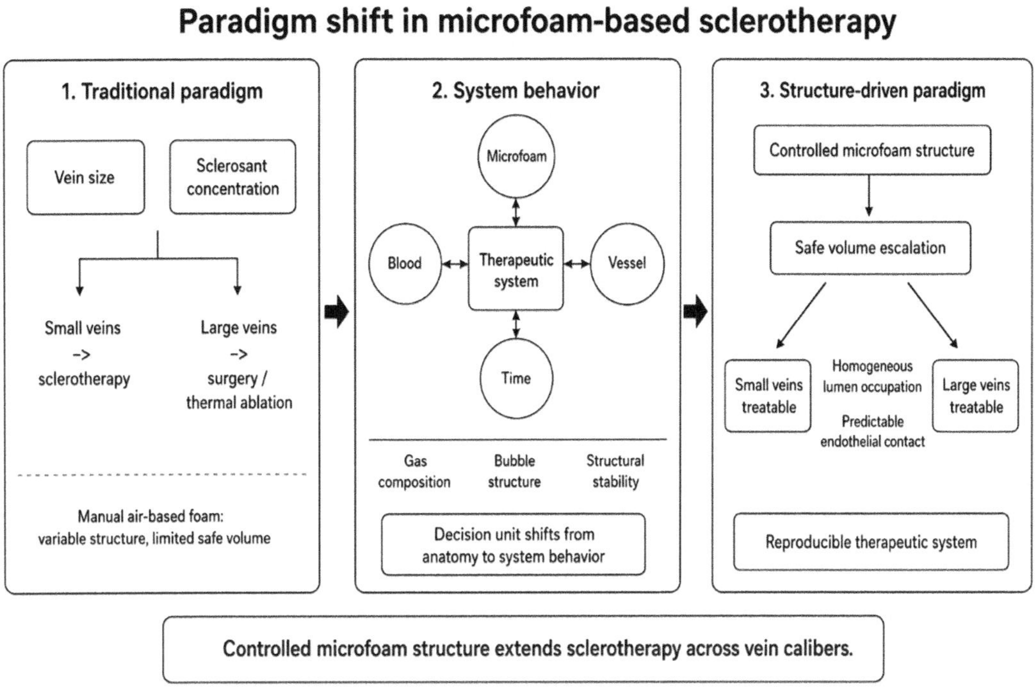

Fig. 5.2 Paradigm shift in sclerotherapy: from technique-limited indication to structure-driven therapeutic systems
Conceptual Illustration of the Paradigm Shift Underlying Modern Microfoam-Based Sclerotherapy
In the traditional indication paradigm, treatment decisions were primarily governed by vein size and sclerosant concentration, confining sclerotherapy to small veins while reserving large truncal veins for surgical or thermal approaches. Foam, when manually prepared and air-based, exhibited variable structure and limited safely injectable volume
The central panel illustrates the paradigm shift from technique to system behavior, where the decision unit changes from static anatomical parameters to the dynamic behavior of a coupled therapeutic system composed of microfoam, blood, vessel geometry, and time. Within this framework, gas composition, bubble structure, and structural stability jointly determine how the system behaves once activated in vivo
Controlled microfoam structure enables safe volume escalation without increasing sclerosant concentration, allowing homogeneous lumen occupation and predictable endothelial contact. As a result, both small veins and large truncal veins become treatable within the same structure-driven pharmacological paradigm, transforming sclerotherapy from an empirical, operator-dependent technique into a reproducible therapeutic system

physiology, this approach converts a large, high-capacity vein into a precisely controlled therapeutic environment, marking a conceptual and practical milestone in the evolution of modern sclerotherapy.

This conceptual transition is summarized in Fig. 5.2, which illustrates the shift from technique-limited sclerotherapy to a structure-driven therapeutic paradigm.

3.2 Viscosity and Mechanical Action

In the treatment of large-caliber varicose veins (≥8 mm), where high intraluminal flow and gravitational forces challenge controlled sclerosant delivery, the mechanical properties of pharmaceutical microfoam play a decisive role. In this context, foam behavior cannot be understood as that of a simple liquid, but rather as that of a semi-viscous, structured system whose rheological properties govern intravascular performance.

Foam drainage, coalescence and mechanical stability are governed by interfacial forces and viscosity, which together determine how bubbles interact with each other and with the surrounding blood under shear conditions [13]. A viscosity higher than that of liquid sclerosants allows pharmaceutical microfoam to advance slowly and uniformly through the venous lumen, limiting premature blood–foam mixing and preserving structural coherence long enough to establish effective endothelial contact.

Unlike low-viscosity liquids, pharmaceutical microfoam behaves as a cohesive continuum: it resists rapid drainage, adheres transiently to the venous wall and maintains homogeneous contact along the endothelium despite high-flow conditions. Experimental studies have shown that microfoams generated with physiological gases (CO_2/O_2) maintain cohesion under shear stress and resist coalescence more effectively than air-based, manually prepared foams, resulting in more predictable intravascular behavior and reproducible rheological performance [3, 14].

This mechanical behavior translates directly into a piston-like action within the vessel. As the foam advances, it displaces blood efficiently while distributing the sclerosant evenly along the endothelial surface. Such controlled mechanical propagation helps ensure that each treated venous segment experiences a comparable effective dose, reducing spatial heterogeneity in endothelial injury and improving treatment predictability.

From a clinical standpoint, structure-driven viscosity links the physician's hand directly to intravascular dynamics. The microfoam does not merely flow: it can be guided. It advances deliberately, displacing blood without turbulence and occupies the lumen in a predictable, laminar fashion. In this setting, viscosity emerges not merely as a physical parameter, but as an enabling property that supports mechanical precision, pharmacological stability, and hemodynamic predictability in the treatment of large veins.

3.3 Bubble Echogenicity and Ultrasound Visibility

Echogenicity, the ability of a structure to reflect ultrasound waves, plays a central role in the visualization and control of sclerotherapy procedures. In the treatment of large-caliber veins (≥8 mm), where high-volume injections of microfoam (≥20 mL) are frequently required, ultrasound visibility becomes a critical determinant of procedural precision and safety.

Each microbubble within pharmaceutical microfoam acts as a discrete ultrasound reflector. The gas–liquid interface of bubbles in the micrometric range generates a pronounced acoustic impedance mismatch, making microfoam highly echogenic under duplex ultrasound. This physical property allows clinicians to follow foam propagation in real time, assess its intraluminal distribution, and verify complete lumen occupation while monitoring for unintended passage into deep venous systems [12].

Unlike liquid sclerosants, which are essentially sonographically invisible, microfoam provides continuous visual feedback throughout injection. The advancing foam column can be observed as it displaces blood, induces vasospasm, and initiates sclerosis, enabling dynamic adjustment of injection rate and volume. This real-time visualization constitutes a key safety feature when treating large venous segments.

From a biophysical standpoint, echogenicity reflects the density and persistence of gas–liquid interfaces within the foam. A stable and homogeneous ultrasound signal corresponds to a coherent population of microbubbles, maintaining their structure under intravascular conditions. Experimental studies comparing pharmaceutical-grade microfoam with manually prepared, air-based foams have demonstrated that physiologic gas microfoams produce uniform, sustained ultrasound reflections, whereas hand-made foams generate irregular and rapidly fading signals due to heterogeneous bubble size and early collapse [7, 15].

Clinically, this visibility enhances operator control and confidence. Under ultrasound guidance, foam progression can be paused, redirected, or confined in response to visual cues, ensuring that therapeutic action remains limited to the intended venous territory. In this context, echogenicity is not merely a diagnostic convenience but an intrinsic pharmacotechnical feature, linking acoustic physics, foam structure, and the controlled execution of sclerotherapy in large veins.

3.4 Exclusive Vessel Occupation

One of the defining mechanical advantages of pharmaceutical microfoam is its ability to achieve complete and homogeneous occupation of the venous lumen, particularly in large-caliber veins treated with high-volume injections. This property transforms the treated vein from a passive conduit into a controlled therapeutic chamber, in which sclerosant action can be spatially and temporally regulated.

Unlike liquid sclerosants, which mix freely with blood and are rapidly diluted or deactivated by circulating erythrocytes and plasma proteins, pharmaceutical microfoam behaves as a deformable intravascular piston. Its structured organization, characterized by a coherent population of microbubbles and a balanced gas–liquid architecture, allows it to displace blood effectively and establish direct, uninterrupted contact with the endothelial surface. By excluding blood from the reaction space, microfoam minimizes premature sclerosant neutralization and maximizes pharmacological efficiency.

This piston-like behavior enables uniform endothelial exposure even in tortuous, dilated, or irregular venous segments. Exclusive vessel occupation thus functions not only as a pharmacological enhancer, but also as a safety mechanism: by isolating the treatment segment, it limits uncontrolled mixing with circulating blood and reduces the risk of distal migration of active bubbles. In practical terms, the vein becomes a transient, closed therapeutic environment optimized for controlled chemical injury.

Clinical and experimental observations support this principle. In ex vivo and in vivo models, pharmaceutical-grade microfoam has been shown to maintain structural coherence and uniform displacement along the venous segment under variable pressure conditions, resulting in homogeneous endothelial contact. In patients with great saphenous vein incompetence, real-time ultrasound imaging confirms complete lumen filling during injection and reproducible vein closure outcomes.

From a clinical perspective, exclusive vessel occupation represents both a pharmacological advantage and a procedural safeguard. By confining sclerosant action to a well-defined intravascular space, both concentration and contact time can be controlled at the endothelial target, largely free from the "blood noise" that otherwise interferes with chemical injury. In this state, dilution, uneven distribution, and restricted access to the vessel wall are minimized or eliminated. The result is a precise, localized endothelial insult leading to predictable fibrosis and safe therapeutic resolution—an operational realization of the concept of *controlled therapeutic injury* that underpins the microfoam paradigm.

4 Intravascular Gas Bubbles Within the Human Circulatory System

4.1 Systemic Neutralization of Bubbles After Action

As the microfoam piston exits the treated venous segment and enters vessels of larger caliber, the physical conditions that once sustained its cohesion progressively change. The foam, which behaved as a compact and laminar front within the confined geometry of the target vein, now encounters a wider lumen, reduced wall friction, and increasingly turbulent blood flow. In this new environment, the balance between surface tension and viscous confinement is lost, and the microfoam gradually disassembles into its elementary bubbles, thereby leaving the TBK regime imposed by the confined geometry of the treated vein.

This transition is continuous and self-regulating. Fragmentation begins at the leading edge of the piston: the outermost bubbles, exposed to direct contact with venous blood, lose their shared lamellae and detach from the collective matrix. Each bubble becomes an independent entity surrounded by plasma proteins and erythrocytes that immediately adsorb the amphipathic sclerosant molecules remaining at its surface. As a result, the foam packet progressively dissolves into individual bubbles, each losing its sclerosing capacity at the moment it abandons the structural protection of the piston.

In physical terms, this process represents a shift from collective stability to individual dissolution. The structured ensemble that once moved as a single therapeutic entity disperses into transient components undergoing deactivation through dilution, adsorption, and diffusion. In physiological terms, it marks the safe termination of the therapeutic action, the precise moment when localized pharmacologic activity yields to systemic neutrality.

The same amphipathic nature of polidocanol that enables its strong interaction with endothelial membranes also ensures rapid inactivation once the foam begins to mix with circulating blood beyond the treatment zone. Because amphipathic molecules show no specificity for endothelial membranes, they bind indiscriminately to the abundant erythrocyte membranes and plasma proteins present in the bloodstream. As demonstrated by Wright and colleagues, once microfoam enters the circulation there is no measurable enrichment of polidocanol at the bubble interface, confirming that the agent is rapidly stripped from the foam and redistributed into plasma and erythrocyte membranes [16].

As bubbles become enveloped by red blood cells that adsorb the remaining sclerosant into their lipid membranes, each bubble is progressively deprived of pharmacologic activity, leaving only transient spheres of inert gas. Experimental and theoretical analyses of microbubble behavior have shown that such gas spheres, once separated from their stabilizing structure, rapidly lose biological relevance and traverse the circulation without inducing tissue injury [13].

From a clinical perspective, this self-limiting behavior is particularly relevant in the treatment of large vessels (≥8 mm) using high-volume microfoam injections (≥20 mL). Rapid post-contact inactivation of the sclerosant ensures systemic safety even when extensive venous territories are treated. This chemical neutralization occurs concurrently with dissolution of the gas phase, governed by Henry's and Laplace's laws simultaneously. The physiological CO_2/O_2 gas mixture used in pharmaceutical microfoam dissolves rapidly in blood: smaller bubbles, characterized by higher internal pressure, collapse first, releasing minute amounts of polidocanol that are immediately bound and rendered inert. Within seconds to minutes, the initially cohesive piston transforms into a diffuse suspension of inert gas remnants and blood-bound detergent molecules, completing the transition from pharmacologic activity to physiological clearance [5].

In pharmacologic terms, pharmaceutical microfoam behaves as a self-limiting system. Although the plasma half-life of polidocanol ranges from approximately 100–150 min, its sclerosing activity is extinguished within seconds once diluted in circulating blood. In parallel, the CO_2/O_2 gas mixture employed in pharmaceutical microfoam is absorbed within minutes and eliminated through pulmonary exhalation, completing systemic clearance [5, 12].

In summary, the interplay between amphipathic chemistry, controlled geometry and physiologic dissolution ensures that the sclerosant acts precisely where intended and nowhere else. The bloodstream, often viewed solely as a source of dilution, reveals its dual role as both a competitor and an antidote. Controlled degradation of microfoam thus marks the natural conclusion of the therapeutic cycle: action, effect, and resolution. In large-vessel, high-volume sclerotherapy, this mechanism constitutes the cornerstone of safety, allowing potent local efficacy while preventing systemic adverse effects.

The behavior of pharmaceutical smicrofoam can be understood as a time-ordered therapeutic journey, summarized in Fig. 5.3.

4.2 Gas Composition, Nitrogen, and Intravascular Safety

The composition of the gas phase is a critical determinant of the intravascular behavior and safety profile of sclerosing microfoam. Although

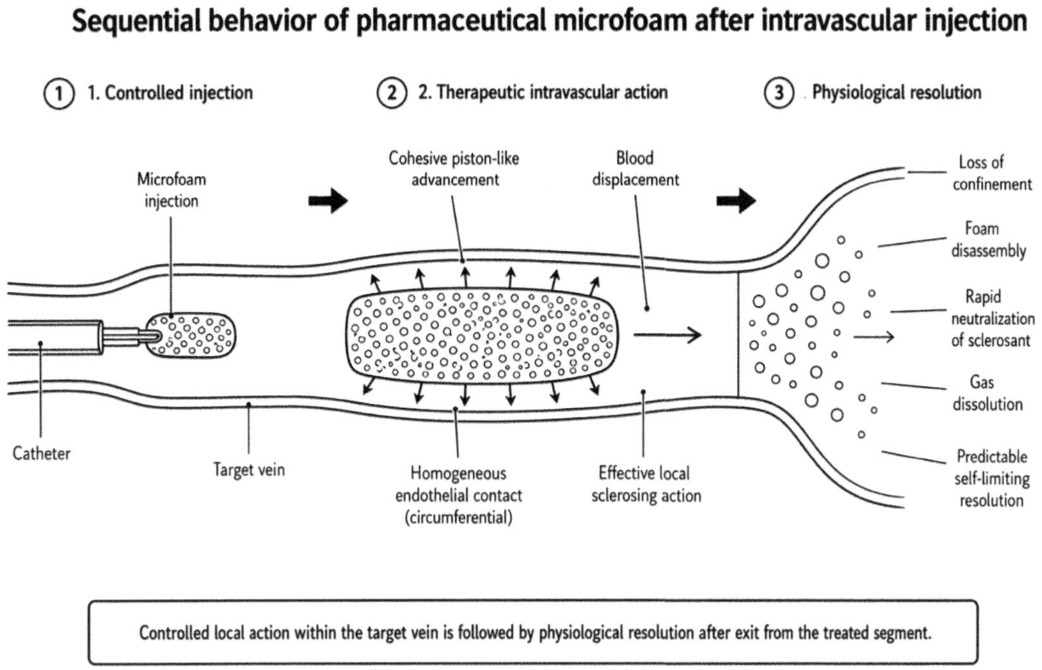

Fig. 5.3 The therapeutic journey of injectable microfoam
Schematic Representation of the Sequential Behavior of Pharmaceutical Microfoam Following Intravascular Injection
After controlled injection, microfoam advances as a cohesive, piston-like structure that displaces blood and occupies the venous lumen. This enables homogeneous endothelial contact and effective local sclerosing action within the target segment
Upon exiting the treated vein, loss of structural confinement leads to disassembly of the foam, rapid neutralization of the sclerosant, and dissolution of the gas phase. The therapeutic system thus transitions from controlled action to physiological resolution in a predictable and self-limiting manner

gas volume and bubble size influence mechanical performance, it is the physiological solubility of the gas itself that ultimately governs systemic fate once the foam exits the treatment zone.

Carbon dioxide and oxygen, the gases used in pharmaceutical-grade microfoam, are highly soluble in blood and rapidly diffuse across the alveolar membrane according to Henry's law. In contrast, nitrogen exhibits markedly lower solubility and persists intravascularly for longer periods. This fundamental physicochemical difference has direct clinical implications: bubbles composed of physiological gases dissolve quickly, whereas nitrogen-rich bubbles remain stable and detectable for prolonged intervals [13].

Experimental studies of microbubble behavior have shown that nitrogen-containing air-based foams generate bubbles that resist dissolution and maintain intravascular integrity well beyond their therapeutic window. These persistent gas emboli may traverse the circulation as intact entities, producing detectable embolic signals and, in susceptible anatomical contexts, raising safety concerns [14]. By contrast, microbubbles composed of CO_2/O_2 collapse rapidly once structural confinement is lost, leading to efficient systemic clearance.

The preferential dissolution of physiological gases introduces an inherent safety gradient. Smaller bubbles, characterized by higher internal pressure as described by Laplace's law, dissolve first, accelerating the breakdown of the foam structure into biologically inert components. This process is self-amplifying: as bubbles shrink, dissolution accelerates, ensuring that residual gas is eliminated before it can exert mechanical or embolic effects [12].

Clinical observations corroborate these physical principles. In studies comparing pharmaceutical-grade microfoam with air-based foams, the former demonstrate rapid disappearance of intravascular gas signals and an absence of sustained embolic activity, even following high-volume injections. This behavior contrasts with the prolonged persistence observed with nitrogen-containing foams, reinforcing the central role of gas composition in determining safety [14, 17].

From a pharmacotechnical perspective, the deliberate exclusion of nitrogen from pharmaceutical microfoam formulations represents a decisive design choice rather than a secondary optimization. Gas composition does not merely influence how long bubbles persist; it defines whether the foam behaves as a self-limiting therapeutic system or as a potentially persistent intravascular gas phase.

Thus, the use of physiological CO_2/O_2 mixtures ensures that microfoam stability is confined to the therapeutic interval and that systemic exposure to gas is transient and clinically silent. In this context, gas solubility becomes a central safety mechanism, complementing the geometric and chemical controls described in the preceding sections.

4.3 Cerebral Safety, Patent Foramen Ovale, and Regulatory Oversight

The safety of foam sclerotherapy has been debated since the widespread adoption of manually prepared air-based foams for the treatment of venous insufficiency. Central to this discussion is the behavior of injected microbubbles within the circulation, a topic that has been rigorously investigated in preclinical and translational studies, most notably by Eckmann and colleagues.

These investigations demonstrated that the intravascular fate of microbubbles depends critically on gas composition, bubble size, and structural stability. Microbubbles composed of physiological gases such as carbon dioxide and oxygen dissolve rapidly in blood due to their high solubility, thereby minimizing intravascular residence time and reducing the risk of microvascular obstruction. In contrast, nitrogen—the predominant component of ambient air—is markedly less soluble. Nitrogen-rich microbubbles generated by manual agitation techniques may therefore persist intravascularly for prolonged periods.

In the presence of a right-to-left shunt, such as a patent foramen ovale (PFO), persistent nitrogen-containing bubbles may bypass the pulmonary filter and enter the arterial circulation. This mechanism provides a plausible explanation for the rare but well-documented neurological events reported in association with air-based, physician-compounded foams. Importantly, these events have been described exclusively in the context of manually prepared foams, lacking control over gas composition and bubble size.

The mechanistic basis for this distinction was incorporated into the regulatory evaluation of pharmaceutical-grade polidocanol microfoam. Preclinical studies cited by the U.S. Food and Drug Administration (FDA) demonstrated that nitrogen content and bubble heterogeneity were key determinants of microvascular lodging and delayed clearance, whereas low-nitrogen, physiologic gas mixtures produced rapidly dissolving microbubbles with limited embolic potential. These findings formed part of the toxicological rationale underlying the FDA's differentiation between standardized pharmaceutical microfoam and room-air manually prepared foams.

Clinical imaging studies have directly addressed this issue. Prospective investigations using diffusion-weighted magnetic resonance imaging have demonstrated no increase in new cerebral lesions following treatment with pharmaceutical-grade polidocanol microfoam, even after high-volume injections. Importantly, these findings extend to patients with known PFO, in whom transient microbubbles may bypass the pulmonary circulation without producing detectable ischemic injury [7, 17].

The absence of cerebral injury is consistent with the physicochemical properties of pharma-

Table 5.2 Comparative structural and safety features of pharmaceutical microfoam and manually prepared foams

Feature	Pharmaceutical microfoam	Manually prepared (air-based) foams
Gas composition	CO_2/O_2 with minimal N_2	High N_2 content
Bubble size	Small, controlled, narrowly distributed	Large, heterogeneous
Structural coherence	Engineered, reproducible	Variable, operator-dependent
Interfacial behavior	Stable endothelial contact	Rapid fragmentation
Elimination pathway	Rapid dissolution and exhalation	Prolonged persistence
Safety profile	Predictable and validated	Variable and uncertain

ceutical microfoam described in the preceding sections. Microbubbles composed of physiological gases dissolve rapidly once they leave the structured environment of the treated vein. As a result, even when transiently present in the arterial circulation, these bubbles lack the persistence and mechanical stability required to occlude cerebral microvasculature or sustain tissue ischemia [13].

Transcranial Doppler studies further support this interpretation. Although embolic signals may be detected transiently following foam injection, these signals do not correlate with structural brain injury or clinical neurological sequelae when physiological gas mixtures are used. The presence of Doppler-detectable signals therefore reflects acoustic phenomena rather than pathological embolization, underscoring the distinction between signal detection and clinical harm [12].

From a regulatory perspective, these safety considerations have been rigorously evaluated. Unlike manually prepared foams, pharmaceutical-grade microfoam underwent dedicated preclinical toxicological assessment and controlled clinical trials prior to approval. Regulatory agencies required explicit demonstration of systemic safety, including pulmonary and cerebral endpoints, before authorizing its clinical use for the treatment of truncal vein incompetence [4].

Taken together, these data support a coherent safety narrative: when generated with physiological gases and delivered within a controlled structural framework, microfoam sclerotherapy does not confer an increased risk of cerebral injury, even in anatomically susceptible patients and large microfoam volumes. Cerebral safety is therefore not an incidental observation, but an emergent consequence of deliberate structural and physicochemical design.

A comparative overview of the structural and safety features of pharmaceutical microfoam and manually prepared foams is provided in Table 5.2.

5 Pharmacologic and Physicochemical Properties

5.1 Structure Delivers Function

Within a structure-driven therapy framework, clinical intuition reflects underlying physical organization rather than chance or technique alone.

In everyday phlebology, the term "foam" encompasses materials with profoundly different physical properties, stability, and safety profiles. In a majority of clinical settings, access to pharmaceutical-grade microfoam has historically been limited by regulatory and market constraints. As a result, standardized injectable microfoam has remained virtually available only in the United States, while most other regions have relied on manually prepared foams with variable and poorly controlled characteristics. These hand-made mixtures represent uncontrolled colloidal systems whose behavior differs fundamentally from that of engineered pharmaceutical microfoam.

In physical systems, structure precedes function; in sclerotherapy, this relationship becomes clinically explicit. *The wrong structure inevitably leads to the wrong function.* This conceptual confusion extends far beyond physics and into clinical language itself. *Foam sclerotherapy* is often used interchangeably to describe anything from the cosmetic treatment of small telangiectasias to the occlusion of major truncal veins traditionally reserved for surgery, EVLA, or radiofrequency. Similarly, the term *varicose vein* may refer to vessels differing by orders of magnitude in diameter and volume, yet treated under the same linguistic umbrella. Such terminological flattening has blurred the boundaries between aesthetic, functional, and surgical-level interventions.

In this disorderly landscape, outcomes vary widely and so does perception.

Many physicians think sclerotherapy "sometimes works, sometimes doesn't," without realizing that they are not using the same physical agent.

A true pharmaceutical microfoam is a designed material: monodisperse bubbles, tangent contact geometry (TBK), physiological gases (CO_2/O_2), and verified rheological stability. It behaves as a coherent piston, displacing blood, coating endothelium and then dissolving safely. An *artisanal foam*, by contrast, behaves as a transient emulsion: it breaks, it mixes and it leaves uncertainty.

The first principle of structure and function is distinction. Not every foam is a microfoam, not every sclerotherapy is equivalent, and not every varicose vein belongs to the same universe of treatment. The availability of reproducible fully automated microfoam platforms, capable of producing pharmaceutical-grade microfoam with full reproducibility, represents an opportunity to restore clarity. If all practitioners can access a standardized pharma-grade structure, then outcomes can finally be judged by skill, not by chemistry. To achieve this, we must first understand what defines a "good foam day": the measurable parameters that transform intuition into science and make every treatment safe, effective, and reproducible.

The following clinical perceptions, often described informally as a "good foam day," correspond to specific and measurable structural parameters of pharmaceutical microfoam:

- "*The Foam Looks and Feels Right*"
  corresponds to small, uniform bubbles with no excess liquid at the bottom of the syringe; neither too wet nor too dry, flowing smoothly through the needle.
- "*It Behaves as a Cohesive, Piston-Like Column*"
  corresponds to a microfoam that is coherent, controllable, and responsive under the physician's hand as it fills the vein and displaces blood cleanly.
- "*The Image Is Clear to Follow*"
  corresponds to properly sized microbubbles that finely scatter ultrasound waves, generating a bright and stable trace showing complete, laminar occupation of the vessel.
- "*The Vein Reacts with Elegance*"
  corresponds to a homogeneous microfoam that properly displaces blood in a large vessel, producing an immediate and "welcoming" vasospasm that confirms contact and effective action.
- "*The Experience Feels Safe and Reproducible*"
  corresponds to a pharmaceutical-grade microfoam with small bubble size and physiological gases, producing consistent results across patients without cough, chest tightness, or neurological signs—only the calm sense that dose, position, and concentration were appropriate, with excellent metabolism of the drug.

Experienced clinicians often describe the behavior of pharmaceutical microfoam using qualitative terms derived from real-time observation during ultrasound-guided injection. These perceptions, while expressed in informal language, consistently reflect underlying structural properties of the foam rather than subjective impressions.

For example, when foam is perceived as advancing smoothly and uniformly within the lumen, this typically corresponds to a high degree of structural coherence and a relatively homogeneous distribution of bubble sizes. Similarly, the clinical impression of stable lumen occupation without premature fragmentation reflects an optimized balance between interfacial surface area and temporal stability. In contrast, foams that appear irregular, rapidly dispersive, or difficult to control under ultrasound commonly exhibit poor geometric organization and early blood-mediated neutralization.

Importantly, such clinical perceptions are not diagnostic endpoints in themselves, but intuitive summaries of complex structural states. What clinicians describe as a "good foam day" is therefore not a matter of chance or technique alone, but the macroscopic manifestation of favorable geometric and physical properties acting within a reproducible structural regime. Clinical observation and quantitative structural descriptors should thus be understood as complementary perspectives on the same underlying organization, rather than as competing modes of assessment.

This distinction preserves the value of clinical expertise while situating it within a broader, physically grounded understanding of microfoam behavior.

What feels like "control" in your hand or looks like "beauty" on ultrasound is the expression of measurable geometry and physics. Fine bubbles, balanced humidity, ordered structure, and physiologic gas composition are not luck: they are quantifiable determinants of stability.

When structure is controlled, operator technique becomes a variable of execution, not of pharmacology. Once structure is recognized as the determinant of function, stability emerges as the key condition that enables that structure to act effectively—and safely—in vivo.

5.2 Stability Factors in Pharmaceutical-Grade Sclerosing Microfoam

In sclerotherapy, stability does not mean lasting longer; it means lasting just long enough.

A stable polidocanol microfoam must simultaneously displace blood effectively, maintain sustained endothelial contact, and self-deactivate once its therapeutic role is complete.

Stability, therefore, should not be regarded as an intrinsic material property, but as the emergent result of three deliberate design choices: the liquid phase, the gas phase, and the geometric structure of the foam.

Beyond its role in drainage control, the liquid phase confers a less obvious but equally critical property to pharmaceutical microfoam: structural resilience under mechanical stress. During injection, microfoam is subjected to repeated compression, shear, and tensile forces as it passes through needles, syringes, and tortuous vascular segments. In most foams, such mechanical work irreversibly accelerates coalescence and structural decay. In contrast, an elastic liquid phase allows temporary deformation while preserving interfacial integrity, enabling the foam to recover a configuration close to its pre-stressed state.

In this sense, elasticity should not be understood as rigidity, but as resistance to entropic drift. Deformable yet non-fusible liquid films can transiently store mechanical energy and release it without triggering irreversible bubble fusion or loss of coherence. This capacity to absorb and return applied work, rather than dissipate it through structural degradation, is a prerequisite for maintaining therapeutic structure throughout injection and early intravascular propagation.

Together, liquid-phase elasticity and controlled viscosity produce interfacial structures that persist long enough to deliver a controlled endothelial lesion without compromising downstream behavior.

The gas phase governs the post-action fate of the foam. Pharmaceutical microfoam is optimally generated using physiological gases (CO_2/O_2) with minimal nitrogen content (<1%).

Carbon dioxide and oxygen dissolve rapidly according to Henry's law, ensuring efficient clearance once endothelial contact has been achieved. Nitrogen, by contrast, dissolves slowly and offers no therapeutic advantage in this context. High gas solubility therefore provides a built-in safety tail: enough structural stability during action, followed by rapid physiological disappearance.

The behavior of pharmaceutical microfoam within the vascular lumen is governed by its geometric organization rather than by isolated procedural factors. When adequately structured, microfoam does not behave as a random dispersion of bubbles, but as a coherent intravascular system whose geometry determines how it occupies space, displaces blood, and interacts with the endothelium. In practical terms, this specification corresponds to maintaining the foam within the TBK regime during its therapeutic interval.

A well-structured foam exhibits a high degree of internal coherence, allowing bubbles to act collectively rather than independently. This collective behavior enables the foam to advance as a continuous column, progressively excluding blood from the lumen and establishing direct, homogeneous contact with the endothelial surface. In this regime, the foam behaves mechanically as a transient piston, translating geometric organization into predictable pharmacological action.

Geometric coherence also underlies the foam's ability to adapt to vessel morphology. Within tortuous or non-uniform segments, a coherent foam redistributes locally without fragmenting, preserving lumen occupation while maintaining sufficient flexibility to conform to vascular anatomy. Conversely, when geometric organization is poor, the foam rapidly disaggregates, mixes chaotically with blood, and loses its capacity to act as a structured therapeutic entity.

Importantly, this geometric specification is not static. It exists within a dynamic window defined by bubble size distribution, interfacial surface area, and temporal stability. Excessive rigidity compromises passive elimination, whereas excessive fragility prevents effective lumen occupation. Pharmaceutical microfoam therefore operates within an intermediate structural regime, optimized to balance guidance, contact, and self-limiting dissolution.

From a clinical perspective, these geometric properties manifest as reproducible and recognizable patterns of behavior under ultrasound guidance: smooth advancement, sustained lumen filling, and controlled retreat as the structure progressively neutralizes. These observable features are not incidental; they are direct expressions of the underlying geometric organization of the foam.

Thus, the geometric specification of pharmaceutical microfoam provides a unifying explanation for its mechanical behavior, pharmacological efficacy, and safety profile. Rather than being an abstract description, geometry constitutes the operational substrate through which structure is translated into therapeutic action.

These geometric constraints not only determine behavior, but also encode the energetic state of the foam.

5.3 Encoding Functionality During Foam Synthesis

This energetic encoding of structure provides a natural bridge between geometric description and more formal energetic representations. Foam synthesis is not a passive mixing process, but an active act of material construction. Stability cannot be achieved by chance at the bedside; it must be encoded during synthesis through the controlled transmission of both information and energy into the forming structure.

In the case of microfoam, material information alone is insufficient. Foam is a metastable material with a higher internal energy than its constituent phases (gas and liquid) and therefore energy must accompany information for the system to reach the desired structural state. The manner in which energy is delivered (its intensity, timing, and spatial distribution) determines how bubbles are progressively formed, divided, and stabilized at the appropriate scale.

The foaming apparatus thus acts as a true synthesizer; the design and operation of the foaming device govern how energy and information are transferred to the material, bubble by bubble, until the target structure is achieved.

Information, energy, structure, and function therefore form a continuous causal chain. Stability emerges only when energy is delivered in a manner informed by the structure that the system is intended to reach.

Operational stability further requires controlled gas-to-liquid ratios, smooth flow transitions, and avoidance of shear spikes that generate satellite microbubbles.

Within these conditions, stable pharmaceutical microfoam is characterized by a narrow bubble size distribution, absence of spray-like sub-bubbles, and a balanced, cohesive texture at the generator outlet.

5.4 From Structure to Bedside: Clinical Translation

At the bedside, the structural principles described above translate into a small number of reproducible clinical observations. Textural coherence and controlled responsiveness reflect low heterogeneity and balanced partitioning, piston-like advancement corresponds to coherent connectivity and uniform curvature, stable echogenicity indicates preserved structure during action, and quiet post-treatment disappearance confirms effective self-limiting dissolution.

In pharmaceutical microfoam, stability is engineered before the needle (through the combined design of liquid, gas, and geometry) and confirmed clinically by two simple signs: a responsive vasospasm and a foam that advances coherently under ultrasound guidance and disappears once its task is complete.

5.5 From Intuition to Orientation: A Formal Language for Navigating Microfoam

Clinical experience teaches that some foam procedures feel controlled, predictable, and almost effortless, while others using the same drug and similar technique quickly lose coherence. Clinicians recognize these moments instinctively: a foam that advances smoothly, fills the lumen cleanly, and behaves as an obedient system, versus one that fragments, disperses, or fades prematurely.

These impressions are familiar to anyone who has practiced sclerotherapy long enough. Yet they remain difficult to articulate, teach, or compare. We can sense when a foam "is right," but we often lack a concise way to describe *what* that "rightness" is, *how close it is to being lost* and *how it changes over time.*

A closer look reveals that the difference does not lie in chemistry. The surfactant is unchanged; the gas–liquid mixture is identical. What evolves is the internal organization of the foam—how bubbles relate to one another, how curvature is distributed, and how energy is stored within the structure. In this sense, structure itself acts as an energetic parameter: it is not merely a descriptor of the material, but a carrier of the forces that govern its evolution.

Conventional descriptors (mean bubble size, variance, lifetime) capture fragments of this behavior but fail to describe the foam as a whole. They tell us what is present, but not where the foam stands among the many possible structural configurations it could adopt, nor how it is moving from one configuration to another. The problem is not a lack of data, but a lack of coordinates.

HyDeF, the Hypervector Description of Foams, was conceived as a response to this gap. Rather than reducing a foam to statistical summaries, HyDeF represents the entire ensemble as a single structural state in a high-dimensional configuration space. Each foam corresponds to a point in that space, encoding not only composition but also the partition of gas among bubbles and the topological relationships that connect them.

Within this framework, clinical behavior is understood as a projection of the underlying structural state rather than as a direct description of the configuration space itself. As the foam evolves in time, through coalescence, drainage, or interaction with the vessel, it traces a structural trajectory through the space of possible configurations. Controlled advancement, stable lumen occupation, and predictable disappearance correspond to motion within a coherent region of that space; fragmentation and loss of control correspond to drift away from it.

The natural next question is how to define "coherence" in geometric terms. Here an ideal reference is useful, not as a physical foam, but as a geometric horizon. HyDeF introduces such a reference in the form of the Eigenschaum: an ide-

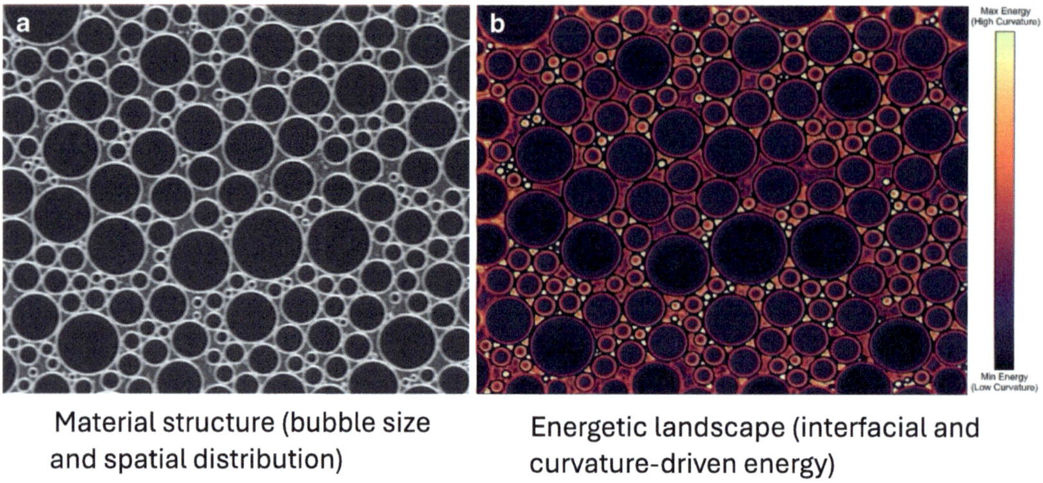

Fig. 5.4 Material and energetic representations of microfoam structure
Comparison Between Material and Energetic Descriptions of the Same Microfoam Configuration
Panel **a** shows the conventional material representation, in which bubble size and spatial arrangement give the impression of a relatively uniform structure. This view corresponds to what is directly accessible through standard imaging and visual inspection
Panel **b** presents an energetic representation of the same region, revealing a highly heterogeneous landscape shaped by surface tension, curvature, and interfacial forces. Smaller bubbles and highly curved interfaces concentrate a disproportionate share of the system's potential energy, reflecting Laplace pressure and related interfacial contributions that are not directly visible in material images
These energetic features are not introduced by the representation itself, but are intrinsic to the construction process of the microfoam. Over time, this stored energy drives structural evolution, coarsening, and decay. Energetic visualization therefore provides an additional conceptual layer for understanding microfoam stability and dynamics, complementing—but not replacing—material descriptions

alized configuration of maximal equipartition. In practice, real foams live in high-dimensional spaces whose dimensionality depends on the number of detected bubbles. Nevertheless, the geometric role of the reference remains the same: it provides a direction and a coordinate system for describing proximity to order and distance to degradation. The formal definition is provided in Appendix B. The key point is conceptual: HyDeF turns "good foam" from a feeling into an orientable region of state space (Fig. 5.4).

5.6 Why Clinicians Should Care

For clinicians, HyDeF provides a bridge between experience and physics by reframing familiar impressions in terms of structural states and structural trajectories. It is important to distinguish this notion from the spatial trajectory of foam within the vein, which describes where the foam moves anatomically under ultrasound. In HyDeF, trajectory refers instead to how the foam's structural state evolves within configuration space over time.

What is perceived clinically as control, smooth advancement, or loss of coherence arises in the physical setting of the vein, but is conditioned by the position of the foam within configuration space and by the direction in which its structure is evolving. In other words, spatial behavior reflects, without being identical to, the underlying structural state.

A well-prepared microfoam occupies a favorable structural state, characterized by coherent geometry, balanced curvature, and ordered energy distribution. As long as the system remains within this region, its structural evolution remains stable, allowing the foam in the vein to advance predictably, displace blood efficiently,

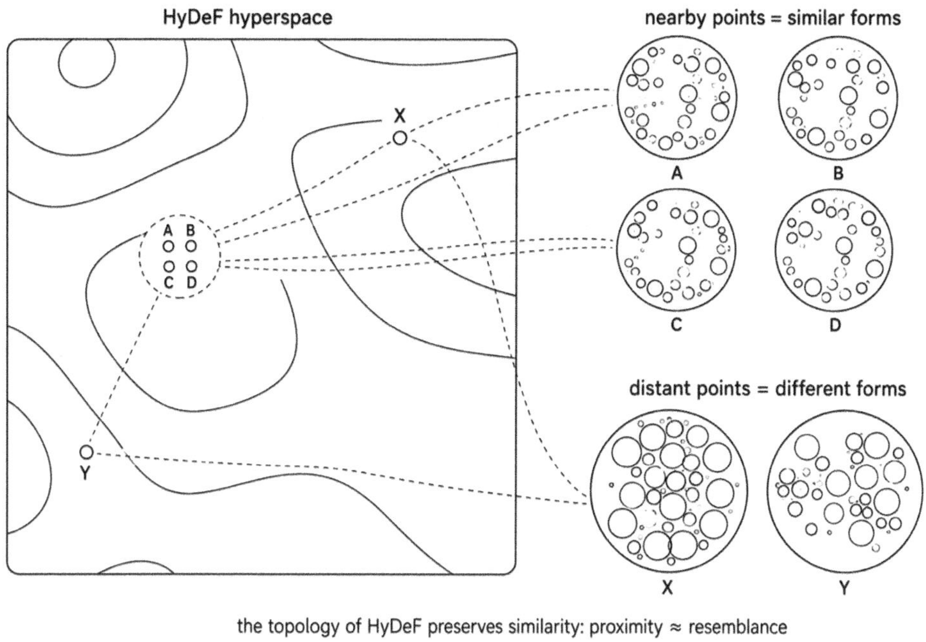

Fig. 5.5 Extended visual journey of the HyDeF framework from material observation to structural orientation Progressive translation from material observation of microfoam to a structural state representation and its placement within configuration space. Foam evolution is interpreted as structural trajectories that may drift toward loss of coherence or be guided toward regions of higher uniformity, illustrating HyDeF as a framework for orientation rather than prescription

and maintain consistent endothelial contact. As structure degrades, the foam moves away from this region, and the clinician observes fragmentation, loss of control, and increasing variability in outcome.

Within this framework, clinical actions, such as preparation conditions, injection rhythm, pauses, or redirection, can be understood as interventions that influence structural evolution, rather than as isolated technical maneuvers. HyDeF thus allows clinicians to think in terms of where the system is and where it is heading, instead of relying solely on retrospective judgment based on outcomes.

Importantly, this perspective makes it meaningful to speak about proximity to an ideal region of structural coherence. Concepts such as the Eigenschaum Proximity Index (EPI) are best understood here not as performance scores or prescriptive metrics, but as examples of how proximity to a region of maximal order can be expressed within a physically grounded framework. Their value lies in orientation and comparison, not in replacing clinical judgment.

In this way, HyDeF does not constrain clinical freedom. It provides orientation: a shared language that allows experienced intuition to be situated within a coherent space of possibilities, enabling comparison, learning, and gradual refinement of practice (Fig. 5.5).

5.7 Structural Synthesis and Control of Foam Trajectories

The preceding sections have established a geometric language in which microfoam behavior can be described in terms of structural states, trajectories, and reference configurations. Within this framework, therapeutic outcomes emerge not from isolated parameters, but from the region of configuration space in which the system evolves.

A natural question follows: *what determines the initial structural state from which a given foam trajectory begins?*

The answer lies upstream of the vein and upstream of clinical technique, in the process by which the foam itself is generated. If structure determines function, *then synthesis determines structure*.

From the HyDeF perspective, foam generation is not a preparatory step external to the therapeutic process, but an integral part of it. The synthesis stage defines the initial partition of gas among bubbles, the adjacency relations between them, and the energetic organization embedded in the structure. These elements jointly determine the starting position of the foam within configuration space, and therefore strongly condition its subsequent trajectory.

In this sense, foam generation acts as a physical operator on the structural state. By shaping the boundary conditions under which gas, liquid, and energy interact, the synthesis process imprints information into the foam at the moment of its creation. That information is not symbolic: it is embodied in geometry, curvature, and connectivity, and it governs how the foam will respond to pressure gradients, contact-mediated exchange, and physiological constraints.

Importantly, this view reframes the role of control. Control does not act primarily by correcting behavior downstream, but by positioning the system upstream in a region of configuration space from which stable and predictable trajectories naturally emerge. When synthesis is poorly controlled, the foam may begin its evolution already close to regions associated with rapid loss of coherence. When synthesis is controlled, the system may start within a basin of structural robustness, where small perturbations do not immediately lead to degradation.

This distinction helps clarify a long-standing clinical observation: two foams prepared with the same chemical composition and injected with similar technique may behave very differently. Within the HyDeF framework, such differences are not attributed to chance or operator intuition alone, but to differences in the initial structural state set by the synthesis process.

The implication is not prescriptive, but conceptual. HyDeF does not mandate a specific method of foam generation, nor does it define an optimal device or protocol. Rather, it provides a language in which different synthesis approaches can be understood as acting on the same underlying variables, shaping the initial conditions and therefore the space of possible outcomes.

Seen this way, synthesis becomes the first step of structural control. Clinical technique then operates on a system whose trajectory has already been largely determined by its starting point. The therapeutic act is thus distributed across stages: synthesis, injection, interaction, and resolution, all connected through a common geometric description.

This perspective opens a broader view of sclerotherapy as a structure-driven therapy. Instead of selecting treatments solely by vessel size or concentration, attention shifts toward understanding and controlling the behavior of the therapeutic system as a whole. In such a framework, reproducibility, safety, and efficacy emerge from consistent positioning within configuration space rather than from empirical adjustment alone.

The HyDeF language makes this shift explicit. It does not replace clinical expertise, but provides orientation: a way to relate synthesis, structure, and outcome within a coherent conceptual map. As techniques and technologies evolve, this map offers a stable reference against which new approaches can be situated, compared, and refined.

5.8 Take-Home Idea

Structure-driven therapy does not introduce a new technique, but a new way of understanding therapeutic action. It marks a transition from intuition without coordinates to intuition with orientation.

By treating foam structure as a state within a configuration space and its evolution as a trajectory through that space, HyDeF offers a map rather than a prescription. Efficacy and safety no longer emerge from isolated variables or empirical adjustments alone, but from controlled system behavior that can be recognized, compared, and learned collectively.

In this framework, clinical expertise is not replaced: it is amplified. Intuition remains essential, but it is no longer blind. Orientation becomes possible, exploration becomes informed and reproducibility of structure becomes the prerequisite for meaningful clinical comparison and cumulative progress.

Appendix A—Surface Area, Bubble Number, and Endothelial Contact

This appendix provides a quantitative and geometric extension of the concept of active surface area introduced in Sect. 4, for readers seeking a more formal description.

A.1 Geometric Premise

Consider a fixed total volume of gas V_g subdivided into N spherical bubbles of equal radius r. The total gas volume is given by:

$$V_g = N \cdot \frac{4}{3}\pi r^3$$

Solving for r:

$$r = \left(\frac{3V_g}{4\pi N}\right)^{1/3}$$

The total gas–liquid interfacial surface area S is as follows:

$$S = N \cdot 4\pi r^2$$

Substituting for r:

$$S = 4\pi N\left(\frac{3V_g}{4\pi N}\right)^{2/3},$$

which simplifies to:

$$S \propto N^{1/3}$$

Thus, for a constant gas volume, increasing the number of bubbles necessarily increases the total interfacial surface area.

A.2 Pharmacological Consequence

In injectable sclerosing microfoam, therapeutic action occurs exclusively at the *gas–liquid–endothelium interface*. The relevant pharmacological variable is therefore *contact surface*, not gas volume per se.

For a fixed amount of injected gas:

- Fewer, larger bubbles → limited endothelial contact,
- More numerous, smaller bubbles → expanded contact surface and more homogeneous endothelial exposure.

This geometric fact has a direct pharmacological implication: *microbubble subdivision enhances the effective delivery of the sclerosant to the endothelial surface without increasing nominal dose.*

A.3 Structural Limitation and Biological Reality

The relationship described above holds only within a biologically relevant structural regime. Excessive subdivision leads to unstable bubbles that dissolve rapidly or are neutralized before meaningful endothelial contact occurs. Conversely, insufficient subdivision produces large bubbles that fail to uniformly occupy the vascular lumen.

Therapeutic microfoam therefore operates within a *bounded structural window*, where bubble size and number jointly maximize endothelial contact while preserving sufficient stability for local action.

A.4 Transition Toward a Structural Description

These considerations reveal a fundamental limitation of purely volumetric or concentration-based descriptions of sclerotherapy. The same nominal dose of sclerosant may result in profoundly different biological effects depending on how gas volume is partitioned and organized.

This observation motivates the need for a structural descriptor capable of capturing bubble number, size distribution, and interfacial organization—providing the conceptual bridge toward a more general formalism.

Appendix B—HyDeF: A Geometric Language for Foam Structure and Evolution

B.1 Rationale and Conceptual Scope

Injectable microfoam is a structurally complex and dynamically evolving material whose therapeutic behavior cannot be inferred from nominal dose, injected gas volume, or sclerosant concentration alone. As discussed in Appendix A, identical quantities of gas may lead to profoundly different endothelial exposure and clinical outcomes depending on how that gas is partitioned, connected, and allowed to evolve within the foam.

HyDeF (Hypervector Description of Foams) is introduced in this appendix as a geometric language for describing foam structure and its evolution. It does not aim to replace pharmacokinetics or pharmacodynamics, nor to prescribe clinical technique. Rather, it provides a representational space in which foam structure, physical drivers, observable behavior, and intervention can be coherently related.

The conceptual foundation of HyDeF rests on four complementary levels of description, already introduced in the main text and formalized here:

- *Structural State*: What the foam *is* at a given moment, in terms of how gas is partitioned among bubbles and how those bubbles are connected.
- *Structural Evolution*: How that state changes over time under physical drivers such as curvature-induced pressure differences or contact-mediated redistribution.
- *Observables*: Quantities that can be measured or perceived clinically as projections of the underlying structure.
- *Control and Synthesis*: How interventions shape structural trajectories, guiding the system toward regions of higher coherence or robustness.

This appendix focuses on the first two levels (state and evolution) and on the geometric references required to orient them. Its purpose is not to provide an exhaustive model, but to formalize the space in which such models live.

B.2 Foam as a Structural State

At any given instant, a foam can be described by how its total gas content is distributed among individual bubbles and by how those bubbles are connected through physical contact. This instantaneous description defines the structural state of the foam.

HyDeF deliberately adopts this structural viewpoint, shifting the focus away from averaged descriptors and toward configuration. Two foams with identical chemical composition and total gas volume may occupy very different structural states and therefore behave as different materials.

In practice, real injectable foams are heterogeneous and time-evolving systems characterized by the following:

- A distribution of bubble sizes,
- Neighbor (contact) relationships,
- Non-uniform curvature and pressure fields,
- And ongoing structural rearrangement.

Capturing this information requires a representation that preserves both partition and connectivity.

B.3 Hypervector Representation and Configuration Space

Let a foam consist of N bubbles. The partition of gas among bubbles is represented by a normalized hypervector:

$$\tilde{\mathbf{v}} = \left(\tilde{v}_1, \tilde{v}_2, \ldots, \tilde{v}_N\right), \tilde{v}_i \geq 0, \qquad \sum_{i=1}^{N} \tilde{v}_i = 1,$$

where $\tilde{v}_i$ denotes the fraction of total gas contained in bubble i.

This vector lives in a simplex of dimension $N - 1$, which represents the space of all possible gas partitions with fixed total content. Each point in this simplex corresponds to a physically distinct foam configuration at a given resolution.

Connectivity between bubbles is encoded by an adjacency matrix $A \in \{0, 1\}^{N \times N}$, where $A_{ij} = 1$ indicates physical contact between bubbles i and j. Together, the pair $(\tilde{\mathbf{v}}, A)$ defines the structural state of the foam.

Technical Note (Volume vs. Moles)

Strictly, the conserved quantity partitioned among bubbles is the amount of gas (moles), not geometric volume. Under an ideal-gas approximation,

$$n_i = \frac{P_i V_i}{RT}$$

Because smaller bubbles have higher Laplace pressure, volume fractions are a first-order structural proxy rather than a thermodynamic invariant. A molar-weighted formulation can be introduced by replacing V_i-weights with $P_i V_i$ (or directly with n_i) in normalization and distance metrics. The geometric framework remains unchanged.

The configuration space defined in this way is the natural arena in which foam structure can be compared and tracked over time.

B.4 Structural Evolution as Trajectories in Configuration Space

Foams are not static. Curvature-induced pressure differences, gas solubility, and contact-mediated exchange drive the redistribution of gas between bubbles, altering the structural state.

In HyDeF, these physical mechanisms are expressed as operators acting on the structural state. Their action moves the state through configuration space, generating a structural trajectory:

$$\tilde{\mathbf{v}}(t)$$

This trajectory describes how the internal organization of the foam evolves, independently of its spatial displacement within a vessel. Clinically observed behavior, such as stable advancement, uniform lumen occupation, or loss of control, corresponds to projections of this structural evolution.

Different physical drivers define different operators and HyDeF is intentionally operator-agnostic: it provides the space and the grammar in which such operators act, rather than a single closed dynamical law.

B.5 The Eigenschaum: Uniformity as a Geometric Horizon

To orient structural states and trajectories, a reference configuration is required. HyDeF introduces the Eigenschaum as an idealized configuration of maximal uniformity, in which gas is perfectly equipartitioned among bubbles.

For a finite number of bubbles N, the Eigenschaum corresponds to the barycenter of the simplex:

$$\mathbf{e}^{(N)} = \left(\frac{1}{N}, \ldots, \frac{1}{N}\right)$$

This configuration is not physically realizable. Its role is geometric: it defines a direction of maximal uniformity within configuration space.

As the structural description is refined and the number of partition elements increases, this barycenter approaches a geometric horizon corresponding to infinite equipartition. In this asymptotic sense, the Eigenschaum functions not as a physical point, but as a reference at infinity

Table 5.3 Examples of structural descriptors and metrics in microfoam analysis

Descriptor/Metric	What it captures	Structural interpretation	Context of use
PDI	Bubble size heterogeneity	Degree of polydispersity	Comparative characterization
R_{32}	Surface-weighted mean radius	Endothelial contact efficiency	Structural assessment
Var$(1/r)$	Curvature dispersion	Pressure heterogeneity	Stability analysis
Z	Average bubble connectivity	Structural coherence	Packing topology
EPI	Global structural quality index	Projection of structure into scalar form	Comparative descriptor

toward which increasingly uniform structures converge.

B.6 Proximity to the Eigenschaum and the Definition of EPI

The position of a foam state relative to the Eigenschaum provides a natural measure of structural order. For a given resolution N, proximity can be quantified by the Euclidean distance between the state vector and the barycenter of the simplex:

$$d_N = \left\| \tilde{\mathbf{v}} - \mathbf{e}^{(N)} \right\|_2$$

To obtain a dimensionless and comparable index, this distance is normalized by the maximum possible distance within the simplex, which occurs for complete concentration of gas in a single bubble:

$$\mathbf{v}_{\text{collapse}} = (1,0,\ldots,0), d_{N,\max} = \| \mathbf{v}_{\text{collapse}} - \mathbf{e}^{(N)} \|_2 = \sqrt{1 - \frac{1}{N}}$$

The Eigenschaum Proximity Index (EPI) is then defined as follows:

$$EPI_N = 100\left(1 - \frac{d_N}{d_{N,\,\max}}\right)$$

By construction, $\text{EPI}_N = 100$ for the uniform reference configuration and $\text{EPI}_N = 0$ for complete concentration. In high-resolution regimes, where N is large, the normalization term approaches unity, and the index becomes weakly dependent on small variations in N. In this limit, EPI can be interpreted as a coordinate measuring distance to an asymptotic ideal of uniformity rather than to a specific finite-dimensional reference.

Other commonly used descriptors, such as polydispersity indices, surface-weighted radii, curvature dispersion, or connectivity measures, are best understood as projections of the structural state into interpretable scalar quantities. They complement, but do not replace, the geometric description provided by HyDeF.

Examples of structural descriptors that may be used within the HyDeF framework are listed in Table 5.3.

B.7 A Canonical Example of Structural Evolution Within HyDeF

The geometric framework introduced above defines a configuration space and a reference for orientation, but it does not prescribe a unique law of motion. Different physical mechanisms may act on the structural state, generating different trajectories. To illustrate how such mechanisms are expressed within HyDeF, we present here a canonical example of curvature-driven structural evolution, corresponding to gas redistribution mediated by contact and Laplace pressure differences.

This formulation represents one physically relevant generator of trajectories within the HyDeF space. It is not exhaustive, nor exclusive, but serves as a concrete illustration of how operators act on the structural state.

B.7.1 Radius and Internal Pressure

Assuming spherical bubbles, the radius of bubble i is obtained from its gas volume:

$$R_i = \left(\frac{3V_i}{4\pi}\right)^{1/3}$$

Internal pressure is modeled as follows:

$$P_i = P_0 + \Delta P_i, \Delta P_i = C_\gamma \frac{\gamma}{R_i},$$

where P_0 is a base pressure and C_γ is an effective coefficient, reflecting the chosen interfacial model (commonly 2 for a single gas–liquid interface or 4 for a soap-bubble convention). In practice, the product $C_\gamma \gamma$ may be absorbed into an effective constant, provided the modeling assumption is stated explicitly.

This step translates geometric structure into a pressure field defined on the bubbles.

B.7.2 Laplace Difference Operator

Curvature-induced pressure differences between bubbles define the driving potential for gas redistribution. These differences are encoded in a matrix:

$$L_{ij} \propto \left(\frac{1}{R_i} - \frac{1}{R_j}\right) \propto \left(V_i^{-1/3} - V_j^{-1/3}\right)$$

This operator expresses the energetic imbalance associated with non-uniform curvature and serves as the generator of structural change.

B.7.3 Adjacency-Filtered Redistribution

Physical exchange of gas is restricted to bubbles that are in direct contact. This constraint is imposed by filtering the Laplace operator through the adjacency matrix A:

$$W = L \odot A,$$

where $\odot$ denotes entry-wise (Hadamard) multiplication. The resulting operator retains only those pressure differences that correspond to real physical contacts. In this way, the topology of the foam explicitly shapes the pathways along which structural evolution occurs.

B.7.4 Constitutive Transfer Law (Molar Flux)

A simple operational law is used to relate pressure differences to gas transfer across contacts:

$$dn_{ij} = K\left(P_i - P_j\right)dt,$$

where dn_{ij} denotes the amount of gas (in moles) transferred from bubble i to bubble j during the time interval dt, and K is an effective transfer coefficient aggregating film thickness, interfacial area, gas solubility, and diffusivity.

The net molar change for bubble i is given by the local balance:

$$dn_i = \sum_j dn_{ji} - \sum_j dn_{ij}$$

In practical terms, this expression evaluates how much gas enters bubble i from neighboring bubbles with higher internal pressure and how much gas leaves toward neighbors with lower internal pressure. The difference between incoming and outgoing fluxes defines the net molar variation of bubble i over that time step. Exchange is evaluated only across physically adjacent bubbles, ensuring conservation of gas and consistency with the contact topology.

B.7.5 Volume Update and Trajectory Generation

Under an ideal-gas approximation and isothermal conditions, molar exchange is converted into a volume update:

$$dV_i = \frac{RT}{P_i} dn_i, V_i\left(t + dt\right) = V_i\left(t\right) + dV_i$$

Iterating this update generates a structural trajectory $V(t)$ in configuration space. This trajectory describes how the internal organization of the foam evolves under the chosen physical driver. Other mechanisms, such as drainage, rupture, or shear, may be incorporated as additional operators acting on the same state representation.

B.8 Experimental and Clinical Interfaces

The HyDeF framework is designed to interface naturally with experimental observation and clinical practice. Its inputs are not abstract constructs, but quantities that can be inferred from imaging and measurement:

- Segmentation of microscopy images to obtain bubble volumes $\{V_i\}$,
- Construction of the adjacency matrix A from observed contacts,
- Estimation of curvature-derived pressures from geometric data,
- And tracking of structural evolution over time.

Within this framework, commonly used descriptors, such as polydispersity indices, surface-weighted radii, curvature dispersion, or echogenic stability, are understood as observables, that is, projections of the structural state or of its trajectory into lower-dimensional quantities suitable for interpretation.

By mapping measurements into configuration space, HyDeF allows observable behavior to be related back to underlying structure. This connection does not require direct access to every microscopic variable; it relies instead on consistent geometric representation and physically motivated operators.

In this sense, HyDeF functions as an interface between measurement and structure. It provides a common language in which experimental data, clinical perception, and physical interpretation can be compared without conflating observables with the structural state itself.

B.9 Reading Guide

Clinicians and readers primarily interested in conceptual orientation may focus on Appendices B.1, B.2, B.3, B.4, and B.5, which introduce HyDeF as a geometric language for describing foam structure, evolution, and reference configurations. These sections are intended to provide intuition and context rather than operational detail and can be read independently of the formal developments that follow.

Readers with a quantitative, physical, or engineering background may wish to proceed to Appendices B.6 and B.7, where proximity measures, structural trajectories, and a canonical example of curvature-driven evolution are defined within the HyDeF framework. Appendix B.8 describes how these concepts interface with experimental measurement and clinical observation.

The appendix is not meant to be read sequentially. Each section is designed to stand on its own, allowing readers to engage with the level of formalism most relevant to their background and interests.

References

1. Wollmann JCGR. The history of sclerosing foams. Dermatologic Surg. 2004;30(5):694–703.
2. Vandendriessche M, Hobbs JT. The evolution of ultrasound guided foam sclerotherapy. Acta Chir Belg. 2008 Nov-Dec;108(6):660–5.
3. Carugo D, Ankrett DN, Zhao X, et al. Benefits of polidocanol endovenous microfoam (Varithena®) compared with physician-compounded foams. Phlebology. 2016 May;31(4):283–95.
4. U.S. Food and Drug Administration. Summary review and risk assessment for polidocanol endovenous microfoam injection (Varithena®). Silver Spring: U.S. Food and Drug Administration; 2013. Available from: https://www.accessdata.fda.gov
5. Regulatory documentation on pharmaceutical microfoam. Technical and pharmacological dossier. 2017.
6. Cabrera J. Injectable microfoam containing a sclerosing agent. Spanish patent ES9300141; priority date June 23, 1993. Corresponding U.S. Patent: US5676962.
7. Beckitt T, Elstone A, Ashley S. Air versus physiological gas for ultrasound guided foam sclerotherapy

treatment of varicose veins. Eur J Vasc Endovasc Surg. 2011 Jul;42(1):115–9.
8. Coleridge-Smith P. Foam and liquid sclerotherapy for varicose veins. Phlebology. 2009;24 Suppl 1:62–72.
9. Bradbury AW, Bate G, Pang K, Darvall KA, Adam DJ. Ultrasound-guided foam sclerotherapy is a safe and clinically effective treatment for superficial venous reflux. J Vasc Surg. 2010;52(4):939–45. https://doi.org/10.1016/j.jvs.2010.04.077.
10. Bergan J, Cheng V. Foam sclerotherapy for the treatment of varicose veins. Vascular. 2007 Sep-Oct;15(5):269–72.
11. Jia X, Mowatt G, Burr JM, et al. Systematic review of foam sclerotherapy for varicose veins. Br J Surg. 2007 Aug;94(8):925–36.
12. Vassileva E, Schnorf H, Personeni O, et al. Transcranial Doppler detection of microembolic signals in clinical practice. Swiss Arch. Neurol. Psychiatry Psychother. 2000;151(2):74–78.
13. Papadopoulou V, Tang M, Balestra C, et al. Circulatory bubble dynamics: From physical to biological aspects. Advanc Coll Interf Sc. 2014;206:239–49.
14. Omata D, Maruyama T, Unga J, et al. Effects of encapsulated gas on stability of lipid-based microbubbles and ultrasound-triggered drug delivery. J Control Release. 2019 Oct;311–312:65–73.
15. Star P, Connor DE, Parsi K. Novel developments in foam sclerotherapy: Focus on Varithena® (polidocanol endovenous microfoam) in the management of varicose veins. Phlebology. 2018 Apr;33(3):150–62.
16. Eckmann DM. Polidocanol for endovenous microfoam sclerosant therapy. Expert Opin Investig Drugs. 2009 Dec;18(12):1919–27.
17. Sarvananthan T, Shepherd AC, Willenberg T, et al. Neurological complications of sclerotherapy for varicose veins. J Vasc Surg. 2012 Jan;55(1):243–51.

Foam Science in Clinical Practice

6

Sergio Gianesini, Jinsong Wang, and Yung Wei Chi

1 Introduction

Foam sclerotherapy is one of the clearest examples of successful translational application of physical science to clinical vascular medicine. Its efficacy does not primarily arise from novel pharmacological agents, but from the deliberate manipulation of delivery physics, specifically gas–liquid interactions, surface chemistry, and intravascular flow dynamics [1]. For the vascular specialist, foam is therefore not a passive vehicle for a sclerosant but an active therapeutic system whose physical properties directly determine biological effect. At a fundamental level, sclerotherapy foam is a metastable, two-phase colloidal structure composed of a continuous liquid phase (sclerosant solution) and a dispersed gaseous phase (microbubbles). Foam science teaches that such systems are intrinsically unstable, evolving continuously through drainage, coalescence, and gas diffusion. Clinically, this instability is not a limitation but an advantage: the therapeutic window of foam exists precisely during its controlled collapse within the target vein, when endothelial contact is maximized and blood displacement is greatest. The translational leap from physics to practice occurs when these abstract properties are intentionally harnessed. Foams displace intravascular blood rather than mixing with it, thereby preventing sclerosant dilution and enabling homogeneous endothelial exposure. Increased surface area at the gas–liquid interface enhances drug–endothelium interaction while simultaneously slowing intraluminal flow, prolonging contact time even in large-caliber veins. These mechanisms explain, at a mechanistic level, the superior efficacy of foam compared with liquid sclerosants observed in both randomized trials and long-term clinical series [2]. From a clinical standpoint, foam science provides explanations for phenomena that experienced practitioners have historically learned empirically. The importance of patient positioning, the benefit of ultrasound-guided injection, and the superior performance of foam in truncal veins all reflect fundamental physical behaviors such as buoyancy, laminar flow disruption, and shear-dependent bubble fragmentation. Injection speed and pressure, for example, are not merely technical preferences but determinants of bubble integrity and foam wetness at the point of endothelial contact.

S. Gianesini (✉)
Department of Translational Medicine, University of Ferrara, Ferrara, Italy

Department of Surgery, Uniformed Services University of Health Sciences, Bethesda, MD, USA
e-mail: gnssrg@unife.it

J. Wang
Department of Vascular Surgery, Guangdong Provincial People's Hospital, Southern Medical University, Guangzhou, China
e-mail: wangjinsong@gdph.org.cn

Y. W. Chi
Department of Cardiovascular Medicine, University of California, Davis Vascular Center, Sacramento, CA, USA
e-mail: ywchi@ucdavis.edu

S. Gianesini, Y. W. Chi (eds.), *Sclerotherapy*, https://doi.org/10.1007/978-3-032-32794-9_6

The distinction between wet and dry foams further illustrates translational foam science. Dry foams, characterized by a high gas fraction and slow drainage, provide prolonged endothelial contact and extensive luminal coverage, making them particularly effective in large or recurrent veins. Wet foams, with higher liquid content and faster collapse, offer superior injectability and reduced distal migration, which is advantageous in smaller veins and cosmetic indications. These differences arise directly from measurable physical parameters and can be deliberately engineered at the bedside through foam production technique and gas-to-liquid ratio. Safety considerations are also deeply rooted in foam science. Neurological and cardiopulmonary adverse events following foam sclerotherapy correlate with bubble size distribution, gas solubility, and total foam volume rather than with sclerosant dose alone. Rapidly diffusible gases such as carbon dioxide reduce bubble persistence and systemic embolic load, providing a rational basis for gas selection in higher-risk patients. Thus, foam design functions as a risk-modulation strategy, not simply a method of drug delivery. In everyday clinical practice, vascular specialists continuously translate foam science into action, often subconsciously, when adjusting foam consistency, limiting injected volume, or choosing production methods for specific anatomical targets. Making these translations explicit strengthens reproducibility, facilitate training, and align individual practice with evidence-based guidelines. Foam sclerotherapy therefore exemplifies a mature translational pathway: physical principles inform technique, technique shapes biological response, and biological response determines clinical outcome. This chapter builds upon these translational foundations, aiming to equip vascular experts with a mechanistic framework for foam production, selection, and injection. By understanding foam as a tunable therapeutic system rather than a static product, clinicians can refine sclerotherapy into a precise, predictable, and scientifically grounded intervention (Table 6.1).

Table 6.1 Translational aspects in foam sclerotherapy clinical practice

	Basic science	Clinical aspect
Foam-induced blood displacement	No drug dilution Longer endothelial contact time Homogeneous endothelial contact	At the same drug concentration, more powerful and homogeneous sclerotherapy action compared to liquid
Abdominal pressure/ body positioning	Possible variation in foam migration speed Venous emptying/refilling	Avoiding sudden Valsalva Considering leg elevation for reducing blood vein filling
Injection speed and pressure	Bubble integrity	Avoid high speed and pressure to limit foam decay
Dry foams	High gas fraction Slow drainage Prolonged endothelial contact Extensive luminal coverage	To be considered in particular for large or recurrent veins
Wet foams	Higher liquid content Faster collapse Superior injectability Reduced distal migration	To be considered in particular for smaller veins and cosmetic indications
Temperature	Higher temperature increases gas solubility	Colder foam is more stable
Safety	Bubble size distribution Gas solubility Total foam volume	Maximize safety by using: Small bubbles Soluble gas Limited volumes

2 Fundamentals of Medical Foam Science

Foams are thermodynamically unstable by definition. Their continuous evolution through drainage, coalescence, and gas diffusion is not a flaw but the very basis of therapeutic effect. In contrast to stable pharmaceutical formulations, foam efficacy depends on *controlled instability* occurring within a defined temporal and spatial window inside the target vein [3].

The clinician deploys a *time-dependent therapeutic structure* whose biological effect is inseparable from its physical decay profile and the environment from which (syringe/catheter/filter/needle) and in which it is delivered (vein anatomy, histology, and hemodynamics). Foam stability measured in vitro correlates imperfectly with in vivo behavior. In veins, additional destabilizing forces act, such as the pulsatile flow, the vessel compliance, the temperature and the blood constituents are at play [4]. Nevertheless, comparative studies demonstrate that foams with smaller bubbles, optimized liquid fraction, and physiological gases show more predictable in vivo performance [5].

> Understanding stability mechanisms allows clinicians to interpret in vitro data realistically and apply them judiciously at the bedside.

A defining characteristic of foam is its enormous interfacial surface area. By dispersing gas into microbubbles, the sclerosant is distributed over a vastly increased surface compared with a liquid bolus. This has two critical consequences: enhanced endothelial exposure at lower drug concentrations and reduced dilution by blood, as foam displaces rather than mixes.

This interfacial dominance explains why foam achieves superior venous obliteration with smaller sclerosant doses compared with liquid injections [6].

> Clinically, this indicates that foam efficacy depends more on geometry and distribution than on absolute drug quantity.

The simplistic concept of a simple need of increasing the sclerosing drug concentration to obtain a stronger sclerotherapy action must be abandoned, in favor of the full evaluation of all the involved basic sciences parameters involved in foam performance. At the same time, detergent sclerosants, such as polidocanol and sodium tetradecyl sulfate, function as surfactants, reducing surface tension at gas–liquid interfaces and stabilizing foam lamellae. This surfactant activity enables foam formation, influences bubble elasticity and modulates interaction with endothelial cell membranes. At the cellular level, detergent sclerosants disrupt lipid bilayers, leading to endothelial cell lysis or apoptosis depending on concentration and exposure time. This indicates how foam stability and biological potency are inseparable; the same surfactant properties that stabilize bubbles also mediate endothelial injury. Identifying the right sclerosing drug concentration is of paramount importance in order to avoid too aggressive sclerotherapy action on the venous wall.

> Indeed, changing concentration means modifying the foam stability and the related final action on the venous wall.

As reported in Chap. 4, bubble size is a critical determinant of foam behavior. Medical foams produced by manual techniques are polydisperse, containing bubbles ranging from tens to several hundred micrometers [7]. Smaller bubbles provide a greater total surface area, increased resistance to buoyancy-driven separation and a more homogeneous endothelial coverage [8]. However, excessive polydispersity increases the likelihood of Ostwald ripening, whereby gas diffuses from smaller bubbles into larger ones, accelerating foam breakdown.

This means that foams with more uniform bubble size behave more predictably in vivo, improving consistency between operators and reducing unintended distal migration and related heterogeneity in circumferential endothelial interaction.

Apart from the bubble size, also its ratio with the liquid part is of paramount importance in the final clinical choice of the expert practitioner: indeed, it affects foam rheology, stability, and injectability. Dry foams exhibit a higher apparent viscosity, a slower drainage, and a prolonged endothelial contact. Wet foams behave more like viscous liquids with faster collapse, greater control during injection and reduced persistence [9]. Drainage occurs as gravity pulls liquid downward, thinning lamellae and predisposing to rupture.

Adapting the liquid–gas ratio brings the possibility to tailor the treatment in favor of foam persistence depending on vein tortuosity, size, and location. Dry foams are to be considered in particular for large or recurrent veins, while wet ones for smaller and cosmetic treatments.

It should not be forgotten how gases differ markedly in blood solubility and diffusivity: nitrogen-rich air diffuses slowly, prolonging bubble lifespan, while carbon dioxide diffuses rapidly, accelerating foam collapse, with oxygen being in between the two above mentioned gasses [10]. Gas exchange between foam bubbles and blood follows diffusion gradients described by Fick's law (from inside the bubble, where there is more gas, toward the blood, where there is less gas), leading to progressive bubble shrinkage and dissolution.

Gas choice is a safety-modulating decision. Rapidly diffusible gases reduce systemic embolic load and neurological risk, particularly in high-volume treatments, yet they reduce foam stability. The virtual best scenario would provide a nitrogen-free, C02/02 stable foam.

Foams exhibit non-Newtonian rheology, behaving as viscoelastic materials whose apparent viscosity changes with shear rate. Under low shear (static vein), foam maintains structure; under high shear (injection or fast flow), bubbles deform or fragment [11]. Injection pressure and speed directly influence foam architecture as high shear converts dry foam into wet foam, while excessive pressure disrupts lamellae and increases polydispersity.

Based on the above notions, slow, low-pressure injection preserves intended foam characteristics at the target site.

Foam does not mix homogeneously with blood. Instead, it displaces blood as a plug, creating a transient blood-free lumen. At the foam–blood interface, red blood cells aggregate, plasma proteins alter lamellar stability, and gas diffusion accelerates bubble dissolution. In particular, blood proteins bind the sclerosing drug causing rapid inactivation [12].

> The above mentioned explains why foam efficacy decreases in high-flow conditions and why proximal compression and limb elevation can enhance outcomes.

Even more, relatively small blood quantity of blood can inactivate the sclerosant, therefore suggesting to avoid aspirating it in the syringe to confirm the correct needle position, rather using an ultrasound guide if needed. The rapid inactivation also indicates the safety of the procedure, yet requiring some minutes of extreme care in the mobilization of the patient after the procedure.

> Evidently, foam success depends as much on hemodynamic control as on chemical potency.

In conclusion, conceptually, sclerotherapy foam functions simultaneously as a drug carrier, a mechanical blood-displacing agent, and a temporary intravascular scaffold. This multifunctional role distinguishes foam from conventional injectable therapies and explains its high efficacy in large-diameter veins [13]. Foam is not simply "liquid plus gas" but a therapeutic architecture engineered for transient intravascular occupation.

3 Translation into Everyday Clinical Practice

In fluid dynamics, two immiscible phases with different densities and viscosities tend to segregate rather than mix. Gas-containing foams, due to their structure and yield stress, behave as plug-flow systems rather than as freely mixing liquids. When injected into a vein, foam advances as a cohesive bolus that physically displaces blood instead of mixing with it. This creates a transient blood-free lumen in which sclerosant concentration at the endothelial surface is preserved. Liquid sclerosants are rapidly diluted by blood flow, particularly in large or high-flow veins. Foam overcomes this limitation by engineering the intravascular environment before chemical injury occurs.

> The clinician using foam is not increasing drug potency but eliminating the biological confounder of blood dilution.

Detergent sclerosants induce endothelial injury through time- and concentration-dependent membrane disruption. Short exposures may be reversible, whereas sustained exposure leads to irreversible cell death. Liquid sclerosants are cleared rapidly by venous flow, limiting effective contact time. Foam, by increasing apparent viscosity and disrupting laminar flow, slows intraluminal clearance and prolongs sclerosant–endothelium interaction. Prolonged contact allows effective treatment with lower sclerosant concentrations, reducing systemic exposure while maintaining efficacy. Factors influencing foam transit time should always be taken into consideration for the possible sclerotherapy power alteration (for example, injection speed and/or proximity with a fast flow vein confluence) [14, 15].

> Foam transforms time into a controllable therapeutic variable, reducing reliance on higher drug doses.

Foams maximize interfacial surface area and exhibit lateral spreading driven by surface tension and bubble packing geometry. Rather than streaming along preferential flow paths, foam spreads circumferentially, achieving homogeneous contact with the vein wall.

Uniform endothelial injury correlates with higher rates of durable vein closure and lower recanalization rates compared with liquid injections.

Foam converts a localized injection into a three-dimensional therapeutic field [16].

In clinical practice this translates also in the easier diffusion of foam into confluences, junctions, and perforators compared to liquid, for which a careful anatomical and hemodynamics assessment must always be performed.

Another advantage of gas–liquid interfaces is its ability to strongly reflect ultrasound waves due to impedance mismatch, making foams highly echogenic. Foam is readily visible during injection and propagation, allowing real-time tracking of sclerosant distribution. Ultrasound visualization enables precise targeting of refluxing segments, immediate correction of unintended spread, dynamic control of injection volume and speed. Foam converts sclerotherapy from a blind chemical injection into a visually guided interventional procedure. A careful scanning should always parallel the sclerosing act. Foam is created by dispersing gas into a liquid containing surface-active agents (sclerosants) while supplying sufficient mechanical energy to overcome surface tension. The resulting bubble size and distribution depend on shear forces applied, gas-to-liquid ratio, surfactant concentration, duration, and symmetry of mixing. Different foam production techniques apply different shear profiles, leading to predictable differences in foam wetness, stability, and injectability (Table 6.2).

Choosing a foam production method is equivalent to choosing a foam phenotype with defined safety and clinical behavior.

Table 6.2 Relation between foam production type, its physical effect, and the related clinical meaning

Production variable	Physical effect	Clinical meaning
Mixing energy	Bubble size	Endothelial coverage
Connector type/circuit	Polydispersity	Predictability
Gas type	Diffusion rate	Safety profile
Gas/liquid ratio	Wetness	Persistence vs. control

Table 6.3 Dry versus wet foams physical and related clinical features

Foam type	Physical feature	Clinical meaning
Dry	High gas fraction Thin lamellae High bubble density Slower drainage Higher apparent viscosity Close bubble packing Strong surface tension forces	Displace blood more completely Resist rapid collapse Maintain prolonged wall apposition More sensitive to shear forces and injection pressure
Wet	Higher liquid fraction Thicker lamellae Lower bubble density Faster drainage and collapse Similar to viscous liquids, with lower yield stress and easier flow	Easier to inject through small needles or catheters Collapse more rapidly Exhibit reduced intravascular persistence

Foam wetness determines bubble density, lamellar thickness, drainage rate, apparent viscosity. Foams exist on a continuum from very wet (approaching a bubbly liquid) to very dry (polyhedral bubbles with thin lamellae). In sclerotherapy, wetness is primarily determined during foam production by the gas-to-liquid ratio, but it continues to evolve dynamically after injection due to drainage and gas diffusion (Table 6.3).

Wetness is a *designed initial condition* whose clinical effect unfolds over time inside the vein.

Endothelial injury from detergent sclerosants depends on both concentration and exposure time. Foam wetness directly influences exposure time by modulating drainage and collapse kinetics [17].

Dry foams maintain longer endothelial contact, promoting deeper and more uniform injury, while wet foams produce more superficial and localized endothelial damage.

Histopathological studies confirm more extensive endothelial denudation with drier foams at equivalent sclerosant concentrations [18].

> In clinical terms, foam wetness determines how aggressively the vein wall is treated.

Rather than a binary distinction, wet and dry foams define a continuum of therapeutic architectures. Expert practice involves adjusting gas-to-liquid ratio, selecting gas type, modulating injection speed, combining foams within a single session when appropriate. Mastery of foam sclerotherapy lies in graduated control, not rigid categorization.

4 Intravascular Evolution of Foam after Injection

Foam behaves as a cohesive gas–liquid structure that advances as a plug, displacing intravascular blood rather than mixing with it. This behavior is governed by surface tension, lamellar cohesion, and yield stress, distinguishing foam from Newtonian liquids [19]. Immediately after injection blood is mechanically expelled from the treated venous segment, a transient blood-free lumen is created and sclerosant concentration at the endothelium is preserved. This phase occurs over seconds to minutes and is highly sensitive to venous filling, gravity, and flow conditions.

> In everyday practice, this suggests to elevate the limb before and during injection to reduce residual blood volume, perform a proximal compression to enhance foam advancement and containment, while injecting slowly to preserve foam architecture and plug behavior. Early success depends on mechanical control of the intravascular environment before chemical injury begins.

Once stationary or slowly moving, foam bubbles undergo progressive dissolution as gas diffuses into surrounding blood. The rate of dissolution depends on the gas solubility (e.g., CO_2 vs nitrogen), the bubble size, the blood flow, and the pressure gradients. Progressively, bubble volume decreases, foam becomes wetter, the structural integrity proceeds toward collapse. This is the phase in which gas choice directly influences the evolution. Avoidance of early vigorous ambulation reduces premature foam washout, while controlled foam volumes limit systemic gas exposure. In this sense, bubble dissolution defines the safe lifespan of foam within the circulation. Detergent sclerosants induce endothelial injury through membrane solubilization, protein denaturation, and cytoskeletal disruption. Injury severity is governed by sclerosant concentration, exposure time, and uniformity of wall contact. During this phase endothelial cells swell, detach, undergo apoptosis, the basement membrane exposure occurs and pro-inflammatory and pro-coagulant signaling is initiated [20]. Foam prolongs this phase by maintaining lamellar contact even as bubbles dissolve. This phase represents the therapeutic core of sclerotherapy:

timing errors here reduce efficacy. By maximizing exposure time, even low sclerosant concentrations can remain effective.

Clinically, in order to favor the sclerotherapic process, maintaining limb elevation can prolong wall contact and avoiding premature compression release can facilitate adequate injury.

Endothelial denudation exposes subendothelial collagen and tissue factor, triggering platelet adhesion and thrombin generation. Foam-induced injury produces a localized, controlled thrombosis rather than free-flowing clot formation [21]. The intravascular events include the formation of a platelet-rich thrombus along the treated segment, incorporation, or clearance of residual foam fragments, while flow is progressively arrested. This phase develops over hours to days.

Early compression can facilitate vein wall apposition and limit thrombus volume. Ambulation balances thrombosis stabilization with venous thrombosis prevention. Anti-inflammatory and/or thromboprophylaxis management may reduce post-sclerotherapy pain and pigmentation [22, 23].

Thrombus organization triggers fibroblast recruitment, collagen deposition, and vein wall remodeling, resulting in fibrotic obliteration. Over weeks to months thrombus is resorbed and replaced by fibrous tissue, vein lumen collapses permanently, and the treated vein becomes a fibrotic cord. The durability of closure depends on the completeness of earlier phases. Sustained external compression supports fibrotic remodeling: a phenomenon that can be well monitored by ultrasound follow-ups. Early recanalization often reflects inadequate endothelial injury rather than failure of fibrosis.Empirically, post-sclerotherapy compression for some months might facilitate the fibrotic remodeling, yet no strong evidence-based data in support of the statement are currently available up to our knowledge.

Long-term success reflects how well the early physical and chemical phases were executed. Optimal outcomes arise when clinical maneuvers are synchronized with foam biology, not applied indiscriminately (Table 6.4).

Table 6.4 Foam action phases, related dominant mechanism and consequent clinical action

Foam phase	Dominant mechanism	Key clinical action
Blood displacement	Mechanical	Leg elevation Proximal compression
Bubble dissolution	Diffusive	Gas choice Volume control
Endothelial injury	Chemical	Maintain contact time
Thrombotic occlusion	Biological	Compression Controlled ambulation
Fibrotic transformation	Remodeling	Follow-up Sustained support

5 Safety Considerations Rooted in Foam Science

Foam is a metastable, space-occupying system whose biological effects depend on its physical properties, particularly bubble size distribution, gas composition, and stability. Unlike liquid sclerosants, foam introduces a gaseous phase that interacts with blood flow, pressure gradients, and shunts. Many foam-related adverse effects arise not from sclerosant toxicity but from gas bubble behavior within the vascular system.

> Safety management begins at foam construction, not at complication treatment.

Bubble size determines buoyancy, persistence, and the ability to traverse microvascular beds. Smaller bubbles dissolve faster but may pass through arteriovenous or intracardiac shunts; larger bubbles persist longer but are more easily trapped and dissolved locally. Highly polydisperse foams increase the likelihood of systemic bubble passage. Narrow bubble size distributions behave more predictably in vivo. In order to reduce extreme bubble sizes, controlled foam production techniques can help. Avoiding excessive mixing energy means avoiding polydispersity. High-risk patients can benefit from reproducible foam.

> Bubble size control is a primary embolic safety intervention.

Gas solubility and diffusivity in blood determine bubble lifespan. Carbon dioxide dissolves approximately 20 times faster than nitrogen, leading to rapid bubble collapse.

Foams made with room air persist longer in the circulation, whereas CO_2-O_2 based foams show faster intravascular dissolution, reduced systemic bubble load, lower incidence of neurological symptoms [24]. Consequently, CO_2 or CO_2/O_2 mixtures should be preferred in patients with migraine, right-to-left shunts, or prior neurological symptoms, while air-based foams should be limited to situations where prolonged persistence is required and patient risk is low.

> Gas selection is one of the most powerful modifiable safety variables in foam sclerotherapy.

Neurological symptoms following foam sclerotherapy are related to transient cerebral gas and/or microparticle embolization from endothelial disruption, particularly in patients with right-to-left shunts [25]. The most common manifestation includes visual disturbances, migraine aura, transient ischemic symptoms. These events are typically self-limited and correlate with foam volume, gas type and bubble persistence.

> Screening for migraine history and prior neurological symptoms is of fundamental importance to limit such complications, together with the use of CO_2-based foams and with the limitation of foam volume.

Thrombo-embolism is another sclerotherapy possible complication that can be easily prevented by applying the basic science knowledge at the base of the procedure. Endothelial injury combined with stagnant flow promotes thrombosis. Foam-induced thrombosis is intended locally but must be prevented from extending into the deep system [26]. Deep venous extension is uncommon and it is associated with large foam volumes, inadequate compression of the junctional points and proximity to the deep venous system.

Practical strategies that can limit deep venous thrombosis complications are avoiding foam injection too close to the deep venous junctions, applying timely and adequate compression in order to occlude the passage toward the deep veins, and use post-procedure ultrasound surveillance in high-risk cases. Knowing the specific patient individual thrombotic risk is mandatory.

Another significant determinant of foam sclerotherapy safety is its volume. Systemic exposure to foam correlates more strongly with total injected foam volume than with sclerosant concentration. Larger foam volumes increase total gas load and duration of circulation. Yet, total maximum volume values differ in the different guidelines around the world, for which dedicated investigations on the topic should be run, taking care in comparing homogeneous foams [27].

As a general indication, the lowest volume possible should be injected, favoring multiple injection sites and staging treatment of extensive disease rather than treating all segments at once.

Foam stability is reduced by high shear stress and rapid flow, while venous filling increases dilution and washout. Patients with large-diameter refluxing veins, incompetent perforators, and significant hemodynamic overload may require tailored strategies to maintain containment and safety (Table 6.5) [28]. In this scenario, practical safety strategies may include limb elevation and proximal compression.

Table 6.5 Foam property, related scientific risk, and consequent safety strategy

Foam property	Scientific risk driver	Safety strategy
Bubble size	Embolic potential	Controlled production
Gas type	Bubble persistence	Nitrogen-free foam
Volume	Systemic exposure	Limited volume
Wetness	Persistence	Match to anatomy and hemodynamics
Injection pressure	Polydispersity	Slow, controlled injection

6 Foam Sclerotherapy Filters

The introduction of filters into foam sclerotherapy did not arise from technological enthusiasm but from clinical observation guided by foam science. As clinicians gained experience with foam, it became clear that its benefits, enhanced efficacy, reduced drug dose, and improved visualization were inseparably linked to its microstructure, particularly bubble size distribution. Filters emerged as a logical response to a central insight of foam physics: not all bubbles behave equally and extreme bubble sizes carry disproportionate risk [26]. All manually generated foams are inherently polydisperse, containing bubbles that vary widely in size. This variability is a natural consequence of turbulent shear during mixing, asymmetric syringe flow, and local differences in surfactant concentration. From a physical standpoint, polydispersity is expected, while from a clinical standpoint, it introduces uncertainty. Large bubbles tend to persist longer and may migrate further within the venous system, while very small bubbles dissolve rapidly but are more capable of traversing microvascular beds or right-to-left shunts. Improving safety requires structural control of foam, not simply dose reduction. Filtration partially addresses this problem directly by targeting the outliers in the bubble population. When foam is passed through a filter, it is subjected to size exclusion and controlled shear. Bubbles larger than the pore size are fragmented or eliminated, while unstable clusters are disrupted. The result is not the creation of a new foam, but the refinement of an existing one, a narrowing of the bubble size distribution and removal of extreme elements. Clinically, filtered foam appears more homogeneous and behaves more predictably during injection and intravascular propagation. Ultrasound observation often confirms smoother advancement and less erratic distal spread compared with unfiltered foam. This mechanical refinement mirrors a familiar principle in medicine: just as drug purification improves pharmacological predictability, bubble filtration improves foam predictability. An important consequence of filtration is its subtle effect on foam wetness. By fragmenting bubbles and locally increasing liquid redistribution, filtration tends to produce a slightly wetter foam. From a purely physical perspective, this accelerates drainage and shortens foam persistence. Clinically, this effect can be viewed in two ways. In large truncal veins, reduced persistence may necessitate adjustments in gas-to-liquid ratio or injection strategy to maintain efficacy. In contrast, in neurologically sensitive patients or distal venous territories, this same reduction in persistence represents a safety advantage, limiting unintended migration. Thus, filtration exemplifies a recurring theme in foam science: every gain in safety involves a trade-off with persistence, and expert practice lies in managing that balance. The strongest rationale for filters lies in their role as a preventive embolic safety measure. By reducing maximum bubble size, filters lower the probability that any single bubble will persist long enough or remain large enough to cause symptoms. Importantly, filters do not eliminate bubbles altogether, nor do they replace the need for appropriate gas choice or volume limitation. Instead, they reduce the amplitude of risk, smoothing the extremes of foam behavior. In this sense, filters function as a *buffer* between foam production variability and patient physiology. It is tempting to view filtration and gas choice as interchangeable safety strategies, but foam science shows they operate on different dimensions of risk. Gas selection determines how long bubbles persist through diffusion and dissolution, whereas filtration determines how large those bubbles are at the outset. A CO_2-based foam may dissolve quickly but still contain large initial bubbles; a filtered air-based foam may persist longer but with a narrower and safer size distribution. Optimal safety is therefore achieved not by choosing one strategy over the other, but by combining them thoughtfully in patients or procedures where risk tolerance is low. Passing foam through a filter increases resistance and alters flow dynamics. If the clinician responds with excessive injection pressure, the intended benefits of filtration may be partially negated by downstream bubble fragmentation and renewed polydispersity. This highlights an often-overlooked point: filtration requires adaptation of technique. Slow injection, appropriate syringe and needle selection, and real-time ultrasound monitoring remain essential. Filters enhance safety only when integrated into a broader framework of foam-conscious practice. Experience suggests that filters are most valuable in scenarios where the consequences of bubble variability are greatest: high-volume truncal foam treatments, patients with migraine, prior neurological symptoms, or suspected right-to-left shunts, training environments with variable operator technique. The story of filters in foam sclerotherapy is the story of foam science maturing into clinical wisdom. As understanding shifted from "foam as a drug carrier" to "foam as a dynamic physical system," it became clear that controlling structure mattered as much as controlling dose. Filters represent a tangible expression of that insight: a simple mechanical intervention grounded in bubble physics, deployed to improve predictability and reduce risk.

7 Clinical Considerations on Foam Half-Life

When clinicians speak about the "stability" of foam, they are often intuitively referring to its half-life, the time during which foam remains structurally and functionally effective. In foam sclerotherapy, half-life is not a pharmacological concept but a physical–functional one: it describes how long foam retains enough structure to displace blood, maintain endothelial contact, and act as a coherent intravascular entity before collapsing. The half-life of foam is not random. It is largely pre-determined at the moment of foam production, shaped by bubble size distribution, gas content, liquid fraction, and the mechanical energy applied during generation. As experience with foam grew, it became clear that different production techniques create foams with distinct temporal behaviors, which in turn explain their differing clinical performances. In foam science, half-life is most commonly measured in vitro as the time required for 50% of the liquid to drain, or the time until 50% reduction in foam height or bubble count [29, 30]. Clinically, however, half-life should be understood as the duration of effective intravascular behavior, the window during which foam acts as a blood-displacing, endothelial-contacting structure. A foam with a long half-life supports prolonged contact and efficacy in large veins, while a foam with a short half-life favors control and safety in superficial or cosmetic indications. Importantly, neither is better in absolute terms: half-life is a therapeutic variable. In order to compare half-life/stability of the different foams, standardization of the several involved variables is of paramount importance, including drug type/concentration, liquid/gas ratio, temperature, and production materials. A recent investigation standardized the temperature variable and compared Tessari method with the Double Syringe System one, highlighting a longer half-life associated to the latter [31]. Varixio™, Varithena™, and MFoamer™ data are reported in Table 6.6, together with Tessari and DSS methods. The direct comparison of half-life time must take into consideration also the nitrogen content used in the different methods and the related safety consequences. Varithena™ demonstrated lower degradation rate than any physician-compounded foams, even than foams made using room air (high nitrogen levels) [32].

Table 6.6 Different foams production methods half-life: the table report 1% Polidocanol for homogeneity in all production methods analysis

Foam production type	Nitrogen	Half-life (mean)
MFoamer™	<0.8%	NA
Varithena™	<0.8%	NA
Sclerofoam	NA	NA
Varixio™	2%–10%	150 s
EasyFoam™	78%	NA
DSS	78%	148 s ± 37.71
Tessari	78%	90 s ± 8.57

All data were collected in room temperature. It must be noted that the comparison is among foam production methods with totally different nitrogen contents, which means with totally different safety levels. Sources: MFoamer™ (https://m-foamer.com), Varithena™ (https://www.varithena.com/), Varixio™ (https://varixio.com) (Half-life definition: "the time when half the liquid composing the foam had drained in a quiescent upright syringe containing the foam." DSS and Tessari [31]. Half-life definition: «Half-life»: the time taken for half of the volume of the liquid to drain

8 Stabilizers

Increasing liquid viscosity slows gravitational drainage from lamellae, one of the principal causes of foam collapse. In experimental models, viscous additives such as glycerol or glucose significantly prolong foam half-life [33–35]. However, increased viscosity also reduces injectability, alters intravascular spread, and increases shear sensitivity during injection. In everyday clinical practice, this means that viscosity-based stabilizers may improve stability but reduce controllability. High-molecular weight polymers (e.g., cellulose derivatives, poloxamers) stabilize foams by increasing interfacial viscoelasticity, thickening lamellae and slowing coalescence. Such stabilizers are widely used in industrial and pharmaceutical foams but are not routinely used in clinical sclerotherapy due to concerns about biocompatibility, embolic persistence, and regulatory constraints [36]. Also hyaluronic acid demonstrated to increase polidocanol foam stability. Indeed, it demonstrated to increase the liquid's viscosity, reducing bubble size and polydispersity, enhancing the surface elasticity, and slowing the liquid drainage between bubbles, allowing the sclerosant to stay concentrated and deliver a more effective, longer-lasting treatment with better delivery to target cells. It acts as a biopolymer, improving the foam's structure and half-life (time to halve volume) [37]. Yet, hyaluronan acid can cause clot issues whenever injected in the bloodstream. A more recent investigation focused then on Sulodexide, an already available venotonic medication consisted of glycosaminoglycans, reported an increased foam stability, possibly thanks to both a viscosity and electric charge effect. Further benefit of this drug included anti-coagulant and endothelial-protective effect, helping the sclerotherapy act to be confined only to the targeted segment, rather than extending in undesired contiguous vein segments [38].

9 Conclusions

Foam sclerotherapy is an applied science where physics, chemistry, and clinical judgment converge. Mastery requires more than knowing how to make foam: it requires understanding why a particular foam behaves as it does and *when* that behavior is desirable. Translating foam science into daily practice enables vascular specialists to tailor treatment precisely, improving outcomes while minimizing risk of complications.

References

1. Beckitt T, Elstone A, Ashley S. Air versus physiological gas for ultrasound guided foam sclerotherapy treatment of varicose veins. Eur J Vasc Endovasc Surg. 2011;42(1):115–9.
2. Coleridge Smith P. Foam and liquid sclerotherapy for varicose veins. Phlebology. 2009;24(Suppl 1):62–72.
3. Rabe E, Breu FX, Flessenkämper I, et al. Sclerotherapy in the treatment of varicose veins: S2k guideline of the Deutsche Gesellschaft für Phlebologie (DGP) in cooperation with the following societies: DDG, DGA, DGG, BVP. Hautarzt. 2021;72(Suppl 2):23–36.
4. Meghdadi A, Jones SA, Patel VA, et al. Foam-in-vein: a review of rheological properties and characterization methods for optimization of sclerosing foams. J Biomed Mater Res B Appl Biomater. 2021;109(1):69–91.
5. Bottaro E, Paterson JAJ, Quercia L, et al. In vitro and ex vivo evaluation of the biological performance of sclerosing foams. Sci Rep. 2019;9(1):9880.
6. Kanber EM. Comparison of foam and liquid sclerotherapy for the treatment of lower extremity varicose veins and telangiectasia in obese patients. Cureus. 2023;15(7):e42571.
7. Critello CD, Fiorillo AS, Matula TJ. Size of sclerosing foams prepared by ultrasound, mechanical agitation, and the handmade Tessari method for treatment of varicose veins. J Ultrasound Med. 2017;36(3):649–58.
8. Eckmann DM. Polidocanol for endovenous microfoam sclerosant therapy. Expert Opin Investig Drugs. 2009;18(12):1919–27.
9. Bai T, Liu Y, Jiang W, Li Y, Liu J, Yu C, Fan Y. A review of Sclerosing foam stability in the treatment of varicose veins. Dermatologic Surg. 2020;46(2):249–57.
10. Morrison N, Neuhardt DL, Rogers CR, et al. Incidence of side effects using carbon dioxide-oxygen foam for chemical ablation of superficial veins of the lower extremity. Eur J Vasc Endovasc Surg. 2010;40(3):407–13.
11. Roberts TG, Cox S, Lewis AL, et al. Characterisation and optimisation of foams for varicose vein sclerotherapy. Biorheology. 2021;57(2–4):77–85.
12. Dabbs EB, Dos Santos SJ, Mainsiouw LE, Sheikh AA, Gkantiragas A, Shiangoli I, Watkins MR, Nemchand JL, Whiteley MS. Implication of foam sclerosant inactivation by human whole blood in a laboratory setting. Phlebology. 2018;33(5):338–43.
13. Kabnick LS, Jimenez JC, Coogan SM, et al. Comparative effectiveness of non-compounded polidocanol 1% endovenous microfoam (Varithena) ablation versus endovenous thermal ablation utilizing a systematic review and network meta-analysis. J Vasc Surg Venous Lymphat Disord. 2024;12(6):101896.
14. Gianesini S, Sisini F, Di Domenico G, Secchiero J, Malagoni AM, Menegatti E, Gambaccini M, Zamboni P. Lower limbs venous kinetics and consequent impact on drainage direction. Phlebology. 2018;33(2):107–14.
15. Gianesini S, Sisini F, Menegatti E, Di Domenico G, Gambaccini M, Occhionorelli S, Zamboni P. Altered velocity gradient in lower limb chronic venous disease. Phlebology. 2019;34(1):17–24.
16. Hamel-Desnos C, Allaert FA. Liquid versus foam sclerotherapy. Phlebology. 2009;24(6):240–6.
17. Marting B. Understanding sclerotherapy. Plast Surg Nurs. 2000;20(4):209–15, 29.
18. Alder G, Lees T. Foam sclerotherapy. Phlebology. 2015;30(2 Suppl):18–23.
19. Coleridge Smith P. Sclerotherapy and foam sclerotherapy for varicose veins. Phlebology. 2009;24(6):260–9.
20. Whiteley MS, Dos Santos SJ, Fernandez-Hart TJ, et al. Media damage following detergent sclero-

therapy appears to be secondary to the induction of inflammation and apoptosis: an immunohistochemical study elucidating previous histological observations. Eur J Vasc Endovasc Surg. 2016;51(3):421–8.
21. Parsi K, Panozzo B, Bull A, et al. Deep vein sclerosis following sclerotherapy: ultrasonic and d-dimer criteria. Phlebology. 2020;35(5):325–36.
22. Gonzalez Ochoa AJ, Carrillo J, Manríquez D, Manrique F, et al. Reducing hyperpigmentation after sclerotherapy: a randomized clinical trial. J Vasc Surg Venous Lymphat Disord. 2021;9(1):154–62.
23. Bogachev VY, Boldin BV, Turkin PY. Administration of micronized purified flavonoid fraction during sclerotherapy of reticular veins and telangiectasias: results of the national, multicenter, observational program VEIN ACT PROLONGED-C1. Adv Ther. 2018;35(7):1001–8.
24. Wong M. Should foam made with physiologic gases be the standard in sclerotherapy? Phlebology. 2015;30(9):580–6.
25. Gajo EC, Kavinsky CJ, Murphy J, et al. The pivotal role of PFO in paradoxical embolism following venous sclerotherapy: a unique case report with pathological correlations. Eur Heart J Case Rep. 2021;5(8):ytab228.
26. Cavezzi A, Parsi K. Complications of foam sclerotherapy. Phlebology. 2012;27(Suppl 1):46–51.
27. Gianesini S, Obi A, Onida S, et al. Global guidelines trends and controversies in lower limb venous and lymphatic disease: narrative literature revision and experts' opinions following the vWINter international meeting in Phlebology, Lymphology & Aesthetics, 23–25 January 2019. Phlebology. 2019;34(1 Suppl):4–66.
28. Gianesini S, Occhionorelli S, Menegatti E, Malagoni AM, Tessari M, Zamboni P. Femoral vein valve incompetence as a risk factor for junctional recurrence. Phlebology. 2018;33(3):206–21.
29. Bai T, Jiang W, Chen Y, et al. Effect of multiple factors on foam stability in foam sclerotherapy. Sci Rep. 2018;8(1):15683.
30. Cameron E, Chen T, Connor DE, et al. Sclerosant foam structure and stability is strongly influenced by liquid air fraction. Eur J Vasc Endovasc Surg. 2013;46(4):488–94.
31. Buonsante GF, Marques MA, Barros BCS, Assunção VC, Fiorelli SKA, Fiorelli RKA. Impact of temperature on the production of 1% polidocanol foam: comparison between the Tessari and double-syringe techniques in an experimental study. J Vasc Bras. 2025;24:e20250010.
32. Carugo D, Ankrett DN, Zhao X, et al. Benefits of polidocanol endovenous microfoam (Varithena®) compared with physician-compounded foams. Phlebology. 2016;31(4):283–95.
33. Peterson JD, Goldman MP. An investigation on the influence of glycerin on sclerosant foam stability. Phlebology. 2011;26(6):232–4.
34. Rial R, Hervas LS, Monux G, et al. Polidocanol foam stability in terms of its association with glycerin. Phlebology. 2014;29(5):304–9.
35. Sawaby A, Maklad S, Atta I, et al. Evaluation of the efficacy of foam sclerosant after addition of glycerine on human great saphenous vein: histological and immunohistochemical study. Ann R Coll Surg Engl. 2021;103(6):452–8.
36. Baigadilov A, Colombano S, Omirbekov S, et al. Stability and flow behavior of polymer-enhanced foams for improved in-situ remediation of hydrocarbons: effect of polymer-surfactant interactions. J Hazard Mater. 2025;486:137004.
37. Chen AW, Liu YR, Li K, et al. An investigation on the influence of hyaluronic acid on polidocanol foam stability. Dermatologic Surg. 2016;42:56–8.
38. Critello CD, Fiorillo AS, Cristiano MC, et al. Effects of sulodexide on stability of sclerosing foams. Phlebology. 2019;34(3):191–200.

Safety Profiles, Indications, and Contraindications

7

Sergio Gianesini, Ayman Fakhry, and Yung Wei Chi

1 Safety Considerations in Sclerotherapy

Sclerotherapy occupies a distinctive position in the therapeutic spectrum of chronic venous disease. It is at once deceptively simple, often performed in an outpatient setting with minimal equipment and physiologically consequential, because it is designed to provoke a controlled intravascular injury that culminates in fibrosis and durable vein occlusion. That duality explains why the procedure's safety profile is excellent in experienced hands, yet vulnerable to lapses in patient selection, dosing discipline, ultrasound technique, and post-procedural surveillance. Safe sclerotherapy is not merely "injecting a sclerosant," rather executing a standardized intervention with defined indications, contraindications, concentration/volume recommendations, and an explicit awareness of adverse events and their prevention [1]. Over the last two decades, the introduction of ultrasound-guided foam sclerotherapy has further elevated both opportunity and responsibility. Foam improves efficacy in larger-caliber veins by displacing blood and increasing endothelial contact time, yet introduces additional systemic considerations related to the intravascular gas phase [2, 3]. The objective of safety-focused practice is therefore twofold:

1. to prevent avoidable local injury (skin necrosis, nerve irritation, thrombophlebitis, hyperpigmentation) and thromboembolic complications;
2. to minimize rare but high-impact neurological and cardiopulmonary events through careful technique, dose limits, foam standardization, and monitoring [4]. The first safety principle is conceptual: in sclerotherapy, efficacy and harm share a mechanism. The therapeutic endpoint, endothelial disruption leading to vein wall inflammation, thrombotic occlusion, and subsequent fibrotic remodeling, is achieved by a chemical insult that must remain confined to the intended venous segment [5]. When the insult extends beyond the target vein (via extravasation, intra-arterial injection, unintended deep venous propagation, or excessive total dose), complications are not "unexpected"; they are mechanistically predictable. In a modern venous practice, the "safety check" begins well before the

S. Gianesini (✉)
Department of Translational Medicine, University of Ferrara, Ferrara, Italy

Department of Surgery, Uniformed Services University of Health Sciences, Bethesda, MD, USA
e-mail: gnssrg@unife.it

A. Fakhry
Vascular Surgery, Egyptian Venous Forum, Alexandria, Egypt

Y. W. Chi
Department of Cardiovascular Medicine, University of California, Davis Vascular Center, Sacramento, CA, USA
e-mail: ywchi@ucdavis.edu

S. Gianesini, Y. W. Chi (eds.), *Sclerotherapy*, https://doi.org/10.1007/978-3-032-32794-9_7

needle. Sclerotherapy should be preceded by a structured history and a hemodynamic assessment, typically duplex ultrasound, not only to confirm the target vein but to define the reflux source and the relationship of superficial reflux to perforator and deep venous function. Diagnostic duplex is pivotal in choosing the appropriate intervention and sequencing treatments, because treating visible tributaries without addressing the reflux source invites recurrence and repeated exposure to procedural risk. This is particularly evident in case of varicose veins directly draining into the deep system by means of perforating veins, typically in the Hunter canal, in the pelvic escape points and in the below-knee region. From a safety perspective, this mapping accomplishes three things. First, it prevents the operator from injecting a vein that is acting as a collateral pathway in the setting of deep venous obstruction (where obliteration could worsen symptoms or provoke thrombosis) [6]. Second, it clarifies whether the planned sclerotherapy is a primary treatment of truncal reflux, an adjunct after ablation, or a targeted treatment of residual/recurrent varicosities [7]. Third, it anticipates technical hazards (proximity to the deep system, large perforators, aneurysmal segments, and junctional anatomy, etc.) where foam migration or thrombus extension is more likely. In vascular practice, informed consent is not a formality but a safety intervention. A well-consented patient is more likely to report early symptoms, comply with ambulation/compression, and seek timely care if warning signs develop. Side effects and complications mentioning, explaining, and eventual reporting must be part of the standardized practice [8]. Consent discussions should not be proportionate to disease severity and treatment extent: a patient undergoing limited liquid sclerotherapy for reticular veins should enjoy the same emphasis as one undergoing ultrasound-guided foam sclerotherapy of a truncal vein. A typical mistake is indeed to consider aesthetic sclerotherapy of the telangiectasia safer than large vessel foam sclerotherapy. Both conditions demand maximum care. This is particularly evident if we consider how the endothelial surface interested by the sclerotherapy act might be significantly bigger in a telangiectatic network rather than in a large tributary vein. The consent conversation is also where risk-modifiers are identified and acted upon (just to name a few, prior venous thromboembolism, thrombophilia, prolonged immobility, a history suggestive of migraine with aura, known right-to-left shunts, lifestyle, prolonged occupational standing-up/sedentarism, etc.). The key safety principle is not "exclude everyone at risk," but "identify risk, adapt technique, and intensify surveillance." Sclerotherapy is among the most scrutinized vein therapies from a medico-legal standpoint. This scrutiny arises not from a high complication rate, but from the juxtaposition of an often elective or cosmetic indication with a non-zero risk of serious harm. For this reason, the adequacy of informed consent in sclerotherapy must be approached with particular care, intellectual rigor, and professional discipline [9]. Informed consent in this context is not reducible to a signed document. It is a process of communication that must align patient expectations with clinical reality, disclose risks in proportion to their severity and frequency, and document that the patient has been afforded a genuine opportunity to make an autonomous decision. The vascular specialist who underestimates the importance of this process does so at personal, professional, and ethical risk. From an ethical perspective, contemporary standards of informed consent are firmly rooted in patient-centered disclosure. The clinician's obligation is no longer satisfied by reciting what a reasonable physician might disclose, but by communicating what a reasonable patient would consider material to their decision-making. In sclerotherapy, materiality is shaped by several factors: the elective nature of many treatments, the availability of conservative alternatives, the possibility of recurrence or incomplete response, and the existence of rare but potentially devastating complications. Courts and regulatory bodies have consistently held that low-probability events do not become immaterial when their consequences are severe. The consent process must therefore begin with a clear and accurate description of the procedure itself. Patients should understand that sclerotherapy involves the intravascular injection of a chemical agent intended to damage the endothelium, provoke fibrosis, and ultimately obliterate the treated vein. This description should not be mechanistic alone, but contextual, distinguishing between treatment of telangiectasias, reticular veins, and truncal or perforator incompetence. Where ultrasound guidance is employed, or where foam rather than liquid sclerosant is used, these distinctions should be explicitly addressed, as they carry different implications for efficacy and risk. Disclosure must also extend to the sclerosant itself. While most agents used in modern practice are detergent based and well studied, patients should be informed of the specific agent class, the rationale for foam or liquid selection, and any relevant off-label use. This is particularly important in foam sclerotherapy, where systemic distribution and embolic phenomena, though uncommon, are more frequently described than with liquid techniques. Failure to distinguish between these modalities during consent has been a recurring weakness in both expert testimony and adverse legal outcomes. Equally important is a balanced discussion of expected benefits. Sclerotherapy may relieve symptoms such as aching, heaviness, and swelling, and it may improve the appearance of visible veins. However, benefits are often gradual, may be incomplete, and are not permanent. The informed consent must actively counter the implicit promise of cure that patients often infer from minimally invasive procedures. Venous disease is chronic and progressive, and sclerotherapy does not alter the underlying predisposition to venous insufficiency. When cosmetic improvement is a primary goal, this must be stated explicitly, along with the inherent subjectivity of cosmetic outcomes. No consent is adequate without a meaningful discussion of alternatives. These include not only procedural alternatives such as endovenous thermal ablation, mechanochemical ablation, cyanoacrylate closure, phlebectomy, or surgical ligation, but also conservative strategies such as compression therapy, venous active drugs, exercise, weight management, and simple observation. The option of no treatment must be presented as legitimate. Importantly, alternatives should be described in a neutral, non-coercive manner. A consent process that implicitly disparages non-procedural options undermines patient autonomy and exposes the clinician to allegations of bias. Risk disclosure represents the most scrutinized and contested component of informed consent in sclerotherapy. Common and minor adverse effects such as pain, bruising, local inflammation, hyperpigmentation, matting, and pruritus should be disclosed not because they are dangerous, but because they are frequent and often drive dissatisfaction. Patients are more likely to feel misled by an undisclosed cosmetic imperfection than by a rare complication they were warned about. Beyond these predictable effects lie less common complications, including superficial thrombosis, trapped blood requiring evacuation, localized infection, nerve irritation, skin ulceration, and tissue necrosis. These events, while infrequent, have tangible consequences and must be presented as real possibilities rather than theoretical abstractions. Finally, the consent must address rare but serious adverse outcomes. Deep vein thrombosis, pulmonary embolism, transient ischemic attack, stroke, visual disturbances, anaphylaxis, paradoxical embolization, and death are all events with extremely low incidence in experienced hands. Nevertheless, ethical and legal standards require their disclosure, particularly in elective or cosmetic procedures. The use of foam sclerosant warrants explicit discussion of neurological symptoms, especially in patients with migraine disorders or known right-to-left shunts. Minimizing or omitting these risks on the basis of rarity has repeatedly been shown to be indefensible. An often-neglected aspect of informed consent is the articulation of procedural limitations and long-term expectations. Patients must understand that sclerotherapy does not prevent the development of new varicosities, that recurrence is common, and that maintenance treatments may be necessary. These disclosures are not pessimistic: they are essential for aligning expectations with the natural history of venous disease. Adequate consent also encompasses the patient's role in post-procedural care. Compression therapy, eventual anti-inflammatory/thromboprophylaxis/venous active drugs, ambulation, activity modification, and follow-up surveillance are not optional adjuncts but integral components of treatment success. Patients should be informed of warning signs that warrant urgent evaluation, reinforcing the shared responsibility inherent in the therapeutic relationship. Finally, informed consent must be individualized. Pregnancy, thrombophilia, prior thromboembolic events, migraine with aura, hormonal therapy, anticoagulant use, previous venous interventions, and known allergies materially alter risk profiles. Documentation should reflect that these factors were actively reviewed and discussed, rather than passively acknowledged through a generic form. In cases where sclerotherapy is performed primarily for cosmetic reasons, heightened disclosure is warranted. The elective nature of the intervention lowers tolerance for adverse outcomes, and financial considerations, including lack of insurance coverage, should be addressed transparently. Many experienced practitioners favor separate but complementary medical and cosmetic consent documents in such cases. Ultimately, the adequacy of informed consent in sclerotherapy is judged not by the length of the form, but by the quality of the conversation and the integrity of its documentation. A signed consent without evidence of meaningful dialogue is a fragile defense. For the vascular specialist, mastery of sclerotherapy extends beyond technical skill to include mastery of communication, expectation management, and ethical clarity.

Table 7.1 Top five aspects to be included in the sclerotherapy informed consent according to the chapter's authors' experience in the field

Top five aspects to be included in the sclerotherapy informed consent
1. Equal representation of minor and major side effect and complications, highlighting the related severity and prevalence
2. Highlight patient role in post-procedural result optimization
3. Clarify chronic venous disease is chronic indeed
4. Discriminte between therapeutic and aesthetic acts
5. Explain all the possible alternatives, including conservative approaches

The consent process is where these competencies are most visibly tested and most consequential (Table 7.1).

2 Sclerotherapy Clinical Practice Safety Aspects

Because sclerotherapy is frequently performed in office settings, it is easy for procedural discipline to degrade. Yet the setting should not dilute standards. Skin preparation, clean technique, and avoidance of cross-contamination remain basic but non-negotiable. Equally non-negotiable is emergency readiness: availability of medications and protocols for allergic reactions, including rare anaphylaxis. The risk of allergy is explicitly recognized, yet extremely rare (around 1/10.000) [10]. The same applies for cardiac arrest, despite its anecdotal reports and the still uncertain eventual etiology (endothelin-1 release, direct cardiotoxicity, anaphylaxis) [11–15]. A mature sclerotherapy practice is defined by restraint. The aim is to achieve the desired occlusion with the lowest effective concentration and volume, minimizing non-target exposure. Guidelines provide concentration and volume guidance tailored to vein diameter and emphasize dose discipline as a core safety theme. A currently unmet need is the specification not only of the concentration and volume, but also the physical characteristics of the specific eventually foam-based sclerotherapy act (wetness, production method, temperature) (Table 7.2).

Table 7.2 Basics for a safe sclerotherapy act

Basics of safe sclerotherapy
1. Hemodynamic understanding of venous disease, not cosmetic vein targeting alone
2. Mandatory duplex ultrasound assessment before treating non-trivial disease
3. Use of the lowest effective sclerosant concentration and volume
4. Recognition that complications are mechanistically predictable, not random
5. Structured informed consent proportional to treatment extent
6. A procedural environment equipped for emergency management

If sclerotherapy complications had a single dominant predictor, it would be operator-dependent variability. The reason is obvious to the specialists: sclerotherapy is not one procedure but a family of procedures (liquid vs foam, direct-vision vs ultrasound-guided, small tributaries vs truncal veins), each with different error modes and different consequences. The required competence is surely broader than injection skill. Competence includes duplex proficiency; pharmacologic understanding of sclerosant concentration, dose limits, and toxicity; technical mastery of needle/catheter positioning and injection dynamics; judgment in choosing foam vs liquid and selecting gas type; and preparedness to recognize and manage complications. Several competing modalities exist for which the operator must understand comparative risks and how patient factors shift the balance. Large pragmatic randomized trials comparing treatment modalities for varicose veins underscore that "minimally invasive" is not synonymous with "no need for expertise," and that outcomes depend strongly on protocol adherence and follow-up [16]. Expert practice acknowledges the learning curve explicitly. Early experience should focus on low-risk scenarios: small superficial veins, lower concentrations, and modest total volumes. At the same time, the above-described cases should not be considered less prone to complications and/or safer. For example, injecting a too low concentration and/or volume can lead to just a thrombotic rather than fibrotic process. Moreover, telangiectasia presents a wider endothelial area than bigger diameter truncal veins: the consequent endothelial catabolites generated by the sclerotherapy act can paradoxically cause even bigger complications in aesthetic procedures. At the same time, ultrasound-guided foam sclerotherapy of truncal veins and treatment near junctions demand a different level of skill because a small technical misjudgment can translate into deep system exposure or extensive foam propagation. This is not merely an educational issue: it is a safety ethic. A practitioner becomes "safe" not when complications never occur, but when complications are promptly recognized and managed without escalation. This includes the ability to distinguish: expected post-injection discomfort vs evolving skin ischemia, superficial thrombosis vs deep extension, and transient post-foam visual symptoms vs evolving neurologic deficit. Rare but serious events, such as stroke-like presentations after foam, have been reported, including in association with right-to-left shunts, and underscore why operators must have clear escalation pathways [17]. In this context, ultrasound guidance is not simply a convenience: it is a safety technology. As venous specialists know, complications are frequently anatomy problems and ultrasound is the tool that converts anatomy from assumption to observation. In direct-vision sclerotherapy of small superficial veins, non-target injection is still possible but typically limited in scope. A special care must be put in pre-procedure mapping of eventually present deeper refluxing veins feeding the telangiectasia. Whenever treating deeper tributaries, perforators, residual saphenous segments, or recurrent junctional neovascularization, the margin for error narrows. Ultrasound guidance allows the operator to confirm intraluminal needle placement, assess the degree of spasm, and monitor sclerosant travel in real time. The feared complications in sclerotherapy are rare but disproportionately consequential: intra-arterial injection with tissue loss, extensive skin necrosis, and thromboembolic events. Ultrasound reduces risk by providing visual confirmation of vessel identity and flow direction. It also supports a safer injection style: slow, incremental delivery with repeated checks rather than a single large

Table 7.3 Ultrasound safety checklist

Utlrasound safety checklist
1. *Before injection*
(a) Confirm target vein identity and patency (b) Identify proximity to deep veins and junctions
2. *During injection*
(a) Verify intraluminal needle position (b) Monitor sclerosant or foam propagation in real time
3. *After injection*
(a) Assess treated segment for thrombosis and flow (b) Consider early post-procedure duplex in high-risk cases and in hemodynamic overload scenarios

injection based on tactile feel. Foam introduces a distinct safety advantage: it is visible on ultrasound as echogenic material. That visibility allows a skilled operator to observe propagation toward junctions and to terminate injection before foam reaches the common femoral or popliteal vein. Routine post-procedure duplex for every patient may not be necessary in all settings, but expert practice uses selective post-procedure imaging as a safety net. High-risk scenarios include truncal ultrasound-guided foam sclerotherapy, extensive treatment volumes, prior thrombosis, thrombophilia, significant junctional proximity, and unexpectedly severe post-procedure pain/swelling. Early detection of thrombus extension or deep venous involvement changes management and can prevent escalation (Table 7.3).

3 Foam Specific Safety Considerations

Foam sclerotherapy is often described as "liquid sclerotherapy made stronger," but that analogy is incomplete. Foam is a distinct pharmacomechanical entity: a sclerosant delivered within a gas matrix. The choice of gas, the method of preparation, and foam stability alter not only efficacy but systemic exposure risk. The widespread adoption of foam has been facilitated by simple, repeatable manual methods such as the Double System Syringe or Tessari technique [18]. Simplifications on sclerotherapy "simplicity" are a mistake as it is true that, once the experience is acquired, the procedure becomes simple and immediate, but a significant training is needed before becoming able to perform a safe, appropriate, and effective sclerotherapy treatment. In fact, the vascular significance of this convenience is also its danger: foam can be generated easily, but not always consistently. Foam bubble size distribution, stability, and drainage characteristics are influenced by syringe size, number of passes, connector geometry, and the sclerosant-to-gas ratio. Reviews focusing on foam techniques emphasize variability and the need for standardization to improve both outcomes and safety [19]. In practice, the expert approach is to standardize the method: choose a consistent gas, wetness, concentration, volume, and injection timing. Foam that is injected late (after it has degraded) behaves differently: it's never about the foam characteristics inside the syringe, rather inside the vein-specific anatomical and hemodynamic environment. The gas phase is central to systemic safety. As reported in detail in previous Chaps. 4, 5 and 6, room air contains nitrogen, which is relatively insoluble and can persist longer as microbubbles. Physiological gases such as carbon dioxide (CO_2) and CO_2/O_2 mixtures dissolve more rapidly and may reduce the burden of persistent bubbles reaching the central circulation. Gas choice becomes a risk-adaptation tool. In patients with prior migraine with aura, prior transient visual symptoms, or other neurological susceptibility, the rationale for physiological gas foam is compelling, especially when treating truncal veins. Transient visual disturbances, scotoma, dizziness, and migraine-like aura are among the best-recognized systemic side effects of foam sclerotherapy. They are usually self-limited, yet their occurrence is clinically important because it signals systemic bubble passage. Reviews of sclerotherapy safety note that such temporary side effects increase with larger foam volumes [20]. Even rarer, stroke and stroke-like events have been reported after foam sclerotherapy, and although causality can be complex, these reports are the reason expert practice treats neurologic symptoms with seriousness and implements volume limits, careful monitoring, and escalation pathways [21–23]. The presence of a right-to-left shunt, particularly a patent foramen ovale, is a key theoretical risk amplifier because it permits paradoxical embolization. Expert consensus generally does not support routine screening of all patients, particularly considering it has been reported in about a quarter of the healthy population. At the same time, it brings a significantly increased risk of cerebral ischemic events (odds ratio higher than 3) [24]. Known PFO should trigger adaptations, in particular, if symptomatic: reduced foam volume, consideration of liquid or alternative modalities, physiological gas use, and longer observation. An individualized risk–benefit assessment must always be performed (Table 7.4).

An often-overlooked safety aspect deals with single-shot versus multiple-shot overdose. In practice, risk arises less from a single dramatic overdose than from cumulative dosing that creeps upward as multiple tributaries are injected. In the general sclerotherapy practice culture more stress should be dedicated to the physics characterization of the foam limits. For example, currently the European trend is to stay below 10 ml of foam per session, while in Australia dedicated papers mention even 20 ml. For the expert operator, "10 mL" is not a target but a ceiling. Many truncal treatments can be effectively performed with less, particularly when ultrasound-guided delivery is precise and when compression/positioning is optimized to maximize local sclerosant effect. Nevertheless, the indication is incomplete if it does not specify first of all the type of gases involved in the foam production. A ml of nitrogen-free foam is surely not equivalent in terms of safety to a ml of room-air foam.

Table 7.4 Foam safety practical aspects

Foam safety practical rules
1. Standardize your foam preparation technique
2. Use small aliquots rather than large boluses
3. Stop injection if foam approaches deep venous junctions
4. Prefer physiological gases in neurologically susceptible patients
5. Document total foam volume meticulously

Moreover, drug dose and foam volume are two different ceilings. Foam volume is only one axis. The other is total drug dose, which depends on sclerosant concentration and the volume of liquid sclerosant used to generate foam. In practice, safety requires the operator to think like a pharmacologist:

1. How much active drug is being delivered?
2. How much of that drug is likely to remain confined to the target segment?
3. What is the stability of the eventually used foam and the related gas solubility?
4. What is the patient's physiologic reserve and comorbidity burden?
5. How does cumulative dose change as more segments are treated?

Expert centers document sclerosant concentration, total liquid volume, total foam volume, and treated segments, not merely for audit and medicolegal reasons, but because documentation enforces cognitive discipline. If the operator must record cumulative exposure, they are more likely to notice when a session is drifting toward excessive dosing and to stage treatment across multiple visits instead. The final pillar of safety is what happens around the injection: patient positioning, real-time observation, and post-procedure behavior. These elements are sometimes treated as "aftercare," but in venous interventions they are integral to procedural risk reduction. Positioning influences venous filling, hydrostatic pressure, and foam travel. Supine positioning reduces venous pressure and typically facilitates vein spasm and collapse, which can improve local sclerosant effect and limit uncontrolled proximal migration. This is particularly relevant in truncal ultrasound-guided foam sclerotherapy, where junctional propagation is an important hazard. The expert operator often uses slight Trendelenburg positioning when appropriate to reduce proximal flow and to keep foam localized during injection, especially in large-diameter veins and in refluxing trunks. Standing injections, while sometimes used for visualization of small superficial veins, are generally undesirable when delivering foam into larger segments because hydrostatic pressure and higher flow can accelerate non-target distribution. The golden rule is to avoid sudden Valsalva that could displace the foam and stimulate inappropriate vasoconstriction in the periprocedural time. After foam sclerotherapy, most systemic symptoms, if they occur, occur early. For that reason, expert practice includes a structured observation period, commonly 15–30 min, during which visual, neurological, cardiopulmonary, and allergic symptoms are actively queried and assessed. This observation is less critical after small-volume liquid sclerotherapy, but becomes more important as foam volumes increase. This practice is consistent with the broader understanding of foam-related transient symptoms and their relationship to foam burden. Transient scotoma or migraine aura may resolve spontaneously, yet should be documented and should alter future sessions (smaller foam volume, physiological gas, altered technique). Any persistent neurological deficit, atypical headache, or cardiopulmonary symptoms warrants urgent evaluation, because although rare, serious events have been reported [25–27]. Post-procedure management is a safety strategy to reduce thrombosis, hyperpigmentation, and improve clinical outcomes. Early ambulation supports calf-pump function and reduces venous stasis. Compression can reduce inflammation and potentially improve also the aesthetic outcome [28]. Also, venous active drugs such as MPFF and Sulodexide demonstrated a potential in post-sclerotherapy pigmentation control [29, 30]. Finally, a safe sclerotherapy service is one that follows patients. Follow-up is where adverse events are detected in time, residual thrombus is managed, and recurrent reflux patterns are identified. It is also where treatment strategy is eventually refined: this is particularly true in a treatment like sclerotherapy where the skill of the healthcare professional performing the procedure must develop a synergy with the patient compliance with the following indications and with the variability of the anatomy and hemodynamics of each and every venous network. In conclusion, the safety of sclerotherapy is not the product of a single tactic but the convergence of disciplined behaviors: mapping reflux and anatomy, choosing the right tool for the right hemodynamic problem, standardizing foam preparation, respecting dose ceilings, using ultrasound not only to guide needle placement but to monitor propagation, positioning the patient to control flow, and observing patients long enough to detect early systemic symptoms. When these principles are consistently applied, sclerotherapy remains one of the most versatile and safe interventions available to vascular specialists managing chronic venous disease, and the only one that can potentially treat all the different types of veins of the lower limb. A detailed analysis of the possible complications and related management is available in Chap. 8.

4 Indications for Sclerotherapy

Unlike truncal ablation or surgery, which are largely anatomy-driven, sclerotherapy is fundamentally functional. Its indication rests not solely on vein diameter or visibility, but on whether obliteration of a given venous segment will reduce venous hypertension, improve symptoms, promote tissue healing, or enhance quality of life. When used judiciously, sclerotherapy complements other venous interventions and often represents the most efficient and least invasive means of addressing residual or complex disease patterns. At its most fundamental level, sclerotherapy is indicated whenever a superficial or perforating vein contributes to pathological venous reflux or venous hypertension and when its elimination is expected to provide clinical or quality-of-life benefit. This deceptively simple statement conceals considerable complexity, as venous disease is rarely confined to a single segment and often reflects a dynamic interaction between superficial, perforator, and deep systems.

The general indication for sclerotherapy therefore requires three conditions to be met:

1. The target vein is pathological, demonstrating reflux, abnormal dilation, or functional incompetence.
2. The vein is not essential for venous outflow, particularly in the presence of deep venous obstruction (no bypass function in deep venous obstruction).

3. The anticipated benefit outweighs procedural and cumulative risk, considering disease severity, patient comorbidity, and alternative treatments.

Sclerotherapy is particularly well suited to veins that are tortuous, multi-truncal, superficial, or recurrent, all situations in which catheter-based ablation or surgical excision may be impractical or disproportionately invasive. Its ability to be repeated, staged, and combined with other modalities makes it an essential component of comprehensive venous care rather than a competing alternative. Importantly, general indication must always be contextualized. Treating visible veins without understanding their hemodynamic role risks symptom persistence, recurrence, and unnecessary repeat exposure to sclerosants. For this reason, international guidelines emphasize that sclerotherapy should be integrated into a structured management strategy based on duplex ultrasound assessment [1]. The CEAP classification provides a standardized language for chronic venous disease and remains central to rational treatment planning. While CEAP class alone does not dictate treatment choice, it provides an essential framework for understanding disease severity, expected benefits, and therapeutic priorities [31]. At the same time, despite a partial correlation between CEAP and the Venous Clinical Severity Score was reported, it's fundamental not to consider CEAP as a severity score: even histology data confirms the lack of correlation between the same CEAP and the vein wall deterioration [32, 33]. In C0–C1 disease, indications are often dominated by aesthetic concerns, yet symptoms such as burning, itching, and localized discomfort are common and may significantly affect psychosocial well-being. In these patients, sclerotherapy is indicated for both cosmetic and venous hypertension clinical manifestations. It is important to remember how more than a quarter of telangiectasia cases actually present a deeper refluxing feeding vein. Its treatment must be addressed in order to avoid an early recurrence of the spider veins and/or, even worse, a matting phenomenon appearance (Fig. 7.1) [34].

In C2–C6 disease, varicose veins may be the primary manifestation of reflux or may represent tributaries fed by truncal incompetence and/or incompetent perforating veins and/or pelvic sources. An adequate strategy must be put in place, focusing on the suppression of the leaking points by tailored foam features (drug concentrations, wetness, gas types, volume).

In C5–C6 disease, sclerotherapy assumes an adjunctive critical role as it can target multi-truncal perforating veins feeding the same ulcer. A very useful application of sclerotherapy was demonstrated in bleeding varicosities, representing an effective and easy to perform procedure [35, 36]. A 2021 Cochrane on sclerotherapy assessed three randomized comparative trials (RCT) reporting no difference in cosmetic appearance by using different sclerosant agent concentrations. Concentration variation did not influence the rates of thromboembolic complications either. Moreover, no clear improvement in QoL was detected. Two RCTs demonstrated an improved Venous Clinical Severity Score with increasing concentrations of foam, while there was no clear difference in recurrent varicose vein rates. One RCT showed no difference in cosmetic appearance comparing foam with liquid sclerotherapy. No RCT involving liquid and foam sclerotherapy investigated thromboembolic complications, QoL, or persistence of symptoms difference. Very low-certainty evidence was determined for the six studies that showed a potential benefit of polidocanol 3% foam over liquid in reducing residual varicose veins. One study showed no clear difference in recurrent varicose vein rates when comparing sodium tetradecyl sulfate foam or liquid. No strong data demonstrated the superiority of one sclerosant over another [37]. More standardization and high-quality investigations are needed in sclerotherapy for proper comparison among the different sclerosants, in particular in their foam formulation. A detailed analysis of sclerotherapy performance in chronic venous disease is available in Chap. 9. Telangiectasias and reticular veins represent the most traditional and widely recognized indication for sclerotherapy. Despite

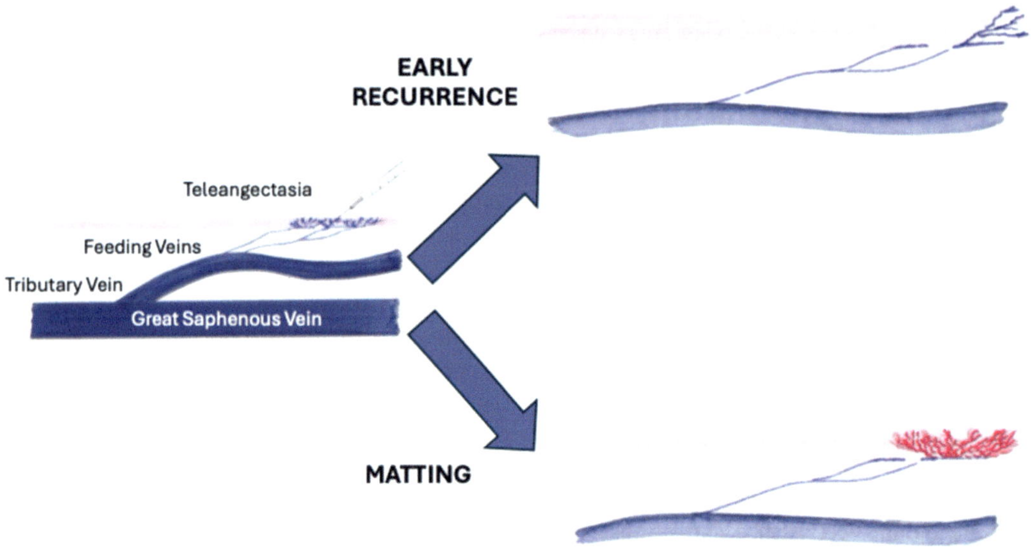

Fig. 7.1 Mistaken telangiectasia treatment without feeding vein ablation: spider veins can be fed by deeper refluxing veins that must be treated in order to avoid early recurrence and/or matting (new telangiectasia generated by the venous hypertension induced by the previous closing of spider veins that were actually draining the underlying refluxing vein). (Picture copyright: Dr. Celine Eggen, (Centrum Oosterwal, Alkmaar (NETHERLANDS)))

their classification as C1 disease, their clinical significance should not be underestimated. Patients frequently report localized pain, burning, itching, and disproportionate psychological distress related to leg appearance [38, 39]. Liquid sclerotherapy remains the treatment of choice for these small-caliber veins. Indication is typically driven by patient-reported symptoms or cosmetic concern, but expert practice recognizes that isolated treatment of telangiectasias without addressing underlying reticular or truncal reflux predisposes to recurrence and matting. For this reason, duplex ultrasound evaluation is increasingly recommended even in apparently minor disease. The V.A.L.I.D. institutional clinical governance document has recently reported the appropriateness of always performing a vascular ultrasound screening before performing even just aesthetic vein treatments, in order to detect eventually underlying refluxes [40]. It should always be remembered that even if of small caliber, telangiectasia and reticular veins are part of a wide network, corresponding to a large endothelial surface. Therefore, sclerotherapy-induced catabolites such as endothelin-1 can reach significant values, potentially leading to the related complications. The endothelin-1 induced post-sclerotherapy complication was first mentioned by Gillet et al. in a valuable publication highlighting how, also for this reason, aesthetic sclerotherapy must be performed with the same expertise and care required for large caliber veins [14]. Foam sclerotherapy has demonstrated particular utility for medium-caliber varices, but limiting it to this context would be a mistake. Indeed, strategy must always proceed with the technique: adequate sclerosant type selection and eventually staged treatments, if performed by expert professionals, can be addressed also to large vessels [41–43]. Moreover, randomized trials comparing foam sclerotherapy with surgery and endovenous ablation demonstrate comparable short-term symptom relief, with higher retreatment rates but lower procedural morbidity. Thus, the indication for sclerotherapy in varicose veins is often contextual rather than absolute, reflecting patient factors, vein anatomy, and treatment goals. Of particular notice, foam sclerotherapy demonstrated competitiveness with endovenous thermal ablation techniques in a recent meta-analysis dedicated to recurrent varicose veins treatment, with a better performance compared to varicose veins surgery [44]. Indeed, residual and recurrent varices constitute one of the strongest indications for sclerotherapy. Repeat surgery in this setting is often technically challenging and associated with higher morbidity. Moreover, in case of multi-truncal recanalization, surgery can become not feasible for a total bonification of the interested area. Sclerotherapy, particularly ultrasound-guided foam sclerotherapy, allows targeted treatment of complex recurrent multi-truncal patterns with minimal trauma. Here, the indication is driven not only by efficacy but by comparative advantage over alternative treatments. Incompetent perforator veins represent another perfect target for sclerotherapy, particularly considering their usual tortuosity and possible multi-channel nature [45]. Their treatment is indicated when reflux is hemodynamically significant and associated with skin changes, ulceration, or recurrent varices. Special care must be paid in considering not only the outward diastolic reflux, rather the net in/outward flow, so to avoid overtreatment [46]. Ultrasound-guided foam sclerotherapy has largely supplanted surgical perforator ligation in many centers due to its minimally invasive nature and repeatability. Indications are strongest in C4–C6 disease, where reducing localized venous hypertension improves tissue perfusion and healing. Endovenous thermal or glue-based techniques can represent an alternative, yet they can not easily address the multi-truncal nature of many perforating veins [47]. Perforator treatment should not be indiscriminate. Isolated perforator reflux without clinical sequelae rarely justifies intervention. Expert practice emphasizes selective treatment based on clinical relevance, not ultrasound findings alone. Ultrasound-guided procedures are to be preferred in order to guarantee adequate procedural performance and post-procedural monitoring [48]. Pelvic sources of lower limb venous reflux can be considered as a special form of perforating veins: the main origin can be from the round ligament vein, the clitoris vein, the Alcock canal vein, the superior and inferior gluteal veins [49, 50]. Sclerotherapy represent an excellent chance of treatment in light of these veins' tortuosity and multi-channel nature. Chapter 13 is entirely dedicated to the topic [51]. Another area of valuable application of sclerotherapy is low-flow venous malformations. In these congenital lesions, chemical ablation induces fibrosis and volume reduction, often providing durable symptom control. Indications include pain, swelling, functional impairment, and cosmetic deformity. Treatment is typically staged, guided by imaging, and performed in specialized centers due to the risks associated with large-volume sclerosant use and proximity to critical structures. In experienced hands, sclerotherapy is considered first-line therapy for most low-flow venous malformations, with surgery reserved for selected cases [52]. Chapter 14 is entirely dedicated to the topic. Modern venous care increasingly prioritizes patient-reported outcome measures (PROMs). Studies consistently demonstrate that sclerotherapy improves disease-specific quality-of-life scores across CEAP classes, including early-stage disease [53]. A 2018 publication by Toniolo J et al. highlighted a cut-off of 6 mm diameter for risk of recanalization after sclerotherapy [54]. Yet, the comparison with the other available techniques showcased a competitiveness of foam sclerotherapy in terms of patient-reported outcomes and potentially also of cost control [55]. Modern technical evolution is aiming at maximizing the performance of foam sclerotherapy also in large vessels to be treated in one single shot. Until the refinement of this research lines, the practitioner should follow adequate ultrasound follow-up and eventually multi-staged sclerotherapy strategic planning in order to cover all the refluxing venous segments possible scenarios. In conclusion, indication to sclerotherapy should therefore integrate symptom severity, functional limitation, psychosocial impact, patient values, and expectations. Shared decision-making aligns treatment with patient goals and improves satisfaction, adherence, and perceived success. Sclerotherapy is indicated across the full continuum of chronic venous disease when applied within a hemodynamically informed, patient-centered framework. Its versatility, from cosmetic treatment to ulcer adjunct therapy, makes it indispensable in modern venous practice. When indications are clearly defined and integrated into comprehensive care, sclerotherapy delivers durable benefit with minimal invasiveness.

Sclerotherapy concentration and volume indications cannot be summed up in a simple table based only on the vein caliber. Indeed, as previously described, many are the variables that can influence the final most appropriate administration. For example, a drier foam will last longer, maximizing its effect. In a similar way a less polydisperse foam will be more powerful and safer. Microfoam increases the contact surface, once again magnifying the sclerotherapy action. Other factors can influence the stability, such as temperature, altitude, syringe geometry, injection speed [56]. In 2014, a consensus recommended specific concentrations, both in liquid and foam formulation [4]. While useful for a general overview, this paper's indications can become too simplistic as several factors can and must influence the final appropriate decision of the expert to increase or lower the drug concentration. Table 7.5 reports this chapter's authors' perspective on the suggested concentrations, together with factors to be taken into account to eventually increase or decrease the related values.

It must be highlighted how the table is generated by years of practical experience of the authors who were not able to identify solid scientific literature comparing the outcomes obtained with the different concentrations in the different formulation possibilities. More comparative studies, both in the lab and in vivo, should be performed to provide a properly standardized indication. It must be noted how the different clinical governances of the different nations can authorize and regulate the drugs in different formulations and concentrations; therefore, the final confirmation is to be aware of own country's authorizations.

Table 7.5 Empirical suggestions on concentration selection based on the author's experience

Vein type	Liquid pol	Liquid sts	Foam pol	Foam sts
Teleangectasia	0.25–0.5	0.2	Up to 0.5	Up to 0.2
Reticular vein	0.5–1	0.5	Up to 0.5	Up to 0.2
Varicose veins	1–3	1–3	Up to 2	Up to 1
Saphenous trunks	3	3	1–3	1–3
Perforating veins	×	×	1–3	1–3
Pelvic varicosities	×	×	1–3	1–3
Factors suggesting to eventually increase the chosen concentration				
Wetness High polidispersity Large size bubbles Manual production method No sylicone free syringes use. Increased temperature High junctional flow Large reflux volume		(Continued)		
Factors suggesting to eventually decrease the chosen concentration				
The opposite of the above Increased altitude Thin subcutaneous thickness above the targeted vein Dark skin phenotype				

It must be noted how the different clinical governances of the different nations can authorize and regulate the drugs in different formulations and concentrations; therefore, the final confirmation is to be aware of own country's authorizations. *Pol* polidocanol, *Sts* sodium tetradecyl sulfate

More recent documents from both USA and Europe, looking for consensus on sclerosant drugs concentrations, did not report specific indications on concentrations and vein types [57, 58]. A recent international clinical governance document highlighted the competitiveness of polidocanol endovenous microfoam with endovenous thermal ablation techniques, yet stressing the importance of considering the national indications of the different regulatory agencies [40]. In conclusion, the indication to sclerotherapy must follow a holistic approach to patient and related venous network features, starting from general standardization principles to be customized on the specific case features. Only in this way sclerotherapy can be assessed at its best and linked to the best outcomes [59].

5 Contraindications

Contraindications to sclerotherapy are often presented as static lists, yet in practice they are anything but static. They are dynamic expressions of patient vulnerability, vascular reserve, and the limits of controlled endothelial injury. Sclerotherapy is fundamentally a paradoxical therapy: it treats venous disease by deliberately inducing thrombosis and inflammation, processes that vascular medicine otherwise seeks to prevent. Contraindications therefore arise when the clinician can no longer reliably confine these processes to their intended anatomical and physiological boundaries. For the expert vascular reader, understanding contraindications requires abandoning a binary mindset. Instead, contraindications should be interpreted as warning signals—markers of reduced tolerance for endothelial injury, impaired capacity to manage thrombosis, or increased susceptibility to embolic or ischemic consequences. All sclerosants act by damaging the venous endothelium. This damage initiates a cascade involving platelet activation, coagulation cascade engagement, leukocyte recruitment, and fibroblast-driven remodeling. In ideal circumstances, this cascade remains localized, self-limited, and therapeutically productive. Contraindications exist when any component of this cascade becomes excessive, uncontrolled, or systemically hazardous. From this perspective, contraindications fall into several mechanistic domains:

- Prothrombotic vulnerability
- Ischemic susceptibility
- Risk of unintended sclerosant migration
- Impaired compensatory physiology
- Inability to adhere to post-procedural requirements

Understanding which domain is dominant in a given patient allows for nuanced, individualized decision-making [60]. Table 7.6 sums up major and minor complications, also including conditions requiring precautions.

Anaphylaxis is among the most feared possible complications of sclerotherapy for which all the practitioners must be trained in the related management. It is an acute, potentially fatal systemic reaction caused by an immunoglobulin E-mediated type I hypersensitivity response that occurs after re-exposure to a specific antigen in a previously sensitized individual. It is typically independent of the dose, and it develops rapidly.

Table 7.6 Sclerotherapy contraindications

Sclerotherapy contraindications	
Absolute	1. Allergy to sclerosing agents 2. Acute venous thrombosis/embolism 3. Severe neurological or cardiological conditions 4. Acute systemic illness 5. Acute infection
Relative	1. Peripheral arterial disease 2. Pregnancy, post-partum, breast feeding 3. Thrombotic risk 4. Neurological risk 5. Patent foramen ovale 6. Cardiac risk
Precautions	1. Skin necrosis 2. Matting 3. Pigmentation 4. Medications (disulfiram, minocycline, tamoxifen and aromatase inhibitors, exogenous estrogen) 5. Psychosocial factors (anxiety, obsessive disorders, unrealistic expectations)

To the contrary, an anaphylactoid reaction is not mediated by IgE, does not require prior sensitization, and demonstrates a dose–response relationship. Both reactions arise from prompt mast cell activation, leading to the release of vasoactive substances such as histamine, along with other mediators including heparin and tryptase, followed by secondary recruitment of inflammatory cells. Clinically, both conditions' manifestations range from generalized urticaria to profound hypotension and cardiovascular collapse. While it is mandatory to be ready to manage the emergency, the literature and clinical practice demonstrate the event is rare (around 0.01%–0.1%), with reports also of extreme rarity, as in Thibault et al.'s paper mentioning only 4 cases out of 2686 treated patients [61, 62]. Yet, deaths attributable to anaphylaxis or anaphylactoid reactions following exposure to detergent sclerosants have been reported [63].

It should be noted that the total number of procedures performed and patients treated during this interval is unknown; consequently, the true incidence of severe adverse reactions cannot be reliably determined. A Cochrane review highlighted no significant differences in the anaphylactic risk associated with polidocanol and sodium tetradecyl sulfate [64]. Hypersensitivity can manifest itself in a lighter way by the occurrence of urticaria and other nonspecific cutaneous reactions following exposure to sclerosants. Also, this happening is rare (about 0.3% in the literature) [65]. All the sclerotherapists with large experience have noticed local skin reactions in the injection site in the form of erythema, urticaria, and pruritus: this should not be considered immediately as an allergic reaction as it could be linked to the simple release of histamine triggered by the injection, independently of the sclerosing agent. Yet, a full evaluation of the patient-specific risk for allergies must be the starting point of every eventual sclerotherapy procedure. It should also be noted that the allergy to either polidocanol or sodium tetradecyl sulfate is not a direct contraindication to use the other detergent as they are not cross-linked. Special attention is required in the assessment of candidates for sclerotherapy in case of asthma, urticaria, and mast cell activation disorders as they are more prone to develop anaphylaxis. Patients at high risk of anaphylaxis should be treated only if strictly necessary and always after a careful expert evaluation, in a context ready to take emergency action if needed. Prophylactic systemic corticosteroids can be taken into consideration. A recent thromboembolic event activates all the venous system, making sclerotherapy a potential trigger of deep venous thrombosis/embolism extension. Up to the knowledge of the authors there is no publication providing evidence on the best timing for sclerotherapy after a venous thromboembolism episode. There is international consensus to wait for at least 3 months after a provoked deep thrombosis, independently of the interested limb [60]. Superficial venous thrombosis represents a questionable scenario as on one side it surely increases the risk of deep venous thrombosis [66], yet, if more distant than 3 cm from the deep venous system and shorter than 5 cm, it can be managed by anti-inflammatories and their eventual sclerotherapy could actually eliminate a further thrombogenic source. For these reasons, superficial venous thrombosis can be considered as a relative contraindication, leaving to the expert physician the assessment of the patient and procedural thrombotic risk, together with the balance between risks and benefits [67]. No strong data show a possible impact of anticoagulation on sclerotherapy performance, for which it is not considered a contraindication and it can actually help managing high-risk patients. While extremely mini-invasive, sclerotherapy represents a significant inflammatory trigger for the whole venous circulation. Therefore, patients already engaged in neurological, cardiac, or general illness should not be treated: a deterioration in their already fragile condition could happen. Obviously, patients who experienced previous transient ischemic attacks or stroke associated with a patent foramen ovale should not undergo sclerotherapy. A history of visual, sensory, and speech disturbances and migraine with or without aurora represents a relative contraindication to be carefully assessed by the physician. If a severe infection is present, a risk of spreading could be developed by the sclerosing injection.

Immunosuppression and frailty require a risk/benefit assessment, representing a relative rather than absolute contraindication. A special assessment is required in indication to sclerotherapy for moderate to severe peripheral arterial disease. On one side there is the concern that post-sclerotherapy compression could hamper the already fragile arterial flow. On the other, data show how appropriate compression can actually be beneficial on the arterial flow, thanks to the venous afterload reduction [68]. While animal data suggest a possible adverse effect on the fetus of both polidocanol and sodium tetradecyl sulfate, no solid publications on human have been found by the authors of this chapter. Both drugs appear in case reports regarding humans treated for conditions different from lower limb chronic venous disease, such as esophageal bleeding and lung development anomalies: no adverse events were reported [69, 70]. During and after pregnancy also the mother is at risk. First of all, the coagulation balance becomes prothrombotic in the last trimester of pregnancy and for the following 3 months, therefore suggesting caution in the eventual decision to practice sclerotherapy during this time [71]. In the absence of clear literature on the topic, the general good practice is to avoid sclerotherapy during pregnancy, unless the risk/benefit assessment suggests otherwise. It's mandatory to always ask the premenopausal patients about possible ongoing pregnancies before proceeding with a sclerotherapy act. Possible scenarios demanding sclerotherapy during pregnancy include highly symptomatic and/or bleeding varices, in particular from the vulvar and anal region. It is appropriate to limit the treatment to the last trimester in order to minimize the risk for the fetus. As mentioned above, this is the time at highest thrombotic risk for the mother, for which proper anticoagulation must be considered. While direct oral anticoagulants cross the placenta, low molecular weight heparin does not and it is to be then preferred [72]. Polidocanol was found in the milk of lactating rats, yet no impact on offspring development was noticed. Moreover, it should also be considered that detergents are rapidly inactivated by the mother's blood plasma proteins [73, 74]. Considering the lack of evidence, it is suggested to avoid breastfeeding for at least 2 days after the administration of detergent sclerosing agents.

6 Venous Thromboembolism Risk

A false myth about sclerotherapy reports that its being more thrombogenic than the other venous procedures, while evidence shows the opposite [75]. Even more, a distinction must be made between real deep venous thrombosis versus parietal sclerosis that represents no particular harm [76]. The incidence of real symptomatic deep venous thrombosis is in between 0.02 and 1.3% according to the literature [77]. From a basic science standpoint, high concentrations of sodium tetradecyl sulfate show anticoagulant properties, while at low concentrations, like polidocanol, demonstrate pro-coagulant features, yet foam sclerosants do not alter clotting times. D-dimer is elevated for up to a week after sclerotherapy, even without thrombotic events [78, 79]. The risk of a real deep venous thrombosis is increased by threefold for larger than 5 mm veins and for more than 10 ml foam injection, therefore proper considerations should be done in terms of thromboprophylaxis and sclerotherapy amount [76]. Special care must be used also in patients who already experienced deep venous thrombosis and/or pulmonary embolism as the risk of recurrence is significant. In this case, thromboprophylaxis should always be taken into detailed consideration. Also, first-degree relatives experiencing unprovoked thrombosis should be reported, particularly if the episode occurred at an early age: this data could suggest hematologic tests for coagulation disorders. Genetic alterations of coagulation can be found in up to 15% of the population [80]. Heterozygous mutations in Factor V Leiden and prothrombin-G20210A are among the most common mutations and they are considered mild. To the contrary, antiphospholipid syndrome is the most common acquired thrombophilia and it represents a high risk for venous thrombosis [81]. Literature shows the feasibility of sclerotherapy in properly anticoagulated subjects affected by genetic coagulation disorders. Certainly, every single case's risk/benefit must be assessed with extreme care [80]. A specific category of patients at risk of venous thromboembolism is the neoplastic one, both for the disease itself and for the eventual therapy related to it [82]. A specific-related drug that could increase post-sclerotherapy thrombosis risk is tamoxifen. Considering the lack of related literature, it's suggested to avoid sclerotherapy during this drug use [83]. Alternative treatments not associated with an increased thrombotic risk are the third-generation aromatase inhibitors, anastrozole, exemestane, and letrozole [84]. Assessing the risk/benefit ratio for sclerotherapy in this kind of patients is of paramount importance and it should always be accompanied by an oncologist/hematologist consultation.

7 Patient Characteristics Leading to Possible Contraindication

Lifestyle and patient characteristics can require special attention in the indication for sclerotherapy.

Immobility is one of the most commonly mentioned in sclerotherapy practice as it is considered dangerous for the possible thrombotic risk associated to it [1]. Yet, an appropriately performed sclerotherapy can sometimes represent the only available option for these fragile patients and, after careful evaluation of the case, it should be considered. This is particularly true considering the possibility of related thromboprophylaxis, eventually also by means of intermittent pneumatic compression. Another form of immobility is the one of the long-haul travels. Trips above 6 and 12 h have demonstrated to increase the venous thromboembolism risk by up to two and fivefold, respectively [85]. In the risk/benefit assessment for a sclerotherapy indication it must be remembered that the risk remains higher up to 4 weeks after the travel [86]. It should also be remembered that it's not an issue related only to economy-class as different factors are involved, including the possible dehydration occurring in the pressurized plane cabin. Up to our knowledge, currently there is no literature dedicated to the investigation of sclerotherapy right before long-haul flights. As general suggestion, if the physician considers appropriate to perform sclerotherapy in the context of a nearby long-haul flight, all the thromboprophylaxis measures should be taken in strong consideration: thrombotic risk assessment, graduated compression, eventual anticoagulant, appropriate hydration, and sedentarism prevention during the travel. Another prothrombotic factor that could be associated to patient habits is to be identified in hormonal therapy and in particular in exogenous estrogen intake. Oral contraceptive pill has been associated to a possible thrombotic risk increase up to 3.5-fold [87]. Other forms of contraception such as the vaginal ring or cutaneous patches still increase the thrombotic risk [88]. Also, hormonal therapy for menopausal syndrome represents a risk factor for thrombosis [89]. This data must be taken into consideration whenever assessing the risk/benefit ratio in sclerotherapy indication. Obesity is another aspect to consider as a thrombotic risk factor in the patient evaluation for possible sclerotherapy. Therefore, adequate thromboprophylaxis must be considered even for mini-invasive sclerotherapy procedures [90].

8 Precautions

Several conditions can represent apparently minor aspects, yet potentially leading to major sclerotherapy complications, therefore requiring caution.

Sclerotherapy can inflame the skin; therefore, a dermatologic evaluation, even if not specialistic, must be performed before performing the sclerosing injection that could worsen already present conditions.

This is the case, for example, of skin necrosis, livedo reticularis, and dermatological conditions leading to subcutaneous sclerosis and fibrosis in general.

Another patient-related aspect to consider for limiting the post-sclerotherapy pigmentation risk is iron metabolism. Data show a possible risk factor in iron deposition conditions such as hemochromatosis. Collecting this information during the history taking is surely valuable [91]. Iron deposition can be involved also after sclerotherapy in patients who are taking the antibiotic minocycline. In the absence of clear literature on the topic, it is suggested to avoid sclerotherapy for at least 4 weeks after the drug intake and to consider doxycycline as an alternative. Pigmentation related to sun-exposure is lacking significant evidence despite being reported in some guidelines [4]. Avoiding excessive exposure, in particular for the darker skin phenotypes is suggested. Among the patients' characteristics, also the use of disulfiram should be reported. It is a drug used to promote abstinence from alcohol. As polidocanol includes an ethanol group, it should not be used in patients using disulfiram. Last but not least, sclerotherapy includes the word "therapy" in itself: an easy way to remember the psychological component of the sclerotherapy office work. Patients with psychosocial and psychiatric comorbidities should be carefully evaluated and eventually not treated in case proper bidirectional trust can be developed between the physician and the same patient. Indeed, sclerotherapy success is to be found in the expertise of the healthcare professional as well as in the adequate compliance of the patient regarding the appropriate measures to be taken in between treatment sessions. Once all the above-mentioned aspects are followed, sclerotherapy can confirm its significant safety and efficacy, potentially in all the chronic venous disease spectrum.

References

1. Gianesini S, Obi A, Onida S, et al. Global guidelines trends and controversies in lower limb venous and lymphatic disease: narrative literature revision and experts' opinions following the vWINter international meeting in Phlebology, Lymphology & Aesthetics, 23-25 January 2019. Phlebology. 2019;34(1 Suppl):4–66.
2. Kanber EM. Comparison of foam and liquid sclerotherapy for the treatment of lower extremity varicose veins and telangiectasia in obese patients. Cureus. 2023;15(7):e42571.
3. Hamel-Desnos C, Allaert FA. Liquid versus foam sclerotherapy. Phlebology. 2009;24(6):240–6.
4. Rabe E, Breu FX, Cavezzi A, et al. European guidelines for sclerotherapy in chronic venous disorders. Phlebology. 2014;29(6):338–54.
5. Green D. Mechanism of action of sclerotherapy. Semin Dermatol. 1993;12(2):88–97.
6. Gianesini S, Occhionorelli S, Menegatti E, et al. CHIVA strategy in chronic venous disease treatment: instructions for users. Phlebology. 2015;30(3):157–71.
7. Goodman EA, Alexander JT, Babrowski TA. Care of patients with chronic venous disease of the legs. jama. 2025;333(19):1722–3.
8. Ng IK. Informed consent in clinical practice: old problems, new challenges. J R Coll Physicians Edinb. 2024;54(2):153–8.
9. Natali J, Farman T. Implications médico-légales au cours du treatment sclérosant des varices [Forensic medical implications in the course of sclerotherapy of varicose veins]. J Mal Vasc. 1996;21(4):227–32.
10. Stricker BH, van Oijen JA, Kroon C, Ovink AH. Anafylaxie na gebruik van polidocanol [Anaphylaxis following use of polidocanol]. Ned Tijdschr Geneeskd. 1990;134(5):240–2.
11. Marrocco-Trischitta MM, Guerrini P, Abeni D, Stillo F. Reversible cardiac arrest after polidocanol sclerotherapy of peripheral venous malformation. Dermatologic Surg. 2002;28(2):153–5.
12. Engelberger RP, Ney B, Clair M, et al. Myocardial infarction after ultrasoundguided foam sclerotherapy for varicose veins: a case report and review of the literature of a rare but serious adverse event. Vasa. 2016;45(3):255–8.
13. Timothy AC, Snow JP, McEntee SC, et al. Myocardial infarction following sclerotherapy in a patient with a patent foramen ovale. N Z Med J. 2012;125:64–7.
14. Gillet JL, Donnet A, Lausecker M, et al. Pathophysiology of visual disturbances occurring after foam sclerotherapy. Phlebology. 2010;25(5):261–6.
15. Stephens R, Dunn S. Non-ST-elevation myocardial infarction following foam ultrasound-guided sclerotherapy. Phlebology. 2014;29(7):488–90.
16. Gianesini S, Chi YW, Agüero C, et al. Fake-news-free evidence-based communication for proper vein-lymphatic disease management. Int Angiol. 2023;42(2):89–189.
17. Rabe E, Breu FX, Flessenkämper I, et al. Sclerotherapy in the treatment of varicose veins: S2k guideline of the Deutsche Gesellschaft für Phlebologie (DGP) in cooperation with the following societies: DDG, DGA, DGG, BVP. Hautarzt. 2021;72(Suppl 2):23–36.
18. Krnić A. Ultrasound guided foam sclerotherapy: the simplest, least invasive and cheapest method for varicose vein treatment. Acta Clin Croat. 2015;54(2):136–42.
19. Cavezzi A, Tessari L. Foam sclerotherapy techniques: different gases and methods of preparation, catheter versus direct injection. Phlebology. 2009;24(6):247–51.

20. Thomasset SC, Butt Z, Liptrot S, Fairbrother BJ, et al. Ultrasound guided foam sclerotherapy: factors associated with outcomes and complications. Eur J Vasc Endovasc Surg. 2010;40(3):389–92.
21. Forlee MV, Grouden M, Moore DJ, et al. Stroke after varicose vein foam injection sclerotherapy. J Vasc Surg. 2006;43(1):162–4.
22. Hanisch F, Müller T, Krivokuca M, Winterholler M. Stroke following variceal sclerotherapy. Eur J Med Res. 2004;9(5):282–4.
23. Picard C, Deltombe B, Duru C, et al. Foam sclerotherapy: a possible cause of ischaemic stroke? J Neurol Neurosurg Psychiatry. 2010;81(5):582–3.
24. Koutroulou I, Tsivgoulis G, Tsalikakis D, et al. Epidemiology of patent foramen ovale in general population and in stroke patients: a narrative review. Front Neurol. 2020;11:281.
25. Bush RG, Derrick M, Manjoney D. Major neurological events following foam sclerotherapy. Phlebology. 2008;23(4):189–92.
26. Hill DA. Neurological and chest symptoms following sclerotherapy: a single centre experience. Phlebology. 2014;29(9):619–27.
27. Sarvananthan T, Shepherd AC, Willenberg T, Davies AH. Neurological complications of sclerotherapy for varicose veins. J Vasc Surg. 2012;55(1):243–51.
28. Nootheti PK, Cadag KM, Magpantay A, et al. Efficacy of graduated compression stockings for an additional 3 weeks after sclerotherapy treatment of reticular and telangiectatic leg veins. Dermatologic Surg. 2009;35(1):53–7. discussion 57–8.
29. Gonzalez Ochoa AJ, Carrillo J, Manríquez D, et al. Reducing hyperpigmentation after sclerotherapy: a randomized clinical trial. J Vasc Surg Venous Lymphat Disord. 2021;9(1):154–62.
30. Bogachev VY, Boldin BV, Turkin PY. Administration of micronized purified flavonoid fraction during sclerotherapy of reticular veins and telangiectasias: results of the national, multicenter, observational program VEIN ACT PROLONGED-C1. Adv Ther. 2018;35(7):1001–8.
31. Lurie F, Passman M, Meisner M, et al. The 2020 update of the CEAP classification system and reporting standards. J Vasc Surg Venous Lymphat Disord. 2020;8(3):342–52. https://doi.org/10.1016/j.jvsv.2019.12.075. Epub 2020 Feb 27. Erratum in: J Vasc Surg Venous Lymphat Disord. 2021;9(1):288.
32. Passman MA, McLafferty RB, Lentz MF, et al. Validation of venous clinical severity score (VCSS) with other venous severity assessment tools from the American Venous Forum, National Venous Screening Program. J Vasc Surg. 2011;54(6 Suppl):2S–9S.
33. Mironiuc A, Palcău L, Rogojan L, et al. Is there a correlation between the CEAP score and the histopathological findings in varicose disease? Romanian J Morphol Embryol. 2011;52(1):117–21.
34. Ruckley CV, Evans CJ, Allan PL, et al. Telangiectasia in the Edinburgh Vein Study: epidemiology and association with trunk varices and symptoms. Eur J Vasc Endovasc Surg. 2008;36:719–24.
35. Tretbar LL. Treatment of small bleeding varicose veins with injection sclerotherapy. Bleeding blue blebs. Dermatol Surg. 1996;22(1):78–80.
36. Bock R, Fontenot D, Bock S, et al. Protocol-based treatment of spontaneous hemorrhage from varicose veins prevents recurrence of bleeding. J Vasc Surg Venous Lymphat Disord. 2025;13(1):101988.
37. de Ávila Oliveira R, Riera R, Vasconcelos V, et al. Injection sclerotherapy for varicose veins. Cochrane Database Syst Rev. 2021;12(12):CD001732.
38. Benigni JP, Bihari I, Rabe E, et al. Venous symptoms in C0 and C1 patients: UIP consensus document. Int Angiol. 2013;32(3):261–5.
39. Nakano LC, Cacione DG, Baptista-Silva JC, et al. Treatment for telangiectasias and reticular veins. Cochrane Database Syst Rev. 2021;10(10):CD012723.
40. https://www.iss.it/it/web/guest/-/gestione-patologia-venosa-e-linfatica.
41. de Groot WP. Practical phlebology. Sclerotherapy of large veins. J Dermatol Surg Oncol. 1991;17(7):589–95.
42. Kanter A, Thibault P. Saphenofemoral incompetence treated by ultrasound-guided sclerotherapy. Dermatologic Surg. 1996;22(7):648–52.
43. Sladen JG, Reid JDS. Compression sclerotherapy for large veins and perforators. In: Ballard JL, Bergan JJ, editors. Chronic venous insufficiency. London: Springer; 2000.
44. Bontinis A, Bontinis V, Koudounas G, et al. Interventions for the treatment of recurrent varicose vein disease arising from the saphenofemoral junction or the great saphenous vein: a systematic review and meta-analysis. Int Angiol. 2024;43(5):485–96.
45. Rinieri J. Perforantes veineuses multi-tronculaires [Multi-vessel venous perforating varices]. Phlebologie. 1991;44(2):281–5. discussion 286–90.
46. Gianesini S, Menegatti E, Sisini F, et al. Comparison between duplex ultrasound and multigate quality Doppler profile software in the assessment of lower limb perforating vein direction. Eur J Vasc Endovasc Surg. 2018;55(5):688–93.
47. Kuyumcu G, Salazar GM, Prabhakar AM, et al. Minimally invasive treatments for perforator vein insufficiency. Cardiovasc Diagn Ther. 2016;6(6):593–8.
48. Masuda EM, Kessler DM, Lurie F, et al. The effect of ultrasound-guided sclerotherapy of incompetent perforator veins on venous clinical severity and disability scores. J Vasc Surg. 2006;43(3):551–6.
49. Barros FS, Storino J, Cardoso da Silva NA, et al. A comprehensive ultrasound approach to lower limb varicose veins and abdominal-pelvic connections. J Vasc Surg Venous Lymphat Disord. 2024;12(3):101851.
50. Ford RW, Winokur RS. Pelvic venous disorders (PeVD). Semin Intervent Radiol. 2022;39(5):483–9.
51. Marcelin C, Le Bras Y, Molina Andreo I, et al. Diagnosis and management of pelvic venous disorders in females. Diagnostics (Basel). 2022; 12(10):2337.

52. Kim KR. Percutaneous sclerotherapy of venous malformations. Tech Vasc Interv Radiol. 2024;27(2):100960.
53. Darvall KA, Bate GR, Bradbury AW. Patient-reported outcomes 5-8 years after ultrasound-guided foam sclerotherapy for varicose veins. Br J Surg. 2014;101(9):1098–104.
54. Toniolo J, Chiang N, Munteanu D, et al. Vein diameter is a predictive factor for recanalization in treatment with ultrasound-guided foam sclerotherapy. J Vasc Surg Venous Lymphat Disord. 2018;6(6):707–16.
55. Davies HO, Popplewell M, Darvall K, et al. A review of randomised controlled trials comparing ultrasound-guided foam sclerotherapy with endothermal ablation for the treatment of great saphenous varicose veins. Phlebology. 2016;31(4):234–40.
56. Bai T, Jiang W, Chen Y, et al. Effect of multiple factors on foam stability in foam sclerotherapy. Sci Rep. 2018;8(1):15683.
57. Gloviczki P, Lawrence PF, Wasan SM, et al. The 2022 Society for Vascular Surgery, American Venous Forum, and American Vein and Lymphatic Society clinical practice guidelines for the management of varicose veins of the lower extremities. Part I. Duplex Scanning and Treatment of Superficial Truncal Reflux: Endorsed by the Society for Vascular Medicine and the International Union of Phlebology. J Vasc Surg Venous Lymphat Disord. 2023;11(2):231.e6–61.e6. https://doi.org/10.1016/j.jvsv.2022.09.004. Epub 2022 Oct 12. Erratum in: J Vasc Surg Venous Lymphat Disord. 2024;12(2):101719.
58. De Maeseneer MG, Kakkos SK, Aherne T, et al. 2022 clinical practice guidelines on the management of chronic venous disease of the lower limbs. Eur J Vasc Endovasc Surg. 2022;63(2):184–267.
59. Liu A, Boen M, Fabi S, et al. Sclerotherapy in aesthetic medicine: myths and realities. Dermatologic Surg. 2022;48(9):972–7.
60. Wong M, Parsi K, Myers K, et al. Sclerotherapy of lower limb veins: indications, contraindications and treatment strategies to prevent complications–a consensus document of the International Union of Phlebology-2023. Phlebology. 2023;38(4):205–58.
61. Goldman MP, Bennett RG. Treatment of telangiectasia: a review. J Am Acad Dermatol. 1987;17:167–82. Research Support, Non-U.S. Gov't Review.
62. Thibault PK. Sclerotherapy of varicose veins and telangiectasias: a 2-year experience with sodium tetradecyl sulphate. ANZ J Phleb. 1999;3:25–30.
63. Nguyen CN, Nguyen Q-BD, Silapunt S. Analysis of adverse events with sclerosants reported to the United States food and drug administration. Phlebology. 2022;37:452–9.
64. Tisi PV, Beverley C, Rees A. Injection sclerotherapy for varicose veins. Cochrane Database Syst Rev. 2006;(4):CD001732. https://doi.org/10.1002/14651858.CD001732.pub2.
65. Goldman MP, Guex JJ, Weiss RA. Sclerotherapy: treatment of varicose and telangiectatic leg veins. 5th ed. Philadelphia: Saunders Elsevier; 2011.
66. Piazza G, Krishnathasan D, Hamade N, et al. Superficial vein thrombosis: a review. JAMA. 2025;334(22):2020–30.
67. Lee JT, Kalani MA. Treating superficial venous thrombophlebitis. J Natl Compr Cancer Netw. 2008;6(8):760–5.
68. Rother U, Grussler A, Griesbach C, et al. Safety of medical compression stockings in patients with diabetes mellitus or peripheral arterial disease. BMJ Open Diabetes Res Care. 2020;8(1):e001316.
69. Aggarwal N, Sawhney H, Vasishta K, et al. Non-cirrhotic portal hypertension in pregnancy. Int J Gynaecol Obstet. 2001;72:1–7. Comparative Study.
70. Bermudez C, Perez-Wulff J, Bufalino G, et al. Percutaneous ultrasound-guided sclerotherapy for complicated fetal intralobar bronchopulmonary sequestration. Ultrasound Obstet Gynecol. 2007;29:586–9. Case Reports.
71. Pomp E, Lenselink A, Rosendaal F, et al. Pregnancy, the postpartum period and prothrombotic defects: risk of venous thrombosis in the MEGA study. J Thromb Haemost. 2008;6:632–7.
72. Cohen H, Arachchillage D, Middeldorp S, et al. Management of direct oral anticoagulants in women of childbearing potential: guidance from the SSC of the ISTH. J Thromb Haemost. 2016;14:1673–6.
73. Watkins MR. Deactivation of sodium tetradecyl sulphate injection by blood proteins. Eur J Vasc Endovasc Surg. 2011;41:521–5.
74. Connor DE, Cooley-Andrade O, Goh WX, et al. Detergent sclerosants are deactivated and consumed by circulating blood cells. Eur J Vasc Endovasc Surg. 2015;49:426–31.
75. O'Donnell TF, Eaddy M, Raju A, et al. Assessment of thrombotic adverse events and treatment patterns associated with varicose vein treatment. J Vasc Surg Venous Lymphat Disord. 2015;3(1):27–34.
76. Parsi K, Panozzo B, Bull A, et al. Deep vein sclerosis following sclerotherapy: ultrasonic and d-dimer criteria. Phlebology. 2020;35(5):325–36.
77. Myers KA, Jolley D. Factors affecting the risk of deep venous occlusion after ultrasound-guided sclerotherapy for varicose veins. Eur J Vasc Endovasc Surg. 2008;36:602–5.
78. Connor D, Joseph J, Exner T, et al. Infusion of foam sclerosants results in a distance-dependent procoagulant activity, haemoconcentration and elevation of D-dimerlevels. Phlebology. 2014;29:677–87.
79. Parsi K, Connor DE, Pilotelle A, et al. Low concentration detergent sclerosants induce platelet activation but inhibit aggregation due to suppression of GPIIb/IIIa activation in vitro. Thromb Res. 2012;130:472–8.
80. Hamel-Desnos CM, Gillet JL, Desnos PR, et al. Sclerotherapy of varicose veins in patients with documented thrombophilia: a prospective controlled randomized study of 105 cases. Phlebology. 2009;24:176–82.
81. Makris M. Thrombophilia: grading the risk. Blood. 2009;113:5038–9.

82. Khorana AA, Francis CW, Culakova E, et al. Thromboembolism is a leading cause of death in cancer patients receiving outpatient chemotherapy. J Thromb Haemost. 2007;5:632–4.
83. Hussain T, Kneeshaw PJ. Stopping tamoxifen perioperatively for VTE risk reduction: a proposed management algorithm. Int J Surg. 2012;10:313–6.
84. Fabian CJ. The what, why and how of aromatase inhibitors: hormonal agents for treatment and prevention of breast cancer. Int J Clin Pract. 2007;61:2051–63.
85. Streiff MB, Agnelli G, Connors JM, et al. Guidance for the treatment of deep vein thrombosis and pulmonary embolism. J Thromb Thrombol. 2016;41:32–67.
86. Philbrick JT, Shumate R, Siadaty MS, et al. Air travel and venous thromboembolism: a systematic review. J Gen Intern Med. 2007;22:107–14.
87. Stegeman BH, de Bastos M, Rosendaal FR, et al. Different combined oral contraceptives and the risk of venous thrombosis: systematic review and network meta analysis. BMJ. 2013;347:f5298.
88. Lidegaard O, Nielsen LH, Skovlund CW, et al. Venous thrombosis in users of non-oral hormonal contraception: follow-up study, Denmark 2001–10. BMJ. 2012;344:e2990.
89. Gomes MP a DSR. Risk of venous thromboembolic disease associated with hormonal contraceptives and hormone replacement therapy: a clinical review. Arch Intern Med. 2004;164:1965–76.
90. Kabrhel C, Varraso R, Goldhaber SZ, et al. Prospective study of BMI and the risk of pulmonary embolism in women. Obesity (Silver Spring). 2009;17:2040–6.
91. Thibault PK, Wlodarczyk J. Correlation of serum ferritin levels and postsclerotherapy pigmentation. A prospective study. J Dermatol Surg Oncol. 1994;20:684–6.

Complications of Sclerotherapy

8

Nuttawut Sermsathanasawadi
and Sergio Gianesini

1 Introduction

Sclerotherapy is a well-established minimally invasive procedure that stands as a primary or adjunctive therapy of telangiectasias, reticular veins, and varicose veins [1]. Despite its high safety profile when performed by a trained physician, the procedure is not without risk. The potential for complications, ranging from common, self-limiting cosmetic issues to rare, life-threatening systemic events [2]. Foam sclerosant is created by the turbulent mixing of a liquid detergent sclerosant—polidocanol (POL) or sodium tetradecyl sulfate (STS)—with a gas, typically room air or mixtures of carbon dioxide and oxygen [1]. The foam effectively displaces blood from the vein lumen, allowing prolonged, undiluted contact between the active sclerosant and the endothelium. The increased potency of the foam sclerosant not only enhances the local inflammatory response but also introduces gas microbubbles into the venous circulation, creating a pathway for systemic complications [1]. These bubbles can travel to the central circulation and, in patients with a right-to-left cardiac shunt such as a patent foramen ovale (PFO), may paradoxically embolize to the arterial system, resulting in neurological or cardiopulmonary symptoms [1].

Complication of sclerotherapy is broadly divided based on their anatomical location relative to the treatment site [3].

- *Local Complications*: These events are confined to the treated limb, occurring at or in the immediate vicinity of the injection sites. They can be further subdivided by the tissue type affected, including cutaneous events (hyperpigmentation, telangiectatic matting, cutaneous necrosis) and vascular events (superficial venous thrombosis).
- *Systemic Complications*: These events affect the body remotely from the injection site and are typically caused by the sclerosant or, more commonly, the gas from foam entering the central circulation. This category includes venous thromboembolism (VTE), neurological events, systemic allergic reactions, and cardiopulmonary symptoms.

N. Sermsathanasawadi
Division of Vascular Surgery, Department of Surgery, Faculty of Medicine Siriraj Hospital, Mahidol University, Bangkok, Thailand
e-mail: nuttawut.ser@mahidol.ac.th

S. Gianesini (✉)
Department of Translational Medicine, University of Ferrara, Ferrara, Italy

Department of Surgery, Uniformed Services University of Health Sciences, Bethesda, MD, USA
e-mail: gnssrg@unife.it

S. Gianesini, Y. W. Chi (eds.), *Sclerotherapy*, https://doi.org/10.1007/978-3-032-32794-9_8

2 Local Complications

2.1 Post-Sclerotherapy Pigmentation (PSP)

2.1.1 Incidence

Post-sclerotherapy pigmentation (PSP) is a common and often expected sequela of treatment. The reported incidence is highly variable, ranging from 5% to as high as 30% [4].

2.1.2 Pathophysiology

The primary mechanism underlying PSP is the deposition of hemosiderin in the dermis [4]. Sclerosant-induced endothelial injury and the subsequent inflammatory response increase the permeability of the vessel wall causing the extravasation of red blood cells into the perivascular dermal tissue [5]. The extravasated RBCs are phagocytosed by dermal macrophages. During this process, hemoglobin is broken down, and its iron component is stored as hemosiderin [4]. A secondary component of post-inflammatory hyperpigmentation, involving the transfer of melanin from melanocytes to keratinocytes (melanin incontinence), may also contribute, particularly in patients with darker skin tones [5].

PSP is characteristically not present immediately after the procedure but appears gradually, typically becoming noticeable around 6–8 weeks post-treatment. The natural history is one of spontaneous resolution in the majority of cases; approximately 70% of PSP fades within 6 months, and over 90% resolves within 1 year. However, in a small but significant subset of patients, estimated at 1%–10%, the pigmentation can be permanent [6, 7].

Multiple factors influence the risk of developing PSP. Studies consistently show higher rates of PSP with STS compared to POL [8]. Foam sclerosants carry a higher risk of PSP compared to their liquid counterparts at the same concentration [9]. The use of excessive injection pressures or large volumes of sclerosant, leads to greater endothelial damage, inflammation, and extravasation, all of which promote pigmentation. Patient-specific factors play a major role. Individuals with higher Fitzpatrick skin types (III–IV and above) have a greater propensity for post-inflammatory pigmentary changes [10, 11]. An innate tendency toward pigmentation, vessel fragility, and potentially high total body iron stores, as indicated by elevated serum ferritin levels, have also been identified as risk factors [4]. Furthermore, PSP is more common when treating larger telangiectasias (0.6–1.2 mm) or veins located very superficially beneath the epidermis [10–12]. Inadequate or short-duration post-procedural compression is a significant modifiable risk factor, as compression helps to minimize the extravasation of blood that leads to pigmentation [13].

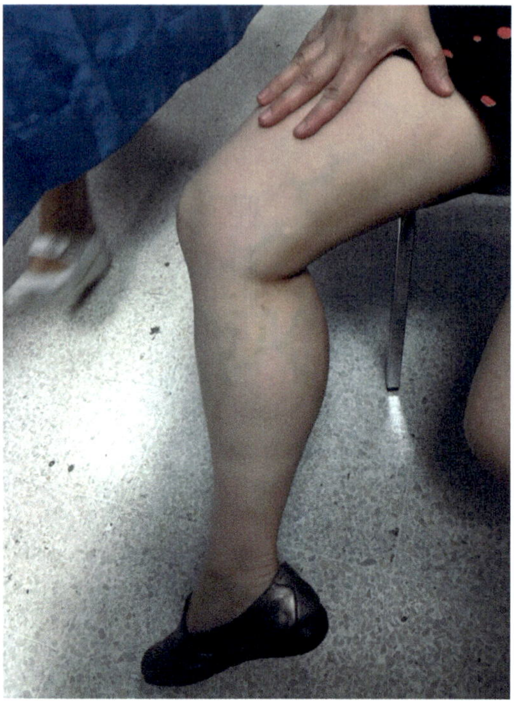

Fig. 8.1 Post-sclerotherapy pigmentation after foam sclerotherapy with 1% polidocanol

2.1.3 Diagnosis

The diagnosis of PSP is clinical, based on the characteristic appearance of linear or punctate brown-black staining that follows the course of a previously treated vein and appears weeks to months after the procedure (Fig. 8.1). It is crucial to differentiate true PSP from a retained coagulum or "microthrombus," which appears as a dark, palpable cord, or lump within the treated vessel. This is trapped blood, not dermal pigment, and it can and should be evacuated.

2.1.4 Management

1. *Observation*: Given the high rate of spontaneous resolution, a "wait-and-see" approach for at least 6–12 months is the standard and most appropriate initial strategy. Patients should be counseled on the expected timeline for resolution at the time of consent.
2. *Microthrombectomy*: This is a key early intervention that also serves as a preventative measure. At a follow-up visit 2–4 weeks after sclerotherapy, any palpable, trapped coagula should be evacuated. This is performed by making a small incision over the vessel with an 18- or 21-gauge needle and expressing the liquefied thrombus (Fig. 8.2). This simple procedure removes a major source of perivenular inflammation and reduces the amount of trapped blood available to become hemosiderin.
3. *Laser and Light Therapies*: For PSP that persists beyond 6–12 months and is of cosmetic concern to the patient, pigment-specific lasers and light sources are the definitive treatment [10]. Q-switched lasers (e.g., 694 nm Ruby, 1064 nm Nd:YAG) and, more recently, picosecond lasers are highly effective. These devices deliver high-energy pulses in extremely short durations (nanoseconds or picoseconds), which creates a photo-acoustic effect that shatters the dermal hemosiderin particles into smaller fragments. These fragments can then be more effectively cleared by the lymphatic system. Multiple treatment sessions are typically required for significant clearing.

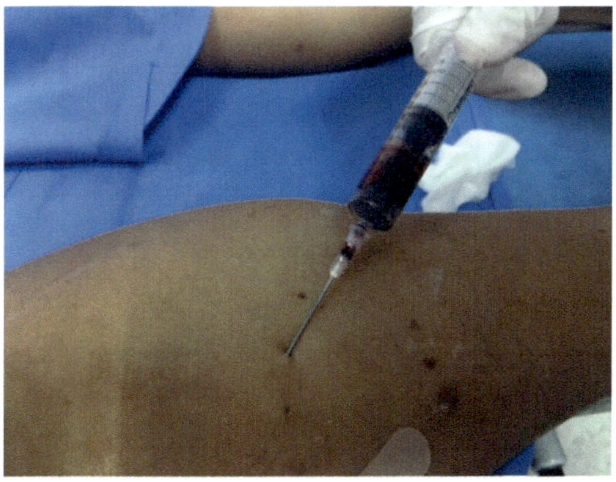

Fig. 8.2 Aspiration of trapped blood 1 week after foam sclerotherapy

2.1.5 Prevention

Prevention is the most effective management strategy for PSP [4, 5, 14]. Key measures include:

1. Adhering to the principle of using the minimal effective sclerosant concentration and volume for the target vessel size.
2. Employing a meticulous injection technique with low, controlled pressure to minimize vessel trauma and extravasation.
3. Routinely performing microthrombectomy of any significant coagula at the 2–4 week follow-up visit.
4. Ensuring the application of adequate, graduated post-procedural compression to minimize blood extravasation.
5. Advising patients to strictly avoid sun exposure on treated areas for several weeks post-procedure, as UV light can exacerbate the melanin component of pigmentation.

2.2 Telangiectatic Matting (TM)

2.2.1 Incidence

Telangiectatic matting (TM) is one of the common cosmetic complications, with a reported incidence in 15%–24% of patients undergoing sclerotherapy [3]. Like PSP, it is a delayed phenomenon, typically appearing 4–6 weeks after a treatment session as a fine "blush" or "mat" of new, red telangiectasias (<0.2 mm in diameter) in or around the treated area [3, 4, 15]. The natural history is also one of spontaneous resolution in most cases, usually over 3–12 months. However, in a minority of patients (estimates range from <1% to 10%), the matting can be permanent [15].

2.2.2 Pathophysiology

The precise etiology of TM is widely believed to be a reactive process involving angiogenesis (the formation of new blood vessels) and the vasodilation of existing, previously subclinical, dermal capillaries. As with PSP, excessive inflammation resulting from overly aggressive sclerotherapy (high sclerosant concentration, high volume, or high injection pressure) appears to be a primary trigger. Sclerosant-induced endothelial damage leads to the degranulation of perivascular mast cells, which release a host of potent angiogenic factors, including fibroblast growth factor and tumor necrosis factor stimulating new vessel growth. Another cause of TM is the inadequate treatment of underlying venous reflux, the persistent proximal hypertension from residual reticular vein can be redirected into the surrounding capillary network, stimulating the formation of TM. Moreover, estrogen is known to promote endothelial cell migration and proliferation, thus encouraging the neovascularization that characterizes TM [16].

Several factors predispose patients to developing TM. TM is significantly more common in women. A family history of telangiectasias, obesity, a history of easy bruising, and possibly underlying allergic conditions or bleeding disorders are also associated with increased risk. The use of exogenous estrogen is a well-established and significant risk factor [4, 16].

2.2.3 Clinical Presentation

The diagnosis of TM is made clinically based on its characteristic appearance: a collection of very fine (<0.2 mm), newly appeared red or purple vessels forming a patch or "mat" in a previous sclerotherapy area [4] (Fig. 8.3). A key step in the workup of TM is to perform a thorough clinical and Duplex ultrasound examination of the affected area to search for any missed proximal sources of reflux, such as an incompetent perforator or reticular feeder vein, that may be driving the process [4].

2.2.4 Management

Conservative Treatment

Observation for 3–12 months is a reasonable first step, as a significant number of cases will resolve spontaneously without intervention [15].

Re-Sclerotherapy

If a proximal source of residual reflux is identified on examination, treating this "feeder" vein with sclerotherapy is the most important step and often leads to the spontaneous resolution of the associated matting [4]. For persistent TM, careful re-sclerotherapy must be done with a very low concentration of a mild sclerosant (0.1–0.25% POL) should be used, injected with minimal pressure through a very fine-gauge (31–33G) needle [16].

Laser and Intense Pulsed Light (IPL)

For TM that are resistant to re-sclerotherapy, pulsed dye laser (585/595 nm) and the long-pulsed 1064 nm Nd:YAG laser target hemoglobin are effective treatment options [4].).

2.2.5 Prevention

Performing a thorough pre-treatment assessment to identify and treat all sources of venous reflux, particularly reticular feeder veins, before or during the same session as the treatment of superficial telangiectasias [4]. Adhering strictly to the principle of using the minimal effective sclerosant concentration, volume, and injection pressure to limit the inflammatory stimulus [4]. Applying adequate, graduated post-procedural

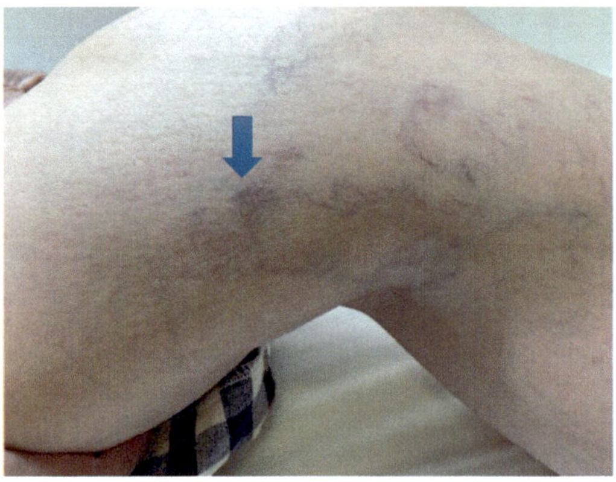

Fig. 8.3 Telangiectatic matting after liquid sclerotherapy of reticular vein and telangiectasia

compression for reducing the incidence of TM. Cryo-assisted laser and cryo-assisted sclerotherapy (CLaCS) might play a role in preventing TM [4]. Counseling patients on estrogen therapy about their increased risk of TM [4].

2.3 Injection Site Reactions

2.3.1 Pain, Ecchymosis, and Edema

Pain and ecchymosis were found in 38% of patients. Severe or persistent pain during injection is suggesting either extravasation of the sclerosant into the perivascular tissue or an inadvertent intra-arterial injection [16]. Ecchymosis is caused by needle trauma to the vessel wall or adjacent capillaries, which allows a small amount of blood to leak into the dermis and subcutaneous tissue [17]. Localized edema, particularly ankle swelling, is common after treatment of veins in the foot or ankle region [4].

Management

Mild post-procedural pain is typically managed with simple analgesics such as acetaminophen or NSAIDs. Application of cold compresses in the first 24–48 h can also help minimize both swelling and bruising. Bruising typically resolves over 1–2 weeks, and edema within a few days. Patients should be advised to avoid medications that can increase bleeding, such as aspirin and NSAIDs, for several days before the procedure [16].

2.4 Superficial Venous Thrombosis (SVT)

2.4.1 Incidence and Pathophysiology

The incidence of clinically significant SVT ranges from 4.4% to 10% following sclerotherapy [3]. The mechanism of sclerotherapy is to induce a controlled chemical phlebitis and subsequent thrombosis within the target vessel. Therefore, the development of a firm, noncompressible, and sometimes tender cord along the treated vein is an expected and desired sign of successful sclerosis. This expected reaction transitions into a clinical complication when the inflammatory response is excessive, leading to significant pain, erythema, and tenderness that is distressing to the patient, or when the thrombus propagates beyond the intended treatment zone, particularly toward the deep venous system.

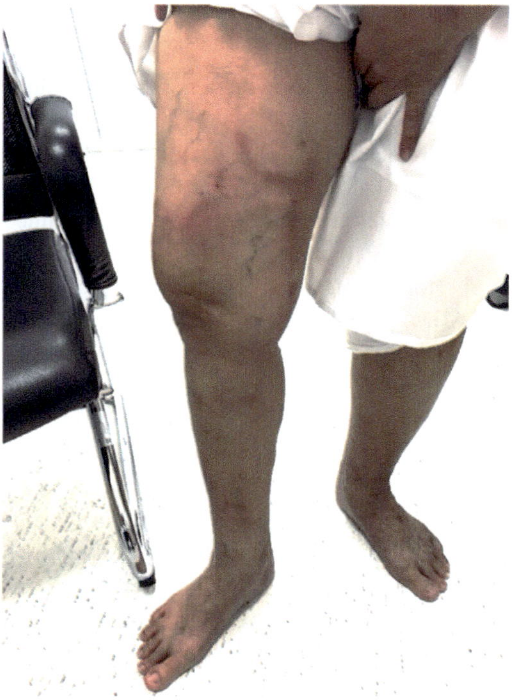

Fig. 8.4 Superficial venous thrombosis after foam sclerotherapy of tributaries of great saphenous vein

2.4.2 Diagnosis

The clinical diagnosis of SVT is based on the presence of a painful, tender, erythematous, and palpable cord along the course of a superficial vein, typically appearing a few days to weeks after the procedure [4] (Fig. 8.4).

Investigation

Duplex ultrasonography confirms the presence of thrombus within the superficial vein. It precisely delineates the extent of the thrombus, measuring its length and, most importantly, its proximity to the deep venous system at the saphenofemoral junction (SFJ) or saphenopopliteal junction (SPJ). Moreover, it is used to rule out a concurrent deep vein thrombosis because a concomitant DVT in up to 18% of SVT patients [4].

2.4.3 Management

Uncomplicated SVT

For patients of SVT that are confirmed by ultrasound to be localized, limited in length (<5 cm), and well-contained within the superficial system at a safe distance (>3 cm) from the SFJ or SPJ, management is primarily symptomatic and aimed at controlling the local inflammatory response [1]. Non-steroidal anti-inflammatory drugs (NSAIDs) are the mainstay of pharmacotherapy to reduce both pain and inflammation. The application of warm compresses can provide symptomatic relief. Use of graduated compression stockings is recommended to reduce symptoms, and patients should be encouraged to maintain normal ambulation to promote venous flow in the deep system. Bed rest should be avoided. Topical preparations containing heparinoids or NSAIDs may provide additional local relief [17].

Complicated SVT

SVT is now recognized as a significant risk factor for VTE, as the thrombus can propagate from the superficial system into the deep system, leading to DVT and potentially PE [1]. Therefore, risk stratification via Duplex ultrasound is the most critical step in management. High-risk factors for VTE extension include thrombus located less than 3 cm from the SFJ or SPJ, a total thrombus length greater than 5 cm and patient-specific VTE risk factors such as personal or family history of VTE known thrombophilia and active malignancy [1].

For SVT patients with any of these high-risk features, symptomatic treatment alone is insufficient, and anticoagulation is recommended to prevent VTE. Current guidelines suggest a prophylactic or intermediate-dose anticoagulation regimen for a period of 45 days [1]. The most evidence-based options are subcutaneous fondaparinux 2.5 mg daily or oral rivaroxaban 10 mg daily [1].

If the thrombus is found to be at or extending into the deep junction more than 50% of lumen of deep vein (endovenous foam-induced thrombosis type 3 or 4), it should be treated as a DVT with full therapeutic-dose anticoagulation for a minimum of 3 months [18].

2.5 Cutaneous Necrosis and Ulceration

Incidence

Cutaneous necrosis is a rare but potentially devastating complication of sclerotherapy. The reported incidence is 0.2%–1.2% [16, 19]. The initial symptom is severe pain or skin blanching, while the evolution to a necrotic eschar and subsequent ulceration is a subacute process. The ulcers are often slow to heal, potentially taking 4 to 6 weeks or longer [16].

Pathophysiology

The leakage of sclerosant into the perivascular tissue was historically considered the main cause of skin necrosis [3, 20, 21]. It remains a significant risk with caustic osmotic agents (hypertonic saline). However, with modern detergent sclerosants (POL, STS), particularly in foam form and at the low volumes used for telangiectasias, extravasation is less likely to cause significant necrosis [3, 20, 21]. Inadvertent intra-arterial injection causes immediate and extensive endothelial destruction, thrombosis, and occlusion of the arterial supply, leading to widespread distal tissue ischemia and necrosis [20, 21]. This is the most catastrophic mechanism. A rapid or high-pressure injection can trigger a powerful veno-arteriolar reflex vasospasm (VAR-VAS). This reflex causes a profound spasm of the associated precapillary arterioles, shutting down blood flow to the overlying skin and causing ischemia. Moreover, it is hypothesized that sclerosant injected into the venous system can pass through arteriovenous anastomoses shunts (AV shunt) into the arterial side, leading to the occlusion of terminal end-arterioles and a subsequent patch of ischemic necrosis [4, 20, 21].

Clinical Presentation

Immediate warning signs during the procedure include the patient reporting unusually severe or

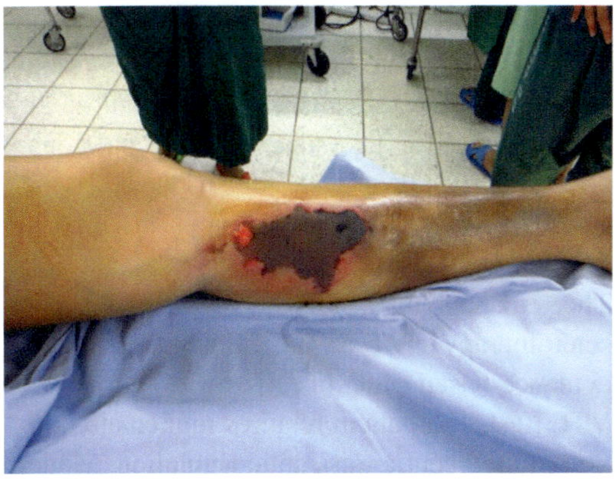

Fig. 8.5 Cutaneous necrosis after foam sclerotherapy

radiating pain, or the clinician observing a distinct area of porcelain-white blanching or a bright erythematous patch at or distal to the injection site. Over the subsequent hours to days, this area progresses to a dusky, cyanotic, or violaceous patch, often with a characteristic retiform or livedoid pattern. This eventually demarcates into a black, necrotic eschar, which will ultimately slough off to reveal an underlying ulcer [21, 22].

The morphological classification of cutaneous necrosis links the physical appearance of the necrosis to its underlying cause. Round necrosis presents as an ulcer with smooth, regular, and non-geographic borders is characteristic of a localized chemical injury and is typical of necrosis caused by extravasation of the sclerosant. Stellate necrosis presents with irregular, jagged, angulated, or geographic borders, often following a retiform pattern (Fig. 8.5). This morphology is the hallmark of an ischemic process resulting from arterial or arteriolar occlusion, whether from direct intra-arterial injection, veno-arteriolar reflex vasospasm, or shunting.

Management

Immediate Management

The procedure must be stopped immediately upon recognition of severe pain or blanching. If extravasation (round necrosis pattern) is suspected, the primary goal is dilution. The area should be immediately and aggressively infiltrated with copious amounts of normal saline to dilute the agent. The addition of hyaluronidase to the saline is highly recommended, as it breaks down hyaluronic acid in the extracellular matrix, facilitating the rapid dispersion of the sclerosant away from the injection site. This has been shown to be particularly effective in preventing necrosis from STS extravasation [16, 21, 22].

If ischemia is suspected (stellate necrosis pattern), the primary goals are to reverse vasospasm and prevent thrombosis. Apply vigorous massage and warm compresses to the area to encourage reperfusion [23]. Topical 2% nitroglycerin paste can be applied to induce local vasodilation [23]. Immediate systemic treatment should be initiated. This includes oral aspirin to inhibit platelet aggregation, and consideration of systemic vasodilators. For suspected major arterial injection, immediate initiation of systemic anticoagulation with heparin and high-dose systemic corticosteroids (to combat the intense inflammatory response to ischemia) is recommended [22].

The patient should be immediately transferred to a hospital with vascular and interventional radiology services for further management, which may include intra-arterial vasodilators or thrombolysis.

Long-Term Management

Once an ulcer has formed, management transitions to principles of advanced wound care, with the goal of creating an optimal environment for healing. The necrotic eschar must be removed to allow for the formation of healthy granulation tissue. This can be done surgically, mechanically, or with enzymatic debriding agents. A variety of modern dressings should be used to maintain a moist wound environment, manage exudate, and protect the wound bed.

The wound must be monitored closely for signs of secondary bacterial infection, which should be treated with appropriate topical or systemic antibiotics based on clinical assessment and cultures. For small ulcers (<1 cm), early excision and primary closure can significantly shorten the healing time, reduce pain, and provide a better final cosmetic result compared to healing by secondary intention.

Larger, non-healing ulcers may require more advanced reconstructive techniques, such as skin grafting or local flap coverage [16].

3 Systemic Complications

3.1 Venous Thromboembolism (VTE)

3.1.1 Deep Vein Thrombosis (DVT)

DVT is one of the most serious complications of sclerotherapy. The overall incidence is between 1% and 3% [3]. The vast majority of these cases are asymptomatic, distal (calf or muscular) DVTs detected on routine post-procedural surveillance Duplex ultrasound [18].

Several factors increase the risk of developing post-sclerotherapy DVT. A personal or family history of VTE, a known hypercoagulable state or thrombophilia, active malignancy, estrogen therapy, obesity, and prolonged immobility are all significant risk factors. The risk is higher when treating larger truncal veins (great or small saphenous veins). A study found a 4.6-fold increase in DVT risk when ≥10 mL of foam was used in a single session [18]. Failure to ensure adequate post-procedural ambulation to activate the calf muscle pump and flush the deep veins can also contribute [18].

The diagnosis of DVT should be suspected in any patient presenting with new-onset unilateral leg pain (especially in the calf), swelling, warmth, or erythema after sclerotherapy. The diagnosis must be confirmed with a compression Duplex ultrasound examination of the entire deep venous system of the limb [16].

3.1.2 Pulmonary Embolism (PE)

Pulmonary embolism (PE) is an extremely rare complication of sclerotherapy, almost always occurring as a sequela of a proximal DVT. The estimated risk is approximately 1 in 10,000 procedures [16]. A PE is a medical emergency that presents with the sudden onset of dyspnea, pleuritic chest pain, tachycardia, and in severe cases, hypoxia, hemoptysis, or syncope. Any patient with such symptoms following sclerotherapy requires immediate emergency medical evaluation, including assessment for DVT and definitive imaging for PE, such as a CT pulmonary angiogram (CTPA).

Management

The management of a confirmed post-sclerotherapy DVT or PE follows the standard, evidence-based guidelines for the treatment of VTE [24]. The patient requires immediate initiation of therapeutic-dose anticoagulation. Modern treatment regimens typically involve direct oral anticoagulants (DOACs) or initial treatment with low-molecular-weight heparin (LMWH) bridged to a vitamin K antagonist like warfarin. The standard duration of therapy is a minimum of 3 months. The decision to extend therapy beyond 3 months depends on whether the VTE is considered "provoked" by a transient risk factor (the sclerotherapy procedure) or "unprovoked," and on the patient's individual risk profile for recurrence versus bleeding [24].

3.2 Neurological Events

The advent of foam sclerotherapy has brought to light a spectrum of neurological adverse events. The presence of gas microbubbles, combined with the high prevalence of PFO in the general population creates a distinct pathophysiological pathway for morbidity that requires a fundamental change in pre-procedural screening and patient counseling.

3.2.1 Migraine and Transient Visual Disturbances

These are the most common neurological side effects associated with foam sclerotherapy. The reported incidence of transient visual disturbances is highly variable, ranging from 1.4% to as high as 14% in some series [3]. The clinical presentation is characteristic of a migraine aura, typically occurring during or immediately after the foam injection. Patients describe scintillating scotomas (shimmering lights), fortification spectra (zigzag lines), or blurred vision [3]. These visual symptoms are often, but not always, followed by a headache. The events are almost invariably transient, resolving completely within minutes to a few hours without any lasting deficit.

3.2.2 Transient Ischemic Attack (TIA) and Stroke

TIA and stroke are the most feared neurological complications. The incidence of stroke is estimated to be extremely low, at approximately 0.01% [3]. These events present as a sudden-onset focal neurological deficit, such as unilateral weakness or numbness, aphasia, or facial droop. Unlike a transient visual disturbance, a TIA or stroke constitutes a major medical emergency requiring immediate neurological evaluation and treatment.

Pathophysiology

The mechanism for these neurological events is strongly believed to be paradoxical gas embolism [3]. Microbubbles of gas from the sclerosant foam enter the systemic venous circulation. These bubbles travel to the right atrium of the heart. In patients with a right-to-left shunt, most commonly a PFO, a transient increase in right atrial pressure from a cough or Valsalva maneuver can force these microbubbles across the shunt into the left atrium. From the left side of the heart, the gas microbubbles enter the arterial circulation and can travel to the brain. In the cerebral circulation, these microemboli can cause transient ischemia, leading to the symptoms of a TIA or, in rare cases, a permanent stroke [3]. They can also trigger a wave of cortical spreading depression, the neurophysiological event that underlies migraine aura. The release of the potent vasoconstrictor endothelin-1 from the sclerosant-damaged endothelium may also play a contributing role in these vasospastic phenomena [3].

Prevention

A known symptomatic right-to-left shunt is an absolute contraindication to foam sclerotherapy [3]. A history of migraine with aura is a strong relative contraindication, and these patients should be counseled extensively about the increased risk of triggering an attack or experiencing visual disturbances [3]. Routine screening for PFO with bubble-contrast echocardiography is not currently the standard of care but should be strongly considered in patients with a history of neurological events post-sclerotherapy or other high-risk features.

Several technical modifications can reduce the risk. Adhering to a maximum recommended volume of foam per session (10 mL) is a critical safety measure [4]. Using a mixture of CO_2/O_2 to create the foam instead of room air may reduce risk, as CO2 is significantly more soluble in blood than nitrogen, allowing the bubbles to dissolve more quickly [4]. Instructing the patient to remain still and breathe normally, avoiding any coughing or Valsalva maneuvers for several minutes after injection, can help prevent transient increases in right atrial pressure that promote shunting [4].

3.3 Allergic Reactions

True anaphylaxis is an extremely rare complication of sclerotherapy [3]. Milder hypersensitivity reactions, such as localized or generalized urticaria, are more common. The risk of a reaction may increase with repeated exposure to the same sclerosant over multiple treatment sessions [16]. Historically, anaphylaxis was most associated with sodium morrhuate, followed by STS. Polidocanol is considered to have a lower allergenic potential [3]. Osmotic agents like HTS, being simple salt solutions, carry virtually no risk of true anaphylaxis.

Diagnosis of Anaphylaxis

Anaphylaxis is a life-threatening, multisystem allergic reaction characterized by its rapid onset. Key clinical manifestations include airway compromise (laryngeal edema causing stridor), bronchospasm (wheezing), and cardiovascular collapse (hypotension, tachycardia) [16]. Cutaneous signs like urticaria and angioedema are often present but may be absent in cases of rapid-onset hypotension.

Management of Anaphylaxis
Every facility where sclerotherapy is performed must be equipped with an emergency kit and have staff trained in resuscitation [16].

1. *Stop the Injection Immediately*.
2. *Administer Epinephrine*: The first-line and life-saving treatment is intramuscular epinephrine (0.2–0.5 mL of a 1:1000 solution) administered into the anterolateral thigh.
3. *Position the Patient*: Place the patient in a supine position with legs elevated to manage hypotension.
4. *Airway and Oxygen*: Secure the airway and administer high-flow oxygen.
5. Adjunctive Therapies: After epinephrine, administer IV fluids for hypotension, H1 and H2 antihistamines (e.g., diphenhydramine and cimetidine/famotidine), and systemic corticosteroids. Corticosteroids do not act immediately but help prevent a biphasic or protracted reaction. The patient must be transferred to an emergency department for observation, as biphasic reactions can occur hours after the initial event.

3.4 Cardiopulmonary Events

Transient chest tightness and a dry cough have been reported, particularly following the injection of air-based foam. This is believed to be caused by a bolus of gas microemboli reaching the pulmonary arterial circulation, causing a transient vasospasm or inflammatory reaction. These symptoms are typically mild and self-limiting, resolving within minutes [25]. Anecdotal case reports have linked sclerotherapy to severe cardiac events such as myocardial infarction and Takotsubo (stress) cardiomyopathy [25–27]. However, a direct causal link is difficult to establish. The active sclerosant is rapidly diluted and deactivated by blood components and is highly unlikely to reach the coronary circulation in a pharmacologically active concentration [28]. These events remain exceptionally rare.

4 Conclusions

Sclerotherapy stands as a highly effective, versatile, and generally safe procedure of the modern phlebologist. A comprehensive understanding of the pathophysiology of each potential complication—from the inflammatory cascades that drive cosmetic sequelae to the embolic mechanisms of systemic events—is the fundamental basis of safe and effective practice The majority of complications can be prevented or their severity mitigated through a systematic approach that includes meticulous pre-procedural patient assessment, the selection of appropriate sclerosants and concentrations, precise and judicious injection technique, and diligent application of post-procedural care, particularly compression therapy.

References

1. Gloviczki P, Lawrence PF, Wasan SM, Meissner MH, Almeida J, Brown KR, et al. The 2022 Society for Vascular Surgery, American Venous Forum, and American Vein And Lymphatic Society clinical practice guidelines for the management of varicose veins of the lower extremities. Part I. Duplex scanning and treatment of superficial truncal reflux: endorsed by the Society for Vascular Medicine and the International Union of Phlebology. J Vasc Surg Venous Lymphat Disord. 2023;11(2):231–61 e6.
2. Weiss MA, Hsu JT, Neuhaus I, Sadick NS, Duffy DM. Consensus for sclerotherapy. Dermatologic Surg. 2014;40(12):1309–18.
3. Cavezzi A, Parsi K. Complications of foam sclerotherapy. Phlebology. 2012;27(Suppl 1):46–51.
4. Wong M, Parsi K, Myers K, De Maeseneer M, Caprini J, Cavezzi A, et al. Sclerotherapy of lower limb veins: indications, contraindications and treatment strategies to prevent complications–a consensus document of the International Union of Phlebology-2023. Phlebology. 2023;38(4):205–58.
5. Rabe E, Breu FX, Cavezzi A, Coleridge Smith P, Frullini A, Gillet JL, et al. European guidelines for sclerotherapy in chronic venous disorders. Phlebology. 2014;29(6):338–54.
6. Szczygieł Ł, Juśko M. Hyperpigmentation after sclerotherapy: own experience in therapeutic Q-switched Nd:YAG laser treatment. Phlebol Rev. 2024;32(1):1–7.
7. Gillet JL, Guedes JM, Guex JJ, Hamel-Desnos C, Schadeck M, Lauseker M, et al. Side-effects and complications of foam sclerotherapy of the great and small saphenous veins: a controlled multicentre pro-

spective study including 1,025 patients. Phlebology. 2009;24(3):131–8.
8. Cooley-Andrade O, Jothidas A, Goh WX, Connor DE, Parsi K. Low-concentration detergent sclerosants stimulate white blood cells and release proinflammatory and proangiogenic cytokines in vitro. J Vasc Surg Venous Lymphat Disord. 2014;2(4):433–40.
9. Guex JJ, Allaert FA, Gillet JL, Chleir F. Immediate and midterm complications of sclerotherapy: report of a prospective multicenter registry of 12,173 sclerotherapy sessions. Dermatologic Surg. 2005;31(2):123–8. discussion 8.
10. Seo DJ, Chung B. Low-energy, multi-wavelength long-pulse diode laser for post-sclerotherapy hyperpigmentation in Fitzpatrick skin type III-IV: a case series. Ann Phlebol. 2025;23(1):47–52.
11. Bossart S, Daneluzzi C, Cazzaniga S, Ramelet AA, Uthoff H, Seyed Jafari SM, et al. Skin hyperpigmentation after sclerotherapy with polidocanol: a systematic review. J Eur Acad Dermatol Venereol. 2023;37(2):274–83.
12. Rao J, Wildemore JK, Goldman MP. Double-blind prospective comparative trial between foamed and liquid polidocanol and sodium tetradecyl sulfate in the treatment of varicose and telangiectatic leg veins. Dermatologic Surg. 2005;31(6):631–5. discussion 5.
13. Bayer A, Kuznik N, Langan EA, Recke A, Recke AL, Faerber G, et al. Clinical outcome of short-term compression after sclerotherapy for telangiectatic varicose veins. J Vasc Surg Venous Lymphat Disord. 2021;9(2):435–43.
14. Rabe E, Breu FX, Flessenkamper I, Gerlach H, Guggenbichler S, Kahle B, et al. Sclerotherapy in the treatment of varicose veins: S2k guideline of the deutsche gesellschaft fur Phlebologie (DGP) in cooperation with the following societies: DDG, DGA, DGG, BVP. Hautarzt. 2021;72(Suppl 2):23–36.
15. Goldman MP, Sadick NS, Weiss RA. Cutaneous necrosis, telangiectatic matting, and hyperpigmentation following sclerotherapy. Etiology, prevention, and treatment. Dermatologic Surg. 1995;21(1):19–29. quiz 31–2.
16. Goldman MP. Chapter 15–Complications and adverse sequelae of sclerotherapy. In: Bergan JJ, editor. The vein book. Burlington: Academic Press; 2007. p. 139–55.
17. de Almeida MJ, Guillaumon AT, Miquelin D, et al. Guidelines for superficial venous thrombosis. J Vasc Bras. 2019;18:e20180105.
18. Kulkarni SR, Messenger DE, Slim FJ, Emerson LG, Bulbulia RA, Whyman MR, et al. The incidence and characterization of deep vein thrombosis following ultrasound-guided foam sclerotherapy in 1000 legs with superficial venous reflux. J Vasc Surg Venous Lymphat Disord. 2013;1(3):231–8.
19. Jia X, Mowatt G, Burr JM, Cassar K, Cook J, Fraser C. Systematic review of foam sclerotherapy for varicose veins. Br J Surg. 2007;94(8):925–36.
20. Schuller-Petrović S, Pavlović MD, Neuhold N, Brunner F, Wölkart G. Subcutaneous injection of liquid and foamed polidocanol: extravasation is not responsible for skin necrosis during reticular and spider vein sclerotherapy. J Eur Acad Dermatol Venereol. 2011;25(8):983–6.
21. Kang M, Yang A, Hannaford P, Connor D, Parsi K. Skin necrosis following sclerotherapy. Part 1: differential diagnosis based on classification of pathogenic mechanisms. Phlebology. 2022;37(6):409–24.
22. Kang M, Yang A, Hannaford P, Connor D, Parsi K. Skin necrosis following sclerotherapy. Part 2: risk minimisation and management strategies. Phlebology. 2022;37(9):628–43.
23. King M. This month's guideline: management of necrosis. J Clin Aesthet Dermatol. 2018;11(7):E53–e7.
24. Stevens SM, Woller SC, Baumann Kreuziger L, Bounameaux H, Doerschug K, Geersing GJ, et al. Executive summary: antithrombotic therapy for VTE disease: second update of the CHEST guideline and expert panel report. Chest. 2021;160(6):2247–59.
25. Hill DA. Neurological and chest symptoms following sclerotherapy: a single centre experience. Phlebology. 2014;29(9):619–27.
26. Stephens R, Dunn S. Non-ST-elevation myocardial infarction following foam ultrasound-guided sclerotherapy. Phlebology. 2014;29(7):488–90.
27. Patel S, Nabatian S, Goyfman M. Sclerotherapy induced takotsubo syndrome. Case Rep Cardiol. 2020;2020:5626078.
28. Dabbs EB, Dos Santos SJ, Mainsiouw LE, Sheikh AA, Gkantiragas A, Shiangoli I, et al. Implication of foam sclerosant inactivation by human whole blood in a laboratory setting. Phlebology. 2018;33(5):338–43.

9 Sclerotherapy for Lower Limb Chronic Venous Disease

Sergio Gianesini and Matthieu Josnin

1 Chronic Venous Disease Background

Chronic venous disease (CVD) is best understood not as a single diagnosis but as a continuum of venous structural and functional abnormalities that accumulate over time and express themselves through a recognizably "venous" clinical language: telangiectasias and reticular veins, varicosities, edema, inflammatory skin change, and ultimately ulceration. In day-to-day vascular practice, CVD often presents as a deceptively familiar complaint of "heavy legs," "swelling," "itching," "night cramps," "I can't stand at work anymore," yet beneath this clinical familiarity lies a complex interaction among venous hemodynamics, vein wall biology, valve integrity, microcirculatory failure, and patient perception of symptoms and disability. A useful mental model for the expert is to regard CVD as the phenotype that emerges when ambulatory venous pressures are persistently abnormal, whether from reflux, obstruction, calf pump failure, or combinations thereof, and when the downstream tissues remain exposed long enough for inflammation and remodeling to become self-sustaining [1]. If you follow patients longitudinally, especially those with early disease, the most striking feature is not that CVD exists, but how efficiently it progresses in some individuals and how stubbornly it plateaus in others. This heterogeneity is precisely why modern venous practice requires a common descriptive language, parallel severity metrics, and, crucially, patient-reported outcomes (PROs) that reflect what matters to the person living with the disease, not only what is visible to the clinician [2, 3]. CVD is among the most prevalent chronic conditions in adult populations, and its population footprint is far larger than the subset that reaches a vascular clinic. Large community studies illustrate this clearly: in the Edinburgh Vein Study, trunk varices and chronic venous insufficiency (in the epidemiologic sense of more advanced clinical disease) were common findings even among working-age adults, establishing a baseline reality: CVD is not rare and it is not confined to the elderly [4]. Duplex correlations from the same broad epidemiologic tradition reinforced a practical truth for experts: clinical findings and duplex reflux intersect meaningfully but not perfectly: symptoms, visible signs, and reflux are overlapping circles rather than a single entity [5]. Population-based European data expanded this view by mapping venous reflux across superficial and deep systems in a way that mirrors what vascular laboratories see every day: pathologic reflux is common, its

S. Gianesini (✉)
Department of Translational Medicine, University of Ferrara, Ferrara, Italy

Department of Surgery, Uniformed Services University of Health Sciences, Bethesda, MD, USA
e-mail: gnssrg@unife.it

M. Josnin
Department of Vascular Medicine, St Charles Clinic, La Roche sur Yon, France

S. Gianesini, Y. W. Chi (eds.), *Sclerotherapy*, https://doi.org/10.1007/978-3-032-32794-9_9

distribution varies by age and sex, and its clinical expression ranges from asymptomatic reflux to skin change and ulceration. The Bonn Vein Study program, for example, provided a particularly influential duplex-based epidemiologic frame for reflux prevalence [6]. When you place these findings side-by-side with prospective incidence observations, the story becomes dynamic: new varices and incident chronic venous insufficiency accrue over years in a predictable minority of adults, and risk factors compound rather than merely add [7]. For the expert, the key epidemiologic lesson is not a single prevalence number (which will vary with definitions and sampling), but the scale and distribution:

- Early clinical classes (C0–C1) are extremely common in the general population.
- Varicose veins (C2) are common and often under-treated relative to symptom burden.
- Advanced disease (C4–C6) is less common but disproportionately expensive and disabling.

This "pyramid" is one reason superficial venous interventions can have large public-health implications when appropriately targeted. Yet it is also why venous ulcer services can dominate resource utilization even when ulcers represent a minority phenotype. Epidemiologic studies converge on a familiar risk profile: age, family history, pregnancy exposure, obesity, and occupations with prolonged standing all influence the likelihood of developing visible disease and/or reflux. What matters clinically is how these risks translate into progression: if you track a cohort over years, the incident cases are not random: they are enriched for those already carrying hemodynamic vulnerabilities, connective-tissue predisposition, or both. Longitudinal population follow-up work in community cohorts shows that CVD is not merely prevalent: it is incident and progressive in a measurable way [7]. From a vascular-system perspective, progression should be seen as an evolving imbalance: venous capacitance increases, valve competence decreases, reflux volume grows, ambulatory venous pressures rise, microvascular injury accumulates, and tissue tolerance declines. The epidemiology of symptoms complicates the narrative, because symptoms correlate only modestly with visible signs: one reason patient-reported outcomes have become essential rather than optional. Duplex-clinical correlation work reminds us that "venous symptoms" are real even when the visible phenotype is modest, and conversely, visible disease may be remarkably asymptomatic in some individuals [5]. CVD's socioeconomic impact is defined less by the presence of varicose veins and more by chronicity, recurrence, and downstream complications, especially venous leg ulceration (VLU). Once ulceration enters the picture, the disease becomes a multi-layered cost center: nursing time, dressings, compression systems, wound clinics, infection management, procedural interventions, time off work, caregiving and the psychological burden of long-term visible wounds. Older but still frequently cited health-economic discussions established early that VLU and severe chronic venous insufficiency create large national costs, often quoted in the hundreds of millions to billions annually depending on the country and methodology [8]. More recent multinational estimates (built from published incidence, prevalence, and utilization data) reinforce the same conclusion with updated accounting: venous ulcers consume substantial direct medical resources across multiple health-care systems, and the aggregate burden is enormous when scaled to population level [9]. Yet for the expert clinician, the socioeconomic impact is not only "cost to the system." It is also cost to the patient: work productivity loss, reduced walking capacity, reduced standing tolerance, sleep disturbance from itching or pain, and the quiet attrition of social participation (the patient stops traveling, stops exercising, stops wearing normal clothes). These patient-level consequences are precisely what disease-specific quality-of-life tools were built to capture, because generic instruments frequently underestimate venous-specific disability [10]. A practical way to conceptualize socioeconomic impact is to treat ulceration as a threshold event. Before ulceration, costs are often episodic (consultations, imaging, interventions). After ulceration, costs become continuous and recurrence-prone. Moreover, ulcer healing status is a major determinant of both cost and quality-of-life trajectories in observational work: healed ulcers tend to reduce ongoing cost intensity, whereas unhealed ulcers sustain high utilization and persistent quality-of-life impairment [11]. This is why modern venous services increasingly integrate reflux/obstruction assessment, compression expertise, wound-care pathways, and PRO measurement. CVD is not merely prevalent; it is systemically "expensive" because it is chronic, recurrent, and behaviorally restrictive: exactly the profile that benefits from structured classification and outcomes measurement.

2 Pathophysiology of Chronic Venous Insufficiency

CVD in its pathophysiologic sense is anchored in sustained ambulatory venous hypertension. The venous system is designed to tolerate hydrostatic load only because valves and the calf muscle pump convert a tall fluid column into a segmented, actively emptied conduit. When valve competence fails, when outflow is obstructed, or when pump function is ineffective, the distal venous bed is exposed to abnormal pressures during ambulation, the very time it should be protected. Comprehensive reviews in Circulation emphasize venous hypertension as the sine qua non, linking it to edema, skin change, and ulceration through inflammatory and microcirculatory mechanisms [1]. A key refinement for experts is that "venous hypertension" is not monolithic. Pressure behavior differs between obstruction-dominant and reflux-dominant phenotypes, between supine and erect positions, and across CEAP clinical classes. Contemporary physiologic analyses show that ambulatory venous hypertension tends to worsen as clinical class increases and is strongly associated with reflux severity, while supine venous hypertension aligns more with obstruction [12]. Venous valve failure has long been recognized as a structural finding (tearing, scarring, disappearance), but the modern view treats valve failure as both mechanical and inflammatory. The hypothesis that venous hypertension and inflammation actively damage valves and that this damage promotes further reflux creates the classic self-reinforcing loop: hypertension → inflammation → remodeling → reflux → more hypertension [13]. For the vascular expert, this framing changes how one interprets "primary" disease. Primary varicose veins are not merely passive dilations: they are remodeled tissues. Matrix remodeling, smooth muscle dysfunction, endothelial activation and inflammatory cell infiltration become not downstream epiphenomena but drivers of progression. Mechanistic and translational work on matrix metalloproteinases (MMPs) supports this: increased venous pressures and hypoxia-related signaling can upregulate MMP activity, degrade extracellular matrix, weaken the vein wall, and contribute to dilation and valve degradation [14]. The clinical hallmarks of advanced CVD (hyperpigmentation, eczema, lipodermatosclerosis, atrophie blanche, ulceration) are best understood as manifestations of microcirculatory injury. In this sense, the skin is not merely "affected": it is the target organ in chronic venous hypertension. Microcirculatory dysfunction in CVD has been characterized by capillary morphological change, altered permeability, reduced tissue oxygenation and reduced vascular reserve as disease worsens: features consistent with a chronic inflammatory microangiopathy [15]. This microvascular view is reinforced by physiologic and cellular studies showing that venous hypertension promotes leukocyte activation and sequestration within the leg microcirculation [16]. The downstream logic is coherent: activated leukocytes interact with endothelium, propagate inflammation, and contribute to capillary damage and tissue vulnerability. Venous ulcer pathogenesis has historically been narrated through hypotheses that, rather than competing, can be interpreted as describing different layers of the same process. The "fibrin cuff" hypothesis proposed that pericapillary fibrin deposition forms a barrier to oxygen and nutrient diffusion. Observational work demonstrated the presence of pericapillary fibrin in venous disease and explored its persistence even under compression therapy, keeping the concept alive while also highlighting its complexity. Falanga et al. later reappraisals examined the evidence critically, emphasizing that fibrin cuffs are a reproducible histologic feature but that their precise causal role remains debated [17]. In parallel, the leukocyte trapping/activation concept provided a cellular mechanism linking venous hypertension to endothelial injury and inflammation. Studies demonstrating activated neutrophil and monocyte sequestration in the leg microcirculation during venous hypertension offer a biologically plausible bridge between hemodynamic stress and inflammatory tissue injury [16]. When these concepts are integrated with microcirculatory dysfunction data (reduced oxygenation, altered capillary density, increased permeability) the modern expert view becomes less about choosing a single hypothesis and more about recognizing a convergent path: venous hypertension produces inflammatory microangiopathy and multiple histologic "signatures" (including fibrin deposition) may reflect that injury [15]. Scientific data clearly show how CVD should change its own acronym from chronic venous disease to chronic vascular disease, including a common endothelial inflammation involving veins, but also arteries and lymphatics. Mechanochemical structures like the glycocalyx justify this observation. This structure is indeed a ciliary-like layer that regulates endothelial permeability, while offering protection to it. It is also involved in the coagulation balance and in the vessel contractility. It is a mechanosensory entity translating the physical forces of the fluid dynamics into biochemical pro or anti-inflammatory signals, and it represents an innovative treatment target for arterial, venous and lymphatic disorders [18, 19]. The common endothelial path interesting arteries, veins and lymphatic observed in the lab mirrors with the clinical observation of chronic venous disease patients presenting an increased risk not only of deep venous thrombosis and pulmonary embolism, rather also of arterial conditions [20] and of lymphatic ones [21, 22]. A "pan-endothelial" and "pan-vascular" perspective is fundamental in the correct comprehension and consequent management of the lower limb venous disorder.

3 Chronic Venous Disease Scoring

Clinical–Etiologic–Anatomic–Pathophysiologic (CEAP) is the most renowned classification system in CVD. Yet, it is mandatory not to consider it as a disease severity scoring system: indeed, it is related to the clinical manifestation of the disorder and no correlation has been found between the histology damage and the same CEAP class [23]. The C component grades the outward clinical phenotype, from C0 (no visible signs) through C6 (active ulcer). Advanced classes are subdivided with clinically meaningful nuance (for example, C4a for pigmentation/eczema versus C4b for lipodermatosclerosis/atrophie blanche). The expert should remember that the clinical class captures "what the limb looks like" at a point in time, not necessarily the full hemodynamic burden or symptom severity. Etiology distinguishes congenital, primary, and secondary (often post-thrombotic) causes and allows explicit acknowledgment when no venous etiology is identified. This matters in research reporting and in practice: post-thrombotic disease behaves differently, recurs differently, and often demands different intervention strategies than primary superficial reflux. The A component localizes disease to superficial, deep, and perforator systems and can be expanded segmentally. For experts, the practical value is that it forces precision: "superficial reflux" is not a sufficient description for intervention planning or outcomes reporting; segmental anatomy is. The P component designates reflux, obstruction, or combined mechanisms. This is not mere semantics: in advanced disease, mixed pathophysiology is common, and failure to encode obstruction when present can mislead both treatment strategy and research comparisons. The 2020 update maintained the core structure and preserved the 2004 clinical definitions while introducing refinements intended to improve clarity, incorporate contemporary knowledge, and enhance reporting precision [3].

For the sclerotherapy practitioner, two practical CEAP habits can be recommended:

1. *Document both the "full" CEAP and the "basic" CEAP* when appropriate, full for research-level precision, basic for clinical brevity.
2. *Treat CEAP as descriptive but incomplete*: It tells what is present and where, but not how much it matters to the patient. That missing dimension is where PROs and severity scores enter.

CVD is a condition in which what the patient feels and what the clinician sees may diverge substantially. Two patients with the same CEAP class can have dramatically different symptom burdens, activity limitation, and psychological impact. Conversely, a patient with relatively mild visible disease may report severe heaviness, pain, sleep disturbance, or work impairment. This mismatch is not a failure of clinical observation: it is an intrinsic feature of the disease. Patient-reported outcomes (PROs) exist to measure the lived experience of CVD with tools designed for venous-specific domains: pain/heaviness, physical limitation, social restriction, and emotional distress. The argument for disease-specific instruments was made early and has only become more compelling as venous interventions expanded and outcomes expectations rose [10].

A venous PRO is useful when it is:

- *Valid* (measures what it claims to measure).
- *Reliable* (stable when the clinical state is stable).
- *Responsive* (changes when the patient truly changes).
- *Interpretable* (meaning of a score difference is clinically legible).
- *Feasible* (practical in clinic and in trials).

In venous disease, feasibility matters more than many experts initially assume: if the tool cannot be implemented reliably in routine care, it will not scale, and the outcome story will revert to clinician-centric measures.

The Chronic Venous Insufficiency Questionnaire (CIVIQ) was developed to capture quality-of-life dimensions specific to chronic venous insufficiency that generic tools miss. Its original construction and validation followed a structured psychometric pathway, producing an instrument that became widely adopted and extensively translated [10]. Subsequent international validation work supported its psychometric performance across countries and settings, reinforcing its role as a global venous Health Related Quality of Life instrument rather than a single-language artifact [24]. For the expert, CIVIQ's clinical value is that it converts "venous suffering" into measurable domains that align with what patients actually describe: difficulty standing, leg pain that shapes the day, embarrassment about appearance, frustration with chronic swelling and the erosion of well-being by persistent symptoms. For patients whose primary phenotype is varicose veins (often CEAP C2–C3), instruments tailored to varicosity-related impairment can be especially sensitive. The Aberdeen Varicose Vein Questionnaire (AVVQ) has been used widely and demonstrates reliability and validity in translated validation studies, supporting its utility in measuring treatment impact for varicose vein interventions [25]. Clinically, AVVQ tends to map well to the patient's functional narrative what they can and cannot do comfortably and how much the condition preoccupies them, therefore making it a practical complement to anatomic/hemodynamic assessment.

VEINES-QOL/Sym occupies a distinctive position because it was developed with rigorous methods and explicitly framed as a patient-reported outcome tool for chronic venous disorders of the leg. The original development and psychometric evaluation established it as a practical and scientifically robust instrument for evaluating both symptoms and quality-of-life in venous disease [26]. Additional work evaluating its validity and reliability in relevant populations supports its broader applicability and encourages its use when trials or services require a standardized PRO backbone also for patients affected by deep venous thrombosis [27]. For the expert designing studies or registries, VEINES-QOL/Sym is often attractive because it captures symptom intensity and functional impact with a structure suitable for longitudinal assessment, including responsiveness to change. Once ulceration develops, venous disease is no longer primarily a discomfort-and-function story: it becomes a wound-and-life story. Ulcer pain, exudate, odor, fear, dressing burden, mobility restriction, social withdrawal, and sleep disruption become dominant domains. Ulcer-specific quality-of-life instruments exist precisely because generic venous tools can underrepresent these wound-centered realities. The venous leg ulcer quality-of-life (VLU-QoL) questionnaire was developed and validated to capture ulcer-specific HRQoL burden, grounded in patient-derived content and psychometric validation [28]. In clinical terms, an ulcer-specific PRO can be the difference between describing "ulcer size reduction" and actually quantifying the patient's lived experience of healing versus persistent disease. Venous practice often uses clinician-derived severity scoring systems (for example VCSS) to quantify observable clinical severity and track change. These tools are valuable, but they do not replace PROs: they answer a different question. Validation work supports VCSS as a meaningful clinical assessment tool that can be integrated with other venous measures for global screening and severity characterization [29, 30].

The expert approach is to treat clinician scores and PROs as complementary layers:

- clinician scores quantify *what you observe*,
- PROs quantify *what the patient lives*,
- CEAP encodes *what the disease is and where it is*,
- duplex and physiologic tests explain *how it behaves*.

The most compelling reason PROs matter is simple: CVD is chronic, and chronic disease outcomes are not just technical endpoints. When ulcer healing reduces costs and improves HRQoL that is not merely an economic observation: it is a patient-centered outcome story that aligns clinical success with lived benefit [11]. PROs make that story measurable, comparable, and defensible in both scientific reporting and healthcare policy discussions (Table 9.1).

As general suggestion, CIVIQ is to be chosen whenever a clean, QoL-focused observation is needed, especially in multinational trials or longitudinal observational studies across the full CEAP spectrum. AVVQ can serve well for studying superficial venous disease, particularly when cosmetic impact and visible varicosities are important. VEINES-QOL/Sym is useful granular symptom tracking, eventually also in post-thrombotic syndrome, deep venous disease, or mixed pathology.

Patient-reported outcome measures are frequently treated as if they were interchangeable expressions of a single construct called "venous quality of life." This assumption is convenient, but it is only partially correct. CIVIQ, Aberdeen Varicose Vein Questionnaire (AVVQ), and VEINES-QOL/Sym do correlate with one another but never perfectly and the reasons for this are clinically and methodologically important.

Correlation among PROMs determines whether two instruments are redundant, complementary, or measuring meaningfully different aspects of the venous disease experience. For vascular experts interpreting trials, registries, or longitudinal cohorts, understanding how much these instruments correlate, and why they diverge is essential to avoid false equivalence and misinterpretation of patient-centered outcomes [31]. All three instruments were developed to capture the patient-perceived burden of chronic venous disease and therefore moderate to strong correlations are expected at the total-score level. Indeed, across multiple cohorts, global scores from CIVIQ, AVVQ, and VEINES instruments tend to move in the same direction as disease severity worsens or improves.

However, their conceptual starting points differ:

- CIVIQ was designed explicitly as a health-related quality of life (HRQoL) tool, integrating physical limitation, pain, psychological distress, and social impact.
- AVVQ emerged from surgical varicose vein practice and embeds cosmetic concern and

Table 9.1 Comparison among CIVIQ, Aberdeen Varicose Veins Questionnaire, VEINES-QOL/Sym

Comparison of venous disease specific patient reported outcome measures			
	CIVIQ (Chronic Venous Insufficiency Questionnaire)	AVVQ (Aberdeen Varicose Vein Questionnaire)	VEINES-QOL/ VEINES-Sym
Primary purpose	Measure health-related quality of life (HRQoL) impact of chronic venous disease	Measure disease-specific severity and impact of varicose veins	Measure QoL and symptom burden in venous disease
Target population	Broad chronic venous disease (C1–C6)	Primarily varicose veins (C2–C4)	Broad venous disease (C1–C6, incl. PTS)
Original language/ origin	French/Europe	English/UK	English/North America
Number of items	20 (original CIVIQ-20)	13 questions + leg diagram	26 items total (combined pool)
	Short forms: CIVIQ-14		
Domains covered	Physical, psychological, pain, social	Pain, ankle swelling, ulceration, cosmetic concern, impact on daily life	Symptoms (pain, heaviness, swelling), physical function, emotional impact
Scoring structure	Likert scale (1–5); summed and transformed to 0–100	Weighted scoring; total score 0–100	Standardized T-scores (mean 50, SD 10)
Direction of score	Higher score = worse QoL	Higher score = worse disease impact	Higher score = better QoL/fewer symptoms
Symptom vs QoL emphasis	Primarily QoL	Mix of symptoms + cosmetic + functional	Explicit split: VEINES-Sym (symptoms) and VEINES-QOL (QoL)
Cosmetic sensitivity	Limited	High (unique strength)	Minimal
Ulcer sensitivity (C5–C6)	Moderate	Limited	Good
Responsiveness to intervention	Good for symptom-driven change	Very good after superficial venous interventions	Good, especially for symptom improvement
Use in RCTs/registries	Very common in European trials	Common in varicose vein surgery/ ablation trials	Common in north American trials, PTS studies
Cross-cultural validation	Extensive (many languages)	Moderate	Extensive
Administrative burden	Low–moderate	Moderate (diagram scoring required)	Moderate–high
Strengths	Robust QoL construct, well validated, easy to interpret	Sensitive to cosmetic and visible disease change	Strong symptom measurement, standardized scoring
Limitations	Less sensitive to cosmetic concerns	Less suitable for advanced ulcer disease	Less intuitive scoring for routine clinic use

visual disease burden alongside symptoms and functional impact.

- VEINES-QOL/Sym was developed with a strong emphasis on symptom quantification and standardized QoL measurement, particularly in populations with post-thrombotic syndrome and deep venous pathology.

Because of this, correlations are strongest where constructs overlap most (pain, heaviness, functional limitation) and weaker where one instrument uniquely captures aspects such as appearance or norm-based QoL scaling. When CIVIQ and AVVQ are administered to the same patients, most commonly in cohorts with superficial venous reflux, studies consistently demonstrate moderate to strong correlations, typically in the range of $r \approx 0.6$–0.8. This reflects their shared sensitivity to pain, edema, and activity limitation following interventions such as vein stripping or endovenous ablation.

Yet, the correlation is never perfect. AVVQ includes items that directly assess cosmetic dissatisfaction and visibility of varicosities, including the leg diagram, whereas CIVIQ intentionally avoids explicit aesthetic judgment. As a result, in patients whose primary indication for treatment is cosmetic distress rather than functional impairment, AVVQ scores may remain high despite relatively preserved CIVIQ scores. This divergence has been observed in analyses examining responsiveness of individual questionnaire domains after superficial venous interventions, where AVVQ captures cosmetic improvement that is only weakly reflected in global HRQoL measures [32, 33]. Thus, CIVIQ and AVVQ correlate strongly enough to confirm convergent validity, but not strongly enough to be considered interchangeable, particularly in appearance-driven disease. Among the three instruments, CIVIQ and VEINES-QOL demonstrate the most consistent and strongest correlations. Because both are grounded in HRQoL theory, inverse correlations between CIVIQ total score (higher = worse QoL) and VEINES-QOL score (higher = better QoL) frequently reach absolute values of $r \approx 0.7$–0.85 in mixed venous populations. Domain-level analyses reveal that CIVIQ pain and physical function components correlate particularly well with VEINES-Sym, which focuses on day-to-day symptoms such as aching, heaviness, swelling, and fatigue. These relationships support the view that both instruments are capturing a common latent construct related to symptom-driven impairment, even though their scoring systems and scaling differ. Importantly, VEINES instruments often demonstrate greater sensitivity in populations with post-thrombotic syndrome or combined superficial and deep venous disease, where symptom fluctuation is prominent and global HRQoL tools may be less responsive. This distinction was already evident in the original validation and comparative discussions of venous QoL instruments, which emphasized VEINES as particularly suited to deep venous pathology, eventually also in the elderly [34]. Direct comparisons between AVVQ and VEINES instruments show moderate correlations, generally lower than those observed with CIVIQ. Reported associations typically fall around $r \approx 0.5$–0.7, reflecting partial construct overlap but meaningful divergence. This weaker correlation is conceptually coherent. AVVQ assigns substantial weight to cosmetic impact and localized surface disease, whereas VEINES deliberately excludes appearance-related distress and instead emphasizes symptom frequency, intensity, and functional consequences using standardized scoring. In cohorts dominated by symptom-driven indications, correlations strengthen; in cohorts where cosmetic concern is central, correlations weaken. The implication is clear: AVVQ and VEINES answer related but distinct clinical questions. One captures how the leg looks and feels to the patient, the other how venous disease affects daily functioning and well-being across a broader physiologic spectrum [31]. Three expert-level factors explain why correlations among these PROMs are consistently incomplete. First, they are built on different latent constructs. Even when instruments are labeled "QoL," they operationalize quality of life differently, and AVVQ explicitly integrates domains that HRQoL instruments intentionally exclude. Second, scaling and score direction differ: CIVIQ and AVVQ use intuitive summative

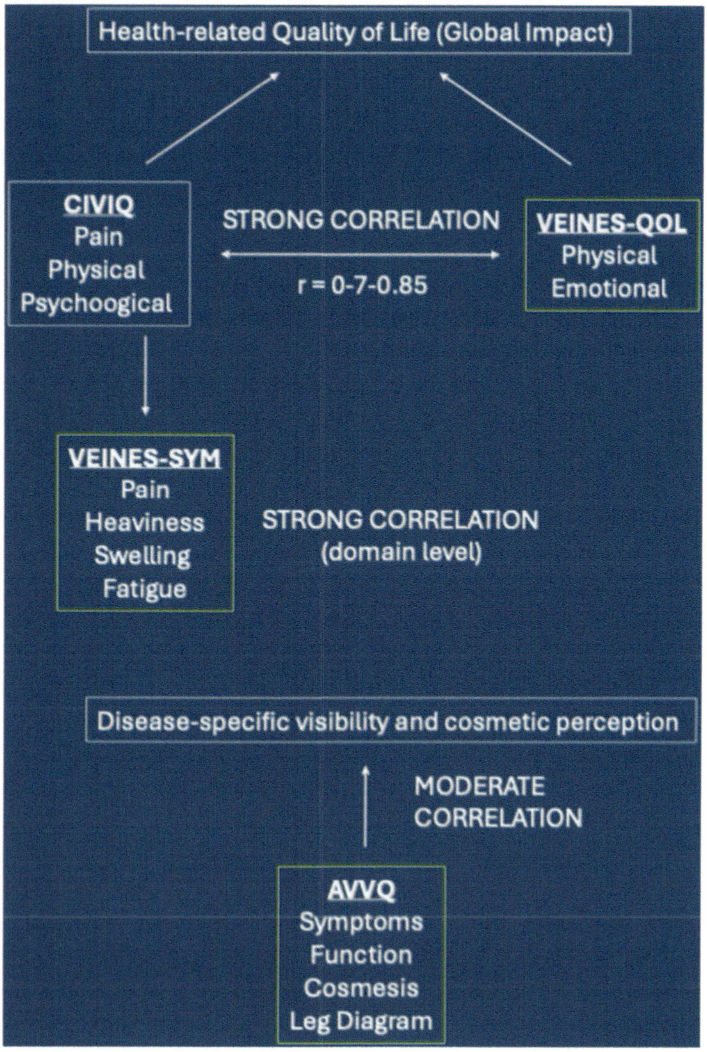

Fig. 9.1 CIVIQ, VEINES-QOL/SYM, AVVQ correlations. CIVIQ is at the center of the global HRQoL construct. VEINES-QOL overlaps most strongly with CIVIQ at the total-score level. VEINES-Sym overlaps strongly at the symptom-domain level, even when QoL scores diverge. AVVQ overlaps only partially with CIVIQ and VEINES because it uniquely captures cosmetic and visual disease burden, which weakens global correlations

scores where higher values indicate worse status, while VEINES uses norm-based standardized scores where higher values indicate better health. This difference introduces nonlinearity and attenuates correlation coefficients, especially at score extremes. Third, disease phenotype matters. Correlations are strongest in C2–C3 superficial reflux, weaker in ulcer-dominant disease, and most variable in post-thrombotic or obstructive venous pathology, where symptom burden and functional impairment may diverge from visible disease. The existing correlation data argue strongly against treating CIVIQ, AVVQ, and VEINES-QOL/Sym as interchangeable. High correlation supports construct validity, not redundancy. Even correlations approaching 0.8 leave substantial non-overlapping variance that can be clinically meaningful. For this reason, expert trial design increasingly favors one carefully chosen PROM, aligned with disease phenotype and intervention, rather than multiple overlapping instruments. CIVIQ or VEINES-QOL/Sym are generally preferred for broad CVD and deep venous disease, whereas AVVQ remains uniquely valuable when cosmetic outcome is a primary endpoint (Fig. 9.1) [35].

The Varicose Vein Symptom Questionnaire (VVSymQ) is another patient-reported outcome measure specifically designed for chronic venous disease patients, but focused only on symptoms

(Heaviness, Aching, Swelling, Throbbing, Itching (HASTI)). Its design was aligned from inception with FDA guidance on patient-reported outcomes, emphasizing direct patient reporting, clear symptom definitions, short recall periods, and responsiveness to intervention Patients record symptoms using a daily electronic diary, minimizing recall bias and enhancing sensitivity to short-term clinical change. Importantly, VVSymQ intentionally excludes clinician interpretation, physical examination findings, cosmetic perception, and broader psychosocial impact. This narrow focus is a strength, not a limitation, when symptom relief is the endpoint of interest. Validation studies demonstrated strong reliability, construct validity, and responsiveness following endovenous and surgical interventions, confirming VVSymQ as a fit-for-purpose PRO for interventional trials [36]. The distinction between VVSymQ and the Venous Clinical Severity Score (VCSS) is fundamental. VCSS is a clinician-reported outcome that integrates observed physical findings (edema, skin changes, ulcer characteristics) with limited patient input (pain, compression use). It quantifies clinical consequence, not symptom experience per se. As such, VCSS is indispensable for longitudinal assessment of disease progression and tissue injury but is inherently constrained in its ability to detect short-term symptom fluctuation.

VVSymQ, by contrast, is entirely patient-reported, insensitive to skin findings and ulcer status, optimized for detecting rapid symptom change after intervention. Thus, VVSymQ and VCSS are complementary rather than competing instruments. VVSymQ answers "how does the patient feel today?"; VCSS answers "what is the clinical severity of the leg?". Their divergent constructs explain why correlations between symptom-only PROs and ClinROs are often modest, even when both improve after treatment. The CIVIQ represents a different philosophical approach. CIVIQ is a HRQoL instrument, integrating physical limitation, pain, psychological distress and social functioning into a single global construct. While symptom improvement contributes to CIVIQ score changes, CIVIQ is not a symptom instrument. A patient may report marked reduction in pain and heaviness (captured by VVSymQ) yet show only modest CIVIQ improvement if psychological or social domains remain unchanged. Conversely, CIVIQ may improve through reassurance or functional adaptation even when day-to-day symptoms persist. The VEINES-QOL/Sym instruments sit conceptually between VVSymQ and CIVIQ. VEINES-Sym captures symptom frequency and intensity, whereas VEINES-QOL measures broader functional and emotional impact using standardized, norm-based scoring.

Despite this overlap, VVSymQ differs in several key respects:

- VVSymQ uses daily recall, whereas VEINES relies on longer recall periods.
- VVSymQ was developed explicitly to satisfy regulatory PRO requirements, whereas VEINES was designed primarily as a clinical research tool.
- VVSymQ focuses on symptom severity and duration, not frequency or general bother.

As a result, VVSymQ is often more responsive to early post-intervention change, while VEINES-QOL provides a broader view of longer-term functional impact, particularly in deep venous or post-thrombotic disease. VVSymQ is a true patient-reported outcome specifically designed to measure symptoms of varicose vein disease. It differs fundamentally from VCSS (ClinRO), CIVIQ and VEINES (HRQoL instruments), and AVVQ (disease-specific, cosmetically sensitive PROM). Its strength lies in regulatory rigor and symptom responsiveness; its limitation is intentional construct narrowness. Used appropriately, VVSymQ adds clarity—not redundancy—to modern venous outcomes assessment. The AVVQ is perhaps the instrument most commonly conflated with VVSymQ, as both are used in varicose vein populations. However, their constructs diverge substantially. AVVQ integrates symptoms, functional limitation, cosmetic concern, and visual disease burden (via the leg diagram). VVSymQ deliberately excludes cosmetic perception and appearance-related distress. Consequently, AVVQ may remain elevated in patients whose symptoms have resolved but who remain dissatisfied with residual varicosities, whereas VVSymQ would register clear improvement. VVSymQ is a true patient-reported outcome specifically designed to measure symptoms of varicose vein disease. It differs fundamentally from VCSS (ClinRO), CIVIQ and VEINES (HRQoL instruments), and AVVQ (disease-specific, cosmetically sensitive PROM). Its strength lies in regulatory rigor and symptom responsiveness; its limitation is intentional construct narrowness. Used appropriately, VVSymQ adds clarity—not redundancy—to modern venous outcomes assessment. From an expert perspective, VVSymQ should be viewed as a precision instrument rather than a global outcome measure. Its optimal use cases include trials where symptom relief is the primary endpoint, early post-intervention assessment, regulatory or industry-sponsored studies requiring FDA-compliant PROs. VVSymQ should not be used in isolation to characterize disease severity or overall patient impact. Best practice pairs VVSymQ with VCSS for clinician-assessed severity, CIVIQ or VEINES-QOL for global QoL impact, AVVQ when cosmetic outcome is central.

4 Natural History and Disease Progression

Understanding the natural history of CVD requires a shift from episodic thinking like "the patient has varicose veins" or "the ulcer healed" to a longitudinal perspective in which venous pathology unfolds over decades. For the vascular expert, natural history is not an abstract epidemiologic construct; it is the explanatory framework that links early venous abnormalities to later disability, informs timing of intervention, and shapes expectations regarding recurrence, progression, and long-term outcomes. CVD is fundamentally a progressive disorder in a subset of patients, but that progression is neither linear nor universal. Some limbs remain clinically stable for years, while others traverse the full CEAP spectrum from C1 to C6 within a working lifetime. The challenge and opportunity for modern venous medicine lies in identifying the trajectories that matter and intervening when modification is still possible [37]. The natural history of CVD begins long before patients seek care. Epidemiologic cohorts reveal that venous reflux and early venous symptoms can exist in the absence of visible disease, suggesting that pathophysiologic processes may precede clinical expression by years. Longitudinal population studies demonstrate incident development of varicose veins and chronic venous insufficiency over time, confirming that CVD is not merely prevalent but actively accruing in adult populations. In the Edinburgh Vein Study, the appearance of new varicose veins and progression to more advanced disease occurred in a measurable proportion of participants over follow-up, particularly among those with baseline reflux, advancing age, and higher body mass index [7]. At this early stage, disease expression is often subtle: leg heaviness at the end of the day, transient ankle swelling, nocturnal cramps, or cosmetic concern without overt disability. Yet even here, the seeds of progression may already be present. Duplex studies in asymptomatic or minimally symptomatic individuals have shown that reflux can exist without overt signs, reinforcing the concept that visible disease lags behind hemodynamic abnormality [5]. From a natural-history standpoint, this lag creates a window of opportunity but also diagnostic ambiguity because not all early reflux will progress to clinically meaningful disease. When natural history is described using CEAP terminology, progression is often conceptualized as movement from lower to higher clinical classes. While intuitive, this simplification masks important nuance. Longitudinal observational data support the reality of such transitions, but also demonstrate that not all patients progress sequentially or predictably. Some patients develop edema early without prominent varicosities, others show extensive varicosities for decades without skin change. In population-based follow-up, progression to skin changes and ulceration is far less common than progression to varicose veins, yet these advanced classes account for a disproportionate share of morbidity and cost [4].

Importantly, CEAP progression is not merely cosmetic. Movement into C4–C6 reflects the accumulation of sustained venous hypertension and microcirculatory injury. Once skin changes appear, the disease biology has crossed a threshold in which inflammatory and fibrotic processes become entrenched, and spontaneous regression is uncommon without intervention. From a mechanistic standpoint, disease progression is best understood as an evolution of hemodynamic burden rather than simply an accumulation of visible signs. Longitudinal physiologic observations indicate that worsening reflux, expansion of refluxing segments, and the development or recognition of venous obstruction all contribute to increasing ambulatory venous hypertension [12]. Superficial reflux may initially dominate the phenotype, particularly in primary disease, but with time, deep venous involvement, whether reflux, obstruction, or both, becomes increasingly relevant in advanced cases. Post-thrombotic disease exemplifies an accelerated natural history: after deep vein thrombosis, valvular damage and residual obstruction can produce chronic venous hypertension within years rather than decades, dramatically shortening the timeline to skin change and ulceration in susceptible individuals [27]. The natural history of mixed disease is particularly important for experts because progression is often underestimated when only superficial pathology is addressed. Persistent or recurrent symptoms after superficial intervention may reflect unrecognized outflow obstruction or deep reflux that continues to drive venous hypertension, underscoring the importance of comprehensive assessment in patients with progressive or recurrent disease. Skin manifestations offer one of the clearest clinical narratives of progression. Edema (C3) represents a functional failure of venous and lymphatic compensation under sustained pressure. With time, repeated episodes of edema and inflammation promote dermal fibrosis, hyperpigmentation, and microvascular damage, culminating in lipodermatosclerosis and atrophie blanche (C4). These changes are not merely markers of severity: they are predictors of future ulceration. Microcirculatory studies show that tissue oxygenation and capillary reserve decline as disease advances, suggesting that once skin changes appear, the limb has entered a biologically vulnerable state [38]. Venous leg ulcers thus represent not an isolated event but the end-stage expression of years of cumulative microvascular injury. Perhaps the most defining feature of advanced CVD natural history is recurrence. Even when venous ulcers heal, recurrence rates remain substantial over long-term follow-up, particularly if underlying hemodynamic abnormalities persist. This recurrent pattern transforms ulcer disease from an episodic condition into a chronic relapsing disorder, with profound implications for quality of life and healthcare utilization. Leg ulcer healing alone does not reset the disease clock, rather the limb remains at high risk unless venous hypertension is durably reduced and compression adherence is maintained [39]. This reality explains why ulcer recurrence dominates long-term cost curves and why prevention of first ulceration or first recurrence is a central goal in venous disease management. Symptoms in CVD exhibit a fluctuating course that can obscure progression when assessed cross-sectionally. Patients may report heaviness, pain, and swelling influenced by activity, climate, hormonal factors, and adherence to compression. Yet longitudinally, symptom burden often increases as disease advances, even if day-to-day variability persists. Patient-reported outcome studies highlight that symptom severity and quality-of-life impairment tend to worsen with higher CEAP classes, but also that substantial heterogeneity exists within classes [40]. This reinforces a key natural-history insight: progression is not solely about moving from one clinical class to another; it is also about deepening functional and psychosocial impact within a given class. One of the most clinically relevant questions for experts is why some patients progress rapidly while others remain stable. Longitudinal studies suggest that progression is multifactorial, influenced by:

- Baseline reflux and extent of venous involvement.
- Obesity and weight gain over time.
- Pregnancy exposure.
- Occupational standing.
- Prior deep vein thrombosis.
- Possibly genetic or connective tissue factors.

However, no single factor reliably predicts progression in isolation. Instead, risk appears cumulative, and disease acceleration often coincides with life events that increase venous load or reduce compensatory capacity [41]. The concept of natural history must be interpreted cautiously in the modern era, because intervention itself modifies disease trajectories. Compression therapy, venous-active drugs use, superficial venous ablation, perforator treatment and correction of venous obstruction can all alter symptom burden, slow progression, and reduce ulcer recurrence when appropriately applied. Observational and interventional data suggest that timely treatment of reflux may reduce progression to skin changes and ulceration, although the magnitude of this preventive effect varies and continues to be refined by ongoing research [7, 42]. From an expert perspective, the most meaningful question is no longer whether CVD progresses as it clearly can, rather when and in whom intervention meaningfully alters that trajectory. This reframing positions natural history not as a passive description of inevitability, but as the baseline against which therapeutic impact must be measured. In synthesis, the natural history of chronic venous disease is best understood as a spectrum of potential trajectories rather than a single pathway. Many individuals will live with mild disease and limited progression, while a significant minority will experience escalating hemodynamic burden, skin injury, ulceration, and recurrence. Disease progression reflects the cumulative effect of venous hypertension on tissues over time, modulated by individual risk factors and altered, sometimes profoundly, by intervention. For vascular experts, mastery of CVD natural history is not academic; it is foundational. It informs prognosis, guides surveillance, frames discussions with patients, and underpins decisions about when to treat early disease aggressively and when to monitor conservatively. Above all, it reminds us that CVD is a lifelong condition whose story unfolds over years, not clinic visits and that our interventions write only part of that story.

5 Patient Selection and Pre-procedure Evaluation for Sclerotherapy of Lower Limb Chronic Venous Disease

Success in sclerotherapy is determined far less by the act of injection than by the rigor of patient selection and pre-procedure evaluation. Indeed, inappropriate selection is the dominant cause of suboptimal outcomes, recurrence, and patient dissatisfaction, whereas careful evaluation allows sclerotherapy to function as a precise, adaptable, and durable intervention across a wide spectrum of CVD. Unlike axial ablation, which often follows relatively standardized pathways, sclerotherapy is inherently individualized. It may be cosmetic or therapeutic, adjunctive or primary, ultrasound-guided or visually directed, liquid or foam. Each of these choices depends on a pre-procedure synthesis that integrates clinical narrative, physical findings, duplex ultrasound, systemic risk, and patient priorities. The evaluation process therefore serves three parallel goals: (1) confirming that the target veins are appropriate for sclerotherapy, (2) excluding conditions in which sclerotherapy may be ineffective or harmful, and (3) aligning procedural intent with realistic, patient-centered outcomes [43]. The clinical history is the foundation upon which all subsequent evaluation rests. CVD is, by definition, chronic and evolving, and the temporal dimension of symptoms often provides insights that imaging alone cannot. A detailed history should establish not only what symptoms are present, but how they behave over time. Venous symptoms classically worsen with prolonged standing or sitting, improve with elevation, and intensify toward the end of the day. Their chronicity, fluctuation, and relationship to activity are essential discriminators between venous and non-venous etiologies [44]. Equally important is symptom burden relative to visible disease. Many patients with extensive telangiectasias or reticular veins are asymptomatic, whereas others with minimal visible change report substantial discomfort, heaviness, or fatigue. This dissociation underscores why history must precede imaging and why sclerotherapy for symptoms should never be justified solely by appearance. Past venous history strongly influences candidacy. For example, prior deep vein thrombosis raises concerns regarding altered deep venous compliance, residual obstruction, and the compensatory role of superficial veins. Previous superficial interventions (surgical stripping, thermal ablation, or sclerotherapy) may alter anatomy, create atypical reflux pathways, or signal aggressive disease biology. In patients with recurrent disease, understanding why prior treatment failed is more important than documenting that it occurred. A comprehensive medical history must address systemic conditions that affect venous tone, healing, or thrombosis risk. Obesity, limited mobility, inflammatory disease, malignancy, and hormonal exposure all modulate outcomes. Medication review is essential, particularly anticoagulants, antiplatelet agents, and vasodilators. While anticoagulation is not an absolute contraindication to sclerotherapy, it influences technique, sclerosant choice, and post-procedure management. Physical examination anchors this history in objective findings. Examination should be performed in the standing position whenever feasible, as venous distension, reflux pathways and edema may be underestimated supine. Inspection documents the distribution and morphology of telangiectasias, reticular veins, varicosities, edema, skin inflammation, hyperpigmentation, lipodermatosclerosis, and ulceration, ideally categorized within the CEAP clinical framework. Palpation provides additional information: tenderness may suggest thrombophlebitis, induration indicates chronic inflammation or fibrosis, temperature changes may hint at infection or arterial compromise. Together, history and examination define the clinical problem that sclerotherapy is being asked to solve and whether it is the appropriate tool to do so. Duplex ultrasound is indispensable in the modern practice of sclerotherapy for lower limb CVD. While purely cosmetic sclerotherapy for isolated telangiectasias may be performed without imaging in selected cases, any therapeutic intent requires duplex confirmation of venous anatomy and function. Duplex ultrasound reveals the hidden architecture of venous disease, often contradicting assumptions based on surface appearance alone. A comprehensive duplex examination evaluates the superficial, perforator, and deep venous systems under physiologic conditions. Reflux testing should be performed with the patient standing or in reverse Trendelenburg, using standardized maneuvers to provoke flow reversal. Documentation of reflux duration, vein diameter, and segmental involvement are important, as well as the leaking reflux points, their re-entry and the hemodynamic load. Indeed, a common mistake is to consider only the diameter of the vein to be treated, without considering the possible flow volume and hemodynamic impact on the specific district. This factor could significantly alter the recurrence risk and the sclerotherapy features choice [45]. For sclerotherapy, duplex ultrasound answers several pivotal questions. Is there axial reflux in the great or small saphenous vein that would overwhelm isolated treatment of tributaries? Is there a hemodynamic overload at the junctions (sapheno-femoral, sapheno-popliteal, perforators/tributary confluence) (Fig. 9.2)? Are the target veins directly connected to refluxing trunks or deep veins, increasing the risk of sclerosant migration? Are there incompetent perforators feeding skin changes or ulcers that require targeted therapy?

Ultrasound is also essential for safety. It identifies vein depth, diameter, tortuosity, and proximity to nerves or arteries, guiding sclerosant concentration, wetness and volume. In ultrasound-guided foam sclerotherapy, duplex imaging becomes an extension of the operator's hands, enabling real-time visualization of sclerosant distribution and early detection of unintended deep venous entry [46].

Perhaps most critically, duplex ultrasound protects against misdirected therapy. Patients with symptoms driven primarily by deep venous

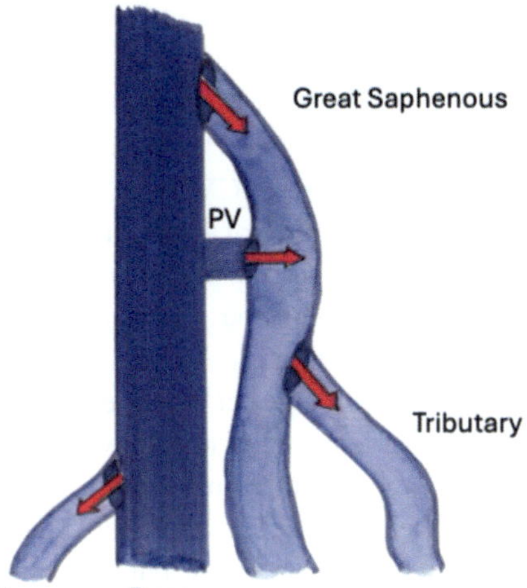

Fig. 9.2 Junctional points (in red) where assessing the hemodynamic overload is of great importance to determine possible recurrence risk and consequently adequate sclerotherapy features

obstruction or advanced post-thrombotic disease are unlikely to benefit from superficial sclerotherapy alone. Identifying these patterns pre-procedure prevents ineffective treatment and redirects care toward more appropriate strategies. Risk stratification in sclerotherapy encompasses procedural safety, thrombotic risk, neurologic events, and long-term disease behavior. Although sclerotherapy has a strong safety record, its risks are not uniform across patient populations. The vascular expert must therefore individualize risk assessment rather than rely on generalized safety profiles. Thrombotic risk is among the most frequently discussed concerns. Factors such as prior deep venous thrombosis, known thrombophilia, malignancy, prolonged immobility, and estrogen exposure increase the likelihood of post-procedural thrombosis, particularly with foam sclerotherapy. While the absolute incidence is low, risk stratification informs decisions regarding sclerosant volume, wetness, biocompatible gasses, session staging, compression intensity and post-procedure surveillance [47]. Evaluation of the deep venous system is mandatory before therapeutic sclerotherapy in symptomatic CVD. Superficial veins are not independent conduits: they function within a pressure-sharing system dominated by deep venous competence and outflow. Treating superficial veins without understanding deep venous behavior risks disrupting compensatory pathways. Duplex assessment should document deep vein patency, compressibility, reflux, and flow patterns. Residual obstruction or valvular incompetence following DVT alters venous compliance and pressure transmission. In post-thrombotic limbs, superficial veins may serve as essential collateral pathways, and their elimination can worsen symptoms rather than relieve them [45]. Recognition of proximal outflow obstruction is particularly important in patients with edema, venous claudication, recurrent ulceration, or poor response to prior superficial therapy. While duplex ultrasound may suggest iliac obstruction, additional imaging may be required in selected cases. In these settings, sclerotherapy should be deferred or used only after addressing the dominant hemodynamic lesion. Ultrasound pre-operative evaluation is fundamental also to identify pelvic escape points. Eventual deeper assessment by trans-vaginal ultrasound can be integrated in the suspect of pelvic venous disorders. It's fundamental to scan the patient in standing or reverse Trendelenburg position in order to avoid masking eventual refluxes. Ultrasound can become extremely useful also in case of echo-guided sclerotherapy treatment of pelvic sources [48]. Chapter 13 is entirely dedicated to the pelvic topic. Assessment of arterial circulation is a critical safety step, particularly when compression therapy accompanies sclerotherapy or when skin changes and ulceration are present. Mixed arterial and venous disease is common in older patients and those with diabetes or smoking history. Clinical evaluation includes palpation of pulses and inspection for trophic changes suggestive of ischemia. When uncertainty exists, objective testing such as ankle–brachial index measurement is warranted. Significant arterial disease does not necessarily preclude sclerotherapy, but it influences compression strategies and healing expectations and must be incorporated into procedural planning. Failure to assess arterial status risks ischemic complications from compression and misinterpretation of non-healing ulcers. Arterial evaluation is an integral component of comprehensive limb assessment. The informed consent process for sclerotherapy is best understood as a continuation of pre-procedure evaluation rather than a separate administrative step. Patients should understand the rationale for sclerotherapy in their specific case and how it integrates with other treatment options. Alternatives, including compression alone, endovenous ablation, surgery, or observation, should be discussed in context, emphasizing why a particular strategy is recommended. Risks should be communicated clearly, distinguishing common, self-limited effects from rare but serious complications. The likelihood of multiple sessions, the potential for recurrence, and the need for ongoing surveillance should be explicit. Equally important is discussion of post-procedure responsibilities: compression use, activity modification, and recognition of warning signs. When informed consent reflects individualized evaluation rather than generic disclosure, it becomes a therapeutic tool, aligning expectations, improving adherence, and strengthening the clinician–patient partnership. Patient selection and pre-procedure evaluation define the success of sclerotherapy more than any sclerosant or technique. Through meticulous history, careful examination, comprehensive duplex ultrasound, thoughtful risk stratification, and system-level vascular assessment, the vascular expert transforms sclerotherapy from a simple injection into a strategic intervention. In doing so, sclerotherapy fulfills its enduring role in venous medicine: precise, adaptable, and effective when guided by deep understanding rather than surface appearance.

6 Special Populations for Sclerotherapy

Sclerotherapy is often described in guidelines and training curricula as a broadly applicable technique, adaptable to a wide range of venous morphologies and clinical presentations. Yet the apparent universality of sclerotherapy can be misleading. In daily vascular practice, the patients most frequently encountered are those whose age, comorbidities, prior interventions or disease severity place them outside the "standard" population on which early evidence and simplified algorithms were built. In these special populations, the biology of CVD, the risks of intervention, and the metrics of success are fundamentally altered. The question is therefore not whether sclerotherapy can be performed, but how it should be modified, contextualized, or subordinated within a broader management strategy. In elderly patients, individuals with prior venous surgery, those with thrombophilia, obese patients, and patients with chronic venous ulcers, sclerotherapy remains relevant, but only when guided by an understanding of altered venous physiology, natural history, and patient priorities. Across all these groups, expert practice is defined by restraint as much as by technical skill. Elderly patients represent one of the fastest-growing populations undergoing evaluation for chronic venous disease and venous intervention. Aging is associated with cumulative exposure to venous hypertension, progressive degeneration of venous valves, reduced calf muscle pump efficiency, and diminished microcirculatory reserve. As a result, elderly patients often present with advanced CEAP classes, long-standing symptoms, and a complex interplay of venous, lymphatic, and systemic contributors to leg morbidity. From a pathophysiologic standpoint, venous disease in the elderly is rarely isolated. Deep venous reflux, residual obstruction from remote thrombosis, reduced mobility, and cardiac or renal contributors to edema frequently coexist. These factors limit the degree to which superficial intervention alone can normalize venous pressures. Skin integrity is a central concern. Age-related dermal thinning, impaired wound healing, and increased susceptibility to hyperpigmentation or necrosis require conservative sclerosant concentrations, meticulous injection technique, and careful post-procedure compression. Foam sclerotherapy may be advantageous in reducing injected volumes, but it also demands heightened vigilance regarding thrombotic and neurologic risks. Equally important is reframing treatment goals. Cosmetic improvement is rarely the primary objective in elderly patients: symptom relief, reduction of recurrent cellulitis or bleeding, facilitation of ulcer healing and preservation of mobility are more meaningful endpoints. When expectations are aligned accordingly, sclerotherapy can significantly improve quality of life even in the presence of advanced disease. Patients who have undergone prior venous surgery or endovenous intervention constitute a distinct and increasingly prevalent subgroup. Recurrence after treatment is not an anomaly but a recognized feature of chronic venous disease progression. Mechanisms include neovascularization, development of new reflux pathways, progression of untreated segments and altered flow dynamics following initial intervention [49]. A recent meta-analysis showcased the competitiveness of foam sclerotherapy in recurrent varicosities management [50]. In this population, sclerotherapy often assumes a central role because recurrent veins are frequently tortuous, superficial, and anatomically unsuitable for repeat thermal ablation or surgical excision. Ultrasound-guided sclerotherapy allows precise targeting of residual refluxing tributaries, neovascular channels, and incompetent perforators that contribute to symptoms or skin changes However, prior surgery profoundly alters anatomy. Scar tissue may tether veins close to the skin, increasing the risk of pigmentation or necrosis. Disrupted fascial planes and atypical venous connections raise the possibility of unintended sclerosant migration. For this reason, comprehensive duplex ultrasound mapping is mandatory, with careful documentation of deep venous connections and residual axial reflux. Treating visible recurrence without addressing persistent proximal drivers is a common cause of repeated failure.

Psychologically, these patients often arrive with frustration and diminished trust in venous interventions. Expert counseling reframes recurrence not as procedural failure but as an expected manifestation of a chronic, progressive condition. When sclerotherapy is presented as part of an ongoing disease-management strategy rather than a definitive "fix," patient satisfaction and adherence improve. Patients with thrombophilia pose one of the most complex decision-making challenges in sclerotherapy. Inherited thrombophilias (such as factor V Leiden or prothrombin gene mutation) and acquired prothrombotic states (including antiphospholipid syndrome, malignancy, or chronic inflammatory disease) increase baseline thrombotic risk and heighten concern regarding procedure-related thrombosis. Importantly, thrombophilia is not an absolute contraindication to sclerotherapy. The critical task is individualized risk stratification. A detailed thrombotic history, number of events, provoking factors, recurrence, and current anticoagulation status are often more informative than laboratory abnormalities alone. Patients with prior unprovoked or recurrent deep vein thrombosis require a higher threshold for intervention than those with isolated laboratory findings and no clinical events. Technical modifications are frequently employed in this population. These include limiting foam volume, staging treatments, avoiding treatment of large axial segments, adequate thromboprophylaxis evaluation and ensuring meticulous ultrasound guidance to prevent deep venous entry. Compression therapy and early ambulation are particularly critical, and post-procedure duplex surveillance may be warranted in selected cases. Equally important is transparent communication. Patients with thrombophilia must understand that sclerotherapy carries incremental risk and that its benefits must clearly outweigh that risk. When this balance is respected, sclerotherapy can be performed safely and effectively, even in high-risk populations and can actually present a smaller prevalence of complications compared to other procedural options. Obesity is a powerful modifier of both chronic venous disease progression and response to intervention. Increased intra-abdominal pressure, impaired calf muscle pump function, systemic inflammation, and reduced mobility contribute to more severe venous hypertension and accelerated disease progression. Obese patients are disproportionately represented among those with edema, skin changes, and recurrent disease. From a technical standpoint, obesity complicates sclerotherapy. Target veins may be deeper and less visible, increasing reliance on ultrasound guidance. Accurate compression, essential for endothelial injury, vein closure, and complication prevention, is often difficult due to limb shape and discomfort, reducing treatment efficacy. These factors partially explain higher recurrence rates and more modest cosmetic outcomes in obese patients. Recent literature confirms the value of sclerotherapy also in this specific type of patients, whenever performed by properly trained healthcare professionals, favoring foam over liquid formulation [51]. Counseling is critical. Weight management, mobility enhancement, and long-term compression use are not ancillary recommendations but central determinants of outcome. When these factors are ignored, technically adequate sclerotherapy may be perceived as ineffective, underscoring the need for holistic disease management. Patients with chronic venous ulcers represent the most severe and biologically complex end of the chronic venous disease spectrum. Ulceration reflects years of sustained venous hypertension, microcirculatory dysfunction, and inflammatory remodeling. In this population, sclerotherapy can bring the advantage of targeting in particular multi-truncular refluxes, including eventually present incompetent perforating veins feeding the ulcer-related hypertension [52]. The rationale for sclerotherapy in ulcer patients is fundamentally hemodynamic. Elimination of refluxing superficial veins or incompetent perforators can reduce venous pressure at the ulcer bed, improve microcirculatory conditions, and facilitate healing when combined with effective compression. However, these patients are uniquely vulnerable. Skin is fragile, infection risk is elevated, and healing capacity is limited. Sclerotherapy must therefore be performed with conservative sclerosant dosing, meticulous ultrasound guidance, and staged treatment plans. Aggressive treatment risks provoking inflammation that may delay healing or precipitate complications.

Expectation management is paramount. Ulcer healing depends on multiple variables, compression adherence, nutrition, mobility, arterial sufficiency, and comorbidity control. Sclerotherapy addresses only one element of this complex pathophysiology. When framed appropriately, however, it can meaningfully alter the long-term trajectory of ulcer disease by reducing recurrence and improving quality of life [53]. Special populations expose the limits of algorithmic thinking in venous medicine. In elderly patients, those with prior surgery, thrombophilia, obesity, or chronic ulcers, sclerotherapy remains a powerful tool, but only when guided by an appreciation of altered physiology, heightened risk, and modified goals. Expert practice lies not in expanding indications indiscriminately, but in integrating sclerotherapy thoughtfully within individualized, long-term management strategies. Across these populations, the defining question is not "Can this vein be sclerosed?" but rather, "How does sclerotherapy serve this patient's overall venous trajectory?" When answered with rigor and humility, sclerotherapy fulfills its most valuable role: targeted, adaptable, and patient-centered care within the lifelong context of chronic venous disease.

7 Outcomes and Efficacy of Sclerotherapy for Chronic Venous Disease Treatment

Assessment of outcomes after sclerotherapy for CVD has matured from an early focus on visual vein disappearance to a sophisticated, multidimensional evaluation encompassing anatomy, symptoms, quality of life, recurrence, and long-term safety. This evolution mirrors the broader conceptual shift in venous medicine: CVD is now understood as a chronic, progressive disorder rather than a collection of isolated veins. Consequently, sclerotherapy outcomes must be interpreted within the context of disease biology, patient selection, and longitudinal management rather than as isolated technical achievements [54, 55]. Outcomes data serve two purposes. First, they inform evidence-based selection of sclerotherapy relative to alternative interventions. Second, they provide a framework for counseling patients realistically, balancing optimism regarding symptom relief and functional improvement with transparency about recurrence and the need for ongoing care. The literature on sclerotherapy is extensive but heterogeneous, reflecting variation in techniques, sclerosants, outcome definitions, and follow-up duration. When synthesized thoughtfully, however, these data describe a coherent efficacy profile that supports sclerotherapy as a durable and adaptable component of modern venous practice, moreover highlighting anatomical cases in which sometimes it can be the only possible option. Anatomical success remains the most traditional and easily quantifiable endpoint in sclerotherapy studies. It is generally defined as complete occlusion or fibrosis of the treated vein segment, assessed either clinically or by duplex ultrasound. Reported anatomical success rates vary widely, ranging from modest to excellent, depending on vein type, diameter, sclerosant formulation, technique, and duration of follow-up. This variability underscores the importance of interpreting success rates in context rather than as absolute benchmarks. For telangiectasias and reticular veins, anatomical clearance rates are consistently high, often exceeding 80–90% after one or more treatment sessions. These outcomes can be influenced by sclerosant concentration, injection technique and post-procedure compression, but are also affected by patient-specific factors such as hormonal exposure and underlying reflux. Even in this seemingly straightforward population, durable anatomical success is contingent upon addressing proximal hemodynamic drivers when present. An entire Cochrane review has been dedicated to sclerotherapy of telangiectasia and reticular veins. Thirty-five randomized comparative trials were included, yet the certainty of evidence was downgraded to moderate or low due to the clinical heterogeneity and imprecision from the wide confidence intervals. In comparison with other sclerosing agents, polidocanol resulted competitive in pain minimization, while sodium tetradecyl sulfate was associated with more hyperpigmentation, matting and possibly pain. Foam vs liquid did not show a significant improvement in terms of telangiectasia resolution or improvement, hyperpigmentation, or pain. With low certainty of evidence, foam was associated with more matting. A possible synergistic effect with transdermal laser was reported [56]. In larger tributaries and saphenous trunks, ultrasound-guided foam sclerotherapy has demonstrated significantly higher occlusion rates than liquid sclerotherapy. Randomized trials and systematic reviews show that foam enhances endothelial contact and displacement of intraluminal blood, leading to improved early closure rates. While thermal ablation techniques often demonstrate higher long-term occlusion in axial veins, foam sclerotherapy remains competitive in selected anatomies, particularly in moderate-diameter veins and recurrent disease. Moreover, sclerotherapy should not be compared in its one-shot performance only, rather in the possible strategic plan of staged procedures. Yet, even in the single-shot option, it remains competitive with surgery and endovenous thermal and nonthermal options. While anatomical recurrence in larger veins such as the saphenous trunks is better controlled by endovenous laser or radiofrequency or properly validated glues, data show that, in terms of patient-reported outcomes, quality of life, and possible cost-control, foam sclerotherapy can show competitive results [55]. Another Cochrane review analyzed ultrasound-guided foam in comparison of the other possible procedures for great saphenous vein reflux management. Endovenous laser ablation showed a better performance in terms of occlusion rate only after the 3-years follow-up. There was no clear difference in recurrence up to 3 years and at 5 years (OR 0.68, 95% CI 0.20–2.36; 2 studies, 443 participants; and OR 1.08, 95% CI 0.40–2.87; 2 studies, 418 participants; very low-certainty evidence, respectively). Foam sclerotherapy versus high ligation and stripping showed a possible benefit of the latter only after 5 years as well: up to 3 years, no clear difference was detected in recurrence (OR 1.81, 95% CI 0.87–3.77; 3 studies, 822 participants; low-certainty evidence) [57]. Two years after the above mentioned Cochrane review, a further meta-analysis highlighted the potentials of appropriate foam sclerotherapy in all CVD CEAP spectrum from C1 to C6. 9670 cases were analyzed, demonstrating how sclerotherapy is the most effective therapy for reducing clinical severity and improving quality of life (VEINES-QOL). Yet the observation time [43]. It must be remembered how the above mentioned data have been produced with whatever kind of foam produced in a real world setting, therefore involving possibly also not appropriate foam production methods making the same foam unstable and/or less performing. In 2024, a meta-analysis assessed the performance of the most standardized Varithena™ foam, demonstrating its competitiveness with laser and radiofrequency techniques in the saphenous vein ablation (OR, 0.65; 95% CI 0.36–1.18; $P = 0.16$). Moreover, it proved the importance of recognizing the difference between physician compounded and automated foam production, showcasing the significant difference in performance among the two (OR, 2.91; 95% CI 1.58–5.37; $P < 0.01$). The median of the follow-up was 4 years, making the publication of great clinical interest regarding the present appropriate treatment of also the more advanced CVD scenarios. This aspect has been included also in the recently published institutional recommendations of the VALID document [58]. A 5-years multi-center follow-up on the performance of ultrasound-guided foam sclerotherapy of the saphenous trunk was published in 2025. The recurrence rate was 26% at a median of 4 years, yet only 14.4% of the patients required treatment because symptomatic. A caliber of more than 8 mm was identified as a risk factor for recurrence (at 5-years follow-up, 91.3% for diameters <8 mm vs 46% for diameters>8 mm; $P < 0.0001$) [59]. Eight years follow-up is the longest the authors of this chapter were able to identify and it deals with the comparison between ultrasound-guided foam sclerotherapy and surgical stripping. In such a long observation time, surgery performed better in terms of reflux-free patients numbers (33·1 vs 49·7%, $P = 0.009$) yet no differences were reported in quality of life, highlighting once again the importance of the outcome measures and of the appropriateness concepts [60]. The heterogeneity found in the literature on sclerotherapy performance mirrors the heterogeneity in the physician-compounded foam methods. Combining homogeneous anatomical and hemodynamic reflux patterns with standardized sclerotherapy injections is mandatory to produce reliable data.

Crucially, anatomical success is time-dependent. Duplex follow-up studies reveal that early occlusion does not necessarily translate into permanent vein fibrosis. Partial recanalization, segmental patency, or development of alternative reflux pathways may occur months or years after treatment, particularly in patients with untreated proximal reflux or deep venous pathology. This temporal dimension reinforces a core expert principle: anatomical success should be viewed as a dynamic outcome rather than a static endpoint. Clinical improvement is often the outcome most relevant to both patients and clinicians. Numerous observational studies and controlled trials demonstrate that sclerotherapy produces significant reductions in symptoms such as heaviness, aching, throbbing, swelling, itching, and localized inflammation. These benefits are most pronounced when refluxing veins contributing to venous hypertension are effectively targeted [2]. Importantly, clinical improvement does not always correlate directly with anatomical outcomes. Some patients experience substantial symptom relief despite partial recanalization or incomplete anatomical closure, while others remain symptomatic despite technically successful vein obliteration. This apparent paradox reflects the multifactorial nature of venous symptoms, which are influenced by calf muscle pump function, deep venous competence, microcirculatory health, and behavioral factors such as activity level and compression adherence [61]. In patients with advanced CVD, particularly those with edema, skin changes, or ulceration, sclerotherapy is rarely the sole determinant of clinical improvement. Instead, it functions as part of a multimodal strategy that includes axial reflux control, compression therapy, venous active drugs, wound care, and lifestyle modification. Within this framework, sclerotherapy contributes to reduced inflammatory episodes, fewer bleeding events, and improved local symptom control. Improvements in validated clinical severity metrics such as the Venous Clinical Severity Score (VCSS) have been documented following sclerotherapy, supporting its role in symptom-driven care, moreover highlighting no difference at 3 years follow-up between 1% and 3% polidocanol [62]. CIVIQ and VEINES-QOL/Sym demonstrated significant post-sclerotherapy improvements in domains related to pain, physical function, social interaction, and emotional well-being. These gains often occur even when anatomical outcomes are modest, highlighting the dissociation between vein closure and patient-perceived benefit [63]. Quality-of-life improvements are particularly striking in patients whose symptoms interfere with occupational standing, daily activity, or sleep. Relief from chronic heaviness or aching can restore functional capacity and participation in work and social roles. In patients with venous ulcers, sclerotherapy-targeting refluxing superficial veins or perforators has been associated with improved ulcer-related QoL when integrated with compression and wound care. Ulcer-specific instruments such as the VLU-QoL capture these benefits more sensitively than generic measures [64–66]. QoL outcomes serve as a critical counterbalance to purely technical success. They reinforce the principle that venous interventions should be judged by their impact on patient well-being rather than by imaging alone. In conclusion, outcomes and efficacy in sclerotherapy for chronic venous disease cannot be captured by a single metric or time point. Anatomical success, symptom relief, quality-of-life improvement, recurrence management, and long-term safety each represent distinct but interdependent dimensions of therapeutic value. The cumulative literature demonstrates that sclerotherapy is effective, safe, and adaptable when applied within a framework of appropriate patient selection and comprehensive venous assessment. For the vascular expert, the true measure of efficacy lies not in short-term vein closure rates but in the sustained ability to reduce disease burden, improve patient well-being, and manage recurrence over time. Viewed through this longitudinal and patient-centered lens, sclerotherapy stands not as a secondary option but as a foundational modality in the modern management of chronic venous disease.

8 Future Perspectives

Sclerotherapy occupies a paradoxical position in modern venous medicine. It is one of the oldest therapeutic modalities still in routine use, yet it remains among the most adaptable and future-facing interventions in CVD. This apparent contradiction reflects the unique nature of sclerotherapy: it is not defined by a single device or fixed protocol, but by a biologic interaction between sclerosant, vein wall, hemodynamics, and patient-specific factors. As understanding of venous biology deepens and technology advances, sclerotherapy is not being replaced, rather, it is being refined, contextualized, and integrated into increasingly sophisticated treatment paradigms. Future perspectives in sclerotherapy therefore extend beyond incremental technical improvement. They encompass a broader rethinking of how venous disease is classified, imaged, treated, and studied, with sclerotherapy evolving from a largely technique-driven intervention into a precision tool within personalized venous care. Advances in sclerosing agents, imaging and guidance technologies, data integration, and clinical research are collectively reshaping both the practice and the evidence base of sclerotherapy. One of the most active areas of innovation involves foam technology. Foam sclerotherapy represented a conceptual leap by enhancing endothelial contact and reducing dilution by intraluminal blood. Ongoing research focuses on optimizing foam characteristics, including bubble size distribution, stability, viscosity, and gas composition. Focusing on fully automated foam production methods allowing the combination of different sclerosing drug concentrations together with several biocompatible gasses combinations is the pillar over which building the present and future of a sclerotherapy that should be as close as possible to the total elimination of the nitrogen components. Only in this way it will be possible to maximize performance and safety at the same time, while guaranteeing proper homogeneous data collection for research and development purposes. Imaging has already transformed sclerotherapy, and further advances are poised to redefine its precision. Duplex ultrasound remains the cornerstone of venous diagnosis and procedural guidance, enabling real-time visualization of anatomy, reflux, and sclerosant distribution. Continuous improvements in ultrasound resolution, Doppler sensitivity, and ergonomics are expanding the range of veins that can be treated safely and effectively, particularly in obese patients, recurrent disease, and deep or atypical venous anatomy. High-frequency probes and enhanced Doppler algorithms allow visualization of smaller perforators, neovascular channels, and subdermal venous plexuses that were previously difficult to assess. These advances improve targeting accuracy and reduce unintended sclerosant migration, directly impacting safety and efficacy. As imaging fidelity improves, the boundary between "visual" and "ultrasound-guided" sclerotherapy continues to blur, with image guidance becoming the default rather than the exception. Beyond conventional duplex, adjunctive imaging modalities are under investigation. Contrast-enhanced ultrasound may allow more precise visualization of venous flow dynamics and sclerosant dispersion, potentially enabling real-time titration of injected volume. Near-infrared and vein-visualization technologies, currently used primarily in cosmetic or cannulation settings, may evolve into complementary mapping tools for complex superficial venous networks. Procedural guidance is also becoming more data-driven. Integration of ultrasound imaging with digital mapping, procedural documentation, and longitudinal outcome tracking supports standardized reporting and facilitates comparison across time and treatments. Looking ahead, artificial intelligence–assisted image interpretation may help identify reflux patterns, predict treatment response, and flag anatomic risk factors, transforming imaging from a diagnostic modality into an active decision-support system [67]. Perhaps the most transformative future direction is the shift toward personalized venous treatment. CVD is increasingly recognized as a heterogeneous condition, with wide variability in onset, progression, symptom expression, and response to intervention. Sclerotherapy, by virtue of its flexibility, is particularly well suited to personalized application, provided that patient phenotyping and outcome measurement continue to advance. Personalization begins with refined clinical and hemodynamic characterization. Advances in severity scoring systems and patient-reported outcome measures enable clinicians to move beyond binary treatment decisions toward nuanced stratification of disease burden and therapeutic goals. In this framework, sclerotherapy may be optimized for symptom relief in one patient, ulcer recurrence prevention in another, and cosmetic improvement in a third, each guided by distinct success metrics. Biologic personalization represents a more speculative but potentially powerful frontier. Genetic predisposition, inflammatory profiles, and connective tissue characteristics likely influence vein wall response to sclerosants and susceptibility to recurrence. Translational studies suggest that variability in extracellular matrix remodeling and inflammatory signaling contributes to differential outcomes after venous intervention. While routine biologic profiling is not yet feasible, future integration of molecular markers could inform sclerosant selection, concentration, and treatment frequency. Equally important is personalization driven by patient priorities. Increasing integration of quality-of-life instruments into routine practice allows outcomes to be aligned with what patients value most: pain reduction, functional improvement, cosmetic appearance, or ulcer prevention. In this model, success is defined not by uniform anatomic endpoints but by concordance between intervention and patient-defined goals. Despite its long history and widespread use, sclerotherapy remains characterized by significant research gaps. Many aspects of contemporary practice are supported by observational studies, expert consensus, or extrapolation rather than by high-quality randomized evidence. Addressing these gaps is essential for refining indications, standardizing techniques and strengthening guideline recommendations. One major gap lies in long-term comparative effectiveness. While short- and mid-term outcomes are well documented, fewer studies provide robust long-term comparisons between sclerotherapy, thermal ablation, and surgical approaches across diverse patient populations. Extended follow-up trials are needed to clarify durability, recurrence patterns, cost-effectiveness, and patient-centered outcomes over more than 5 years. Another critical gap concerns patient selection and prediction of response. Predictors of favorable or unfavorable outcomes, particularly in advanced disease, obesity, post-thrombotic state or special populations are incompletely defined. Prospective studies integrating duplex findings, clinical severity scores, and patient-reported outcomes could yield predictive models that refine candidacy and expectation management. Real-world data collection by means of appropriate global registries are needed in order to develop appropriate precision medicine in this specific context. Safety research also continues to evolve. Although the overall safety profile of sclerotherapy is well-established, ongoing surveillance is needed to refine risk stratification for thrombotic and neurologic events, especially as foam techniques and sclerosant formulations evolve. Large registries and pragmatic trials remain essential complements to randomized studies in capturing rare but clinically meaningful adverse events. In this sense, standardization and automatization of foam production are fundamental steps forward. Finally, there is a growing emphasis on patient-centered endpoints in ongoing trials. Quality of life, functional capacity, ulcer recurrence, and healthcare utilization are increasingly prioritized alongside anatomic closure rates. This shift aligns sclerotherapy research with broader trends in vascular medicine and health policy, emphasizing outcomes that matter to patients and healthcare systems alike. In conclusion, the future of sclerotherapy is defined less by disruption than by refinement. Advances in foam production promise greater precision and safety, improved imaging and guidance will enhance targeting and reproducibility, personalized treatment paradigms will align intervention with individual disease biology and patient priorities, and ongoing research will clarify long-term effectiveness and optimal use. These developments reinforce a central truth: sclerotherapy is not a static technique but a dynamic, evolving modality. As science, technology, and outcomes measurement advance, sclerotherapy is poised to remain a cornerstone of chronic venous disease management, more precise, more personalized, and more firmly anchored in evidence that reflects the complexity of the disease it seeks to treat. The same complexity is present in the appropriate training to perform sclerotherapy. Indeed, even in presence of a perfectly automated foam production device, the physician high expertise in the clinical scenario identification and in the related therapeutic strategy decision is of paramount importance. The technical apparent easiness of an injection should never lower the guard of the healthcare professional approaching sclerotherapy as it remains an act equivalent, if not superior, to more elaborate procedures, therefore requiring the same if not superior training care.

References

1. Eberhardt RT, Raffetto JD. Chronic venous insufficiency. Circulation. 2014;130(4):333–46.
2. Gianesini S, Chi YW, Agüero C, et al. Fake-news-free evidence-based communication for proper vein-lymphatic disease management. Int Angiol. 2023;42(2):89–189.
3. Lurie F, Passman M, Meisner M, et al. The 2020 update of the CEAP classification system and reporting standards. J Vasc Surg Venous Lymphat Disord. 2020;8(3):342–52. https://doi.org/10.1016/j.jvsv.2019.12.075. Epub 2020 Feb 27. Erratum in: J Vasc Surg Venous Lymphat Disord. 2021;9(1):288.
4. Evans CJ, Fowkes FG, Ruckley CV, et al. Prevalence of varicose veins and chronic venous insufficiency in men and women in the general population: Edinburgh Vein Study. J Epidemiol Community Health. 1999;53(3):149–53.
5. Ruckley CV, Evans CJ, Allan PL, et al. Chronic venous insufficiency: clinical and duplex correlations. The Edinburgh Vein Study of venous disorders in the general population. J Vasc Surg. 2002;36(3):520–5.
6. Maurins U, Hoffmann BH, Lösch C, et al. Distribution and prevalence of reflux in the superficial and deep venous system in the general population—results from the Bonn Vein Study, Germany. J Vasc Surg. 2008;48(3):680–7.
7. Robertson L, Lee AJ, Evans CJ, et al. Incidence of chronic venous disease in the Edinburgh Vein Study. J Vasc Surg Venous Lymphat Disord. 2013;1(1):59–67.
8. Simka M, Majewski E. The social and economic burden of venous leg ulcers: focus on the role of micronized purified flavonoid fraction adjuvant therapy. Am J Clin Dermatol. 2003;4(8):573–81.
9. Phillips CJ, Humphreys I, Thayer D, et al. Cost of managing patients with venous leg ulcers. Int Wound J. 2020;17(4):1074–82.
10. Launois R, Reboul-Marty J, Henry B. Construction and validation of a quality of life questionnaire in

chronic lower limb venous insufficiency (CIVIQ). Qual Life Res. 1996;5(6):539–54.
11. Chan DYS, Surendra NK, Ng YZ, et al. Prospective study on the clinical and economic burden of venous leg ulcers in the tropics. J Vasc Surg Venous Lymphat Disord. 2023;11(5):954–63.
12. Raju S, Knight A, Lamanilao L, et al. Peripheral venous hypertension in chronic venous disease. J Vasc Surg Venous Lymphat Disord. 2019;7(5):706–14.
13. Pascarella L, Schmid-Schönbein GW, Bergan J. An animal model of venous hypertension: the role of inflammation in venous valve failure. J Vasc Surg. 2005;41(2):303–11.
14. Chen Y, Peng W, Raffetto JD, et al. Matrix metalloproteinases in remodeling of lower extremity veins and chronic venous disease. Prog Mol Biol Transl Sci. 2017;147:267–99.
15. Jünger M, Steins A, Hahn M, et al. Microcirculatory dysfunction in chronic venous insufficiency (CVI). Microcirculation. 2000;7(6 Pt 2):S3–12.
16. Saharay M, Shields DA, Porter JB, et al. Leukocyte activity in the microcirculation of the leg in patients with chronic venous disease. J Vasc Surg. 1997;26(2):265–73.
17. Van de Scheur M, Falanga V. Pericapillary fibrin cuffs in venous disease. A reappraisal. Dermatologic Surg. 1997;23(10):955–9.
18. Diaz JA, Gianesini S, Khalil RA. Glycocalyx disruption, endothelial dysfunction and vascular remodeling as underlying mechanisms and treatment targets of chronic venous disease. Int Angiol. 2024;43(6):563–90.
19. Gianesini S, Rimondi E, Raffetto JD, et al. Human collecting lymphatic glycocalyx identification by electron microscopy and immunohistochemistry. Sci Rep. 2023;13(1):3022.
20. Chang SL, Huang YL, Lee MC, et al. Association of varicose veins with incident venous thromboembolism and peripheral artery disease. JAMA. 2018;319(8):807–17.
21. Grigorean A, Lindenblatt N, Luchsinger I, et al. Prevalence and prognostic role of lymphedema in patients with deep venous thrombosis and thrombophlebitis. Lymphat Res Biol. 2024;22(1):20–6.
22. Piller N. Phlebolymphoedema/chronic venous lymphatic insufficiency: an introduction to strategies for detection, differentiation and treatment. Phlebology. 2009;24(2):51–5.
23. Mironiuc A, Palcău L, Rogojan L, et al. Is there a correlation between the CEAP score and the histopathological findings in varicose disease? Romanian J Morphol Embryol. 2011;52(1):117–21.
24. Launois R, Mansilha A, Jantet G. International psychometric validation of the Chronic Venous Disease quality of life Questionnaire (CIVIQ-20). Eur J Vasc Endovasc Surg. 2010;40(6):783–9.
25. Garratt AM, Macdonald LM, Ruta DA, et al. Towards measurement of outcome for patients with varicose veins. Qual Health Care. 1993;2(1):5–10.
26. Lamping DL, Schroter S, Kurz X, et al. Evaluation of outcomes in chronic venous disorders of the leg: development of a scientifically rigorous, patient-reported measure of symptoms and quality of life. J Vasc Surg. 2003;37(2):410–9.
27. Kahn SR, Lamping DL, Ducruet T, et al. VEINES-QOL/Sym questionnaire was a reliable and valid disease-specific quality of life measure for deep venous thrombosis. J Clin Epidemiol. 2006;59(10):1049–56.
28. Hareendran A, Doll H, Wild DJ, et al. The venous leg ulcer quality of life (VLU-QoL) questionnaire: development and psychometric validation. Wound Repair Regen. 2007;15(4):465–73.
29. Passman MA, McLafferty RB, Lentz MF, et al. Validation of Venous Clinical Severity Score (VCSS) with other venous severity assessment tools from the American Venous Forum, National Venous Screening Program. J Vasc Surg. 2011;54(6 Suppl):2S–9S.
30. Vasquez MA, Munschauer CE. Venous Clinical Severity Score and quality-of-life assessment tools: application to vein practice. Phlebology. 2008;23(6):259–75.
31. Catarinella FS, Nieman FH, Wittens CH. An overview of the most commonly used venous quality of life and clinical outcome measurements. J Vasc Surg Venous Lymphat Disord. 2015;3(3):333–40.
32. Kuet ML, Lane TR, Anwar MA, et al. Comparison of disease-specific quality of life tools in patients with chronic venous disease. Phlebology. 2014;29(10):648–53.
33. Lattimer CR, Kalodiki E, Azzam M, et al. Responsiveness of individual questions from the venous clinical severity score and the Aberdeen varicose vein questionnaire. Phlebology. 2014;29(1):43–51.
34. Méan M, Limacher A, Kahn SR, et al. The VEINES-QOL/Sym questionnaire is a reliable and valid disease-specific quality of life measure for deep vein thrombosis in elderly patients. Qual Life Res. 2014;23(9):2463–71.
35. de Almeida I, Figueiredo PHS, Silva WT, et al. Reliability and validity of specific quality of life assessment questionnaires related to chronic venous insufficiency: a systematic review. J Vasc Bras. 2022;21:e20210229.
36. Paty J, Turner-Bowker DM, Elash CA, et al. The VVSymQ® instrument: use of a new patient-reported outcome measure for assessment of varicose vein symptoms. Phlebology. 2016;31(7):481–8.
37. Westby D, Nezafat M, McKnight K, et al. Venous disease progression in western Europe (VENPRO): a prospective cohort study. Phlebology. 2025;40(4):275–82.
38. John L, Kota AA, Samuel V, et al. Transcutaneous partial pressure of oxygen measurement in advanced chronic venous insufficiency as a marker of tissue oxygenation. Vasc Specialist Int. 2021;37:21.
39. de Moraes Silva MA, Nelson A, Bell-Syer SE, et al. Compression for preventing recurrence of venous ulcers. Cochrane Database Syst Rev. 2024;3(3):CD002303.
40. Van der Velden SK, Shadid NH, Nelemans PJ, et al. How specific are venous symptoms for diag-

nosis of chronic venous disease? Phlebology. 2014;29(9):580–6.
41. Kostas TI, Ioannou CV, Drygiannakis I, et al. Chronic venous disease progression and modification of predisposing factors. J Vasc Surg. 2010;51(4):900–7.
42. Nicholls SC. Sequelae of untreated venous insufficiency. Semin Intervent Radiol. 2005;22(3):162–8.
43. Dewi DAR, Arimuko A, Norawati L, et al. Effectiveness of sclerotherapy to cure lower limb chronic venous insufficiency grades 1-6: a systematic review and meta-analysis. Cureus. 2023;15(12):e49770.
44. Orhurhu V, Chu R, Xie K, et al. Management of lower extremity pain from chronic venous insufficiency: a comprehensive review. Cardiol Ther. 2021;10(1):111–40.
45. Gianesini S, Occhionorelli S, Menegatti E, et al. Femoral vein valve incompetence as a risk factor for junctional recurrence. Phlebology. 2018;33(3):206–12.
46. Cartee TV, Wirth P, Greene A, et al. Ultrasound-guided foam sclerotherapy is safe and effective in the management of superficial venous insufficiency of the lower extremity. J Vasc Surg Venous Lymphat Disord. 2021;9(4):1031–40.
47. Gianesini S, Obi A, Onida S, et al. Global guidelines trends and controversies in lower limb venous and lymphatic disease: narrative literature revision and experts' opinions following the vWINter international meeting in Phlebology, Lymphology & Aesthetics, 23-25 January 2019. Phlebology. 2019;34(1 Suppl):4–66.
48. Antignani PL, Lazarashvili Z, Monedero JL, et al. Diagnosis and treatment of pelvic congestion syndrome: UIP consensus document. Int Angiol. 2019;38(4):265–83.
49. Brake M, Lim CS, Shepherd AC, et al. Pathogenesis and etiology of recurrent varicose veins. J Vasc Surg. 2013;57(3):860–8.
50. Bontinis A, Bontinis V, Koudounas G, et al. Interventions for the treatment of recurrent varicose vein disease arising from the saphenofemoral junction or the great saphenous vein: a systematic review and meta-analysis. Int Angiol. 2024;43(5):485–96.
51. Kanber EM. Comparison of foam and liquid Sclerotherapy for the treatment of lower extremity varicose veins and telangiectasia in obese patients. Cureus. 2023;15(7):e42571.
52. Cuffolo G, Hardy E, Perkins J, et al. The effects of foam sclerotherapy on ulcer healing: a single-centre prospective study. Ann R Coll Surg Engl. 2019;101(4):285–9.
53. Pihlaja T, Kosunen E, Ohtonen P, et al. Sub-ulcer foam sclerotherapy in patients with venous leg ulcer, analysis and technical aspects of 134 consecutive patients. Int J Low Extrem Wounds. 2024;25:509–14.
54. Guex JJ. Importance of patient-reported outcomes in chronic venous disorders. Phlebology. 2012;27(Suppl 1):136–8.
55. Davies HO, Popplewell M, Darvall K, et al. A review of randomised controlled trials comparing ultrasound-guided foam sclerotherapy with endothermal ablation for the treatment of great saphenous varicose veins. Phlebology. 2016;31(4):234–40.
56. Nakano LC, Cacione DG, Baptista-Silva JC, et al. Treatment for telangiectasias and reticular veins. Cochrane Database Syst Rev. 2021;10(10):CD012723.
57. Whing J, Nandhra S, Nesbitt C, et al. Interventions for great saphenous vein incompetence. Cochrane Database Syst Rev. 2021;8(8):CD005624.
58. Gianesini S, Danese M, AlQedrah D, et al. Multi-specialty recommendations for the appropriate and affordable lower limb vein-lymphatic disorders management. Int Angiol. 2026;45:1–64.
59. Mariani F, Carbone L, Sozio G, et al. Ultrasound-guided foam sclerotherapy of the saphenous trunks is associated with a low 5-year recurrence rate and improved quality of life in patients with chronic venous disease: a multicenter study. J Vasc Surg Venous Lymphat Disord. 2025;13(4):102212.
60. Lam YL, Lawson JA, Toonder IM, et al. Eight-year follow-up of a randomized clinical trial comparing ultrasound-guided foam sclerotherapy with surgical stripping of the great saphenous vein. Br J Surg. 2018;105(6):692–8.
61. Chiesa R, Marone EM, Limoni C, et al. Chronic venous disorders: correlation between visible signs, symptoms, and presence of functional disease. J Vasc Surg. 2007;46(2):322–30.
62. Blaise S, Bosson JL, Diamand JM. Ultrasound-guided sclerotherapy of the great saphenous vein with 1% vs. 3% polidocanol foam: a multicentre double-blind randomised trial with 3-year follow-up. Eur J Vasc Endovasc Surg. 2010;39(6):779–86.
63. Sakugawa LS, Portela FSO, Louzada ACS, et al. Polidocanol-foam treatment of varicose veins: quality-of-life impact compared to conventional surgery. Clinics. 2024;79:100346.
64. Gibson K, Kabnick L, Varithena® 013 Investigator Group. A multicenter, randomized, placebo-controlled study to evaluate the efficacy and safety of Varithena® (polidocanol endovenous microfoam 1%) for symptomatic, visible varicose veins with saphenofemoral junction incompetence. Phlebology. 2017;32(3):185–93.
65. Bacelar ACC, Netto EM, Barreto N, et al. Promising results of ultrasound guided foam sclerotherapy for treating chronic venous ulcers. J Vasc Surg Venous Lymphat Disord. 2025;13(3):102198.
66. Lloret P, Redondo P, Cabrera J, Sierra A. Treatment of venous leg ulcers with ultrasound-guided foam sclerotherapy: healing, long-term recurrence and quality of life evaluation. Wound Repair Regen. 2015;23(3):369–78.
67. Butova X, Shayakhmetov S, Fedin M, et al. Artificial intelligence evidence-based current status and potential for lower limb vascular management. J Pers Med. 2021;11(12):1280.

Sclerotherapy by Saphenous Vein Catheters

10

Sergio Gianesini and Danny Pratama

1 Historical Evolution

Catheter-directed sclerotherapy emerged as a logical progression from ultrasound-guided foam sclerotherapy (UGFS). Early catheter systems were adapted from angiographic devices and introduced in the late 1990s and early 2000s, enabling controlled sclerosant injection along the saphenous trunk. Pullback techniques were developed to standardize sclerosant distribution, reduce dilution effects, and minimize proximal escape of foam into the deep venous system [4]. Gatto documented the first catheter-directed sclerotherapy (CDS) in the abstract book of the International Union of Phlebology 1989 Strasbourg World Congress, using liquid sclerosant [5]. In 1992, Grondin reported technical notes on CDS using ultrasound-guidance [6]. Three years later, a dedicated catheter (Phlebocath™) with three side holes for sclerotherapy was introduced by Robert, yet without dedicated statistics [7]. While Phlebocath™ was echo-guided only for the localization of its tip, the following Extended Long Line Echosclerotherapy (ELLE technique) was reported to be fully echo-guided, with accesses even at ankle level. Pulsed rather than continuous injections of sclerosant were recommended, in the vision of generating turbulence and froth [8]. The contemporary rapid expansion of thermal ablation technologies temporarily overshadowed catheter-based sclerotherapy. Yet, the high initial cost and reimbursement difficulties related to endovenous thermal options allowed CDS to survive [9]. Meanwhile, already in 2007 a balloon catheters aimed to avoid sclerosant migration into the deep system and its confinement into the target tract were already developed [10]. Among these, a well-known one at the time was Varicath™, endowed with a distal occlusion balloon and side holes for sclerosant injection. It reported 87% occlusion rate at 6 months follow-up. Yet, deep venous thrombosis complications, possibly arising from migration of the same sclerosant into the deep system through the perforating veins because of the block of the distal outflow were reported [11]. The utility of adding tumescence also in CDS procedures was clearly stated in 2005, preferring fluids including adrenaline to obtain both the physical and chemical desired compression effect on the targeted vein [12]. Yet, Devereux published a randomized comparative trial highlighting no real benefit in adding tumescence, therefore leaving the topic open for further appropriate investigations [13]. CDS proved to be use-

S. Gianesini (✉)
Department of Translational Medicine, University of Ferrara, Ferrara, Italy

Department of Surgery, Uniformed Services University of Health Sciences, Bethesda, MD, USA
e-mail: gnssrg@unife.it

D. Pratama
Vascular and Endovascular Division, Cardiovascular Department, Fatmawati General Hospital, Indonesian Society for Vascular and Endovascular Surgery – PESBEVI, Jakarta, Indonesia

S. Gianesini, Y. W. Chi (eds.), *Sclerotherapy*, https://doi.org/10.1007/978-3-032-32794-9_10

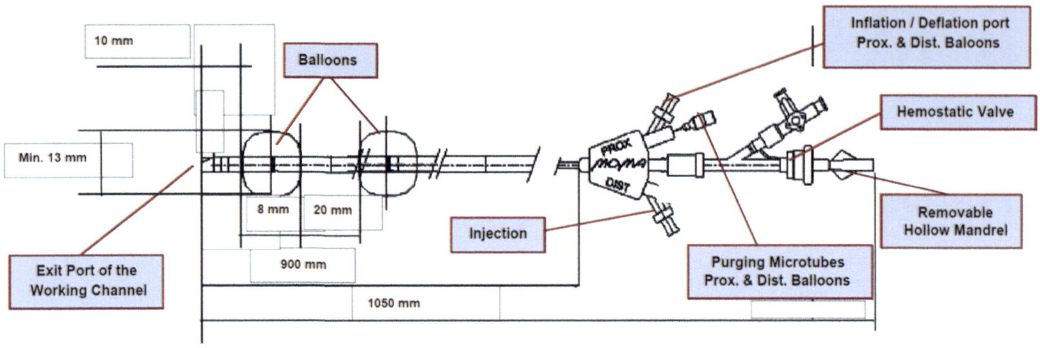

Fig. 10.1 Leu two-balloons catheter. (Open access picture from Leu and Inderbitzi [15])

ful in malformations, under fluoroscopic guidance, already back in 1999, thanks to Donelly work [14]. In 2008, Prof. Leu from Switzerland published about a technical refinement in CDS, adding both a distal and proximal 8-mm balloon, at a 2 cm distance one from the other, with the aim to inject sclerosant into an empty vein tract, moreover allowing the aspiration of the residual sclerosant once the sclerotherapic procedure is concluded. The short distance between the two balloons minimizes the risk of sclerosant migration into the deep venous system (Fig. 10.1) [15].

A similar catheter (Velex™) to inject into an empty vein segment was introduced in 2023, yet presenting a longer distance (12 cm) in between the two occluding balloons, in which a third balloon is lodged to maximize the contact of the liquid sclerosant with the vein wall (Fig. 10.2) [16].

Care in not including saphenous vein tracts with perforating veins in between the two occlusive balloons is recommended in order to avoid sclerosant agent injection into the deep system (Fig. 10.3).

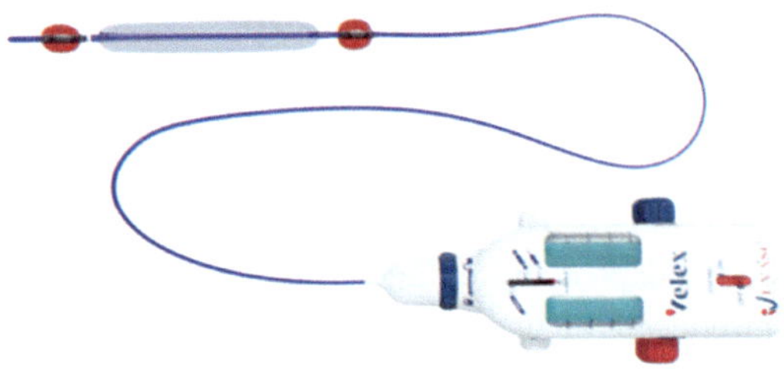

Fig. 10.2 Three balloon catheter aimed to inject into an empty vein. (Picture copyright: Dr. Mario Salerno)

In 2012, mechano-chemical ablation by endothelial cutting through a dedicated catether (Clarivein™) was first reported in the literature [17]. Four years later, a sclerotherapy catheter (Flebogriff™) combining endothelial damage and sclerosant injection was reported in its performance at 3 months observation time [18]. Currently, CDS remains a possible treatment option for chronic venous disease treatment, yet still in need of proper scientific validation before positioning itself as a possible gold-standard.

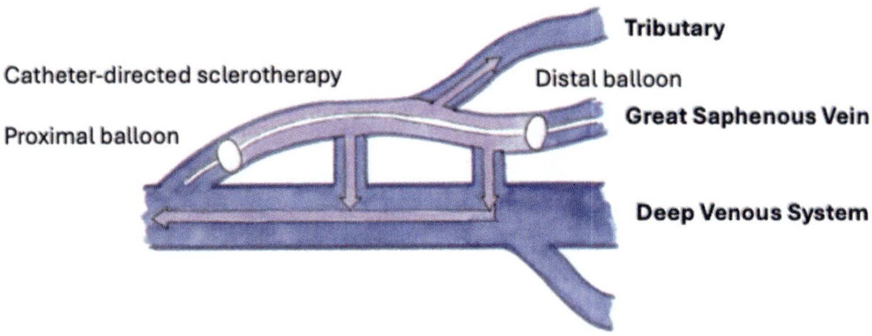

Fig. 10.3 Sclerosant agent direct aspiration into the deep venous system and into saphenous tributaries, after its injection in a saphenous segment closed at both endings by a sclerotherapy catheter balloon. (Figure copyright: Dr. Celine Eggen (Centrum Oosterwal, Alkmaar (NETHERLANDS)))

2 The Rationale of Catheter-Directed Sclerotherapy

The pathophysiology of saphenous vein incompetence is characterized by longitudinal reflux involving extensive segments of the vein, often extending from the saphenofemoral or saphenopopliteal junction to the calf. This continuous disease pattern is poorly addressed by focal or segmental injection techniques, which may leave untreated portions of the vein susceptible to early recanalization. Catheter-based sclerotherapy directly addresses this limitation by enabling uniform treatment of the entire refluxing segment. Foam sclerosants exert their therapeutic effect through endothelial destruction mediated by detergent action, followed by inflammation, fibrosis, and eventual vein obliteration. Experimental and clinical studies have demonstrated that endothelial damage is dependent on sclerosant concentration, contact time, and surface area exposure. Catheter-directed delivery optimizes these variables by maintaining consistent foam density and contact throughout the vein length. Vein diameter is a critical determinant of sclerotherapy success. Large-diameter saphenous veins (>6–7 mm) are prone to incomplete closure when treated with single-point foam injection due to inadequate luminal filling and rapid foam degradation. Catheter-based techniques mitigate this risk by ensuring continuous foam replacement during pullback, improving occlusion rates in larger veins [19]. From a safety perspective, catheter-directed sclerotherapy offers a non-thermal alternative that avoids heat-related complications such as nerve injury, skin burns, and peri-venous fibrosis. The absence of tumescent anesthesia reduces procedural complexity, patient discomfort, and the risk of fluid overload or local anesthetic toxicity. These advantages are particularly relevant in elderly patients, those with peripheral neuropathy, and individuals with superficial or tortuous saphenous veins. Additionally, catheter-based approaches allow precise control of sclerosant volume and injection speed, potentially reducing the incidence of systemic side effects such as visual disturbances, migraine aura, or paradoxical embolic phenomena associated with foam sclerotherapy [20, 21]. Obviously, a balance between endovenous thermal induced and sclerotherapy (drug and gas related) complications must be performed. Within the current spectrum of endovenous therapies, catheter-directed sclerotherapy is classified as a non-thermal, non-tumescent technique, alongside mechanochemical ablation and cyanoacrylate adhesive closure. While EVLA and RFA remain the most extensively studied modalities with high long-term occlusion rates, catheter-directed sclerotherapy offers a distinct risk–benefit profile that justifies its continued use in selected patients. International guidelines acknowledge ultrasound-guided foam sclerotherapy, including catheter-based techniques, as an acceptable treatment for saphenous reflux, particularly in patients unsuitable for thermal ablation or those with recurrent varicose veins after prior surgery or endovenous treatment. These recommendations emphasize the importance of operator expertise and ultrasound surveillance in optimizing outcomes [1, 2]. Catheter-directed sclerotherapy of the saphenous veins requires a precise understanding of venous anatomy, disease progression, and the hemodynamic environment in which sclerosants are delivered. Unlike thermal techniques that rely on circumferential heat-induced vein wall injury, chemical ablation depends on intimate and sustained contact between the sclerosant and the endothelium. Consequently, anatomical variations, reflux patterns, and flow dynamics exert a disproportionate influence on procedural success and durability. Superficial venous disease is not a static condition but a dynamic pathological process involving valve dysfunction, vein wall remodeling, inflammatory signaling, and progressive hemodynamic derangement. Catheter-based techniques must therefore be adapted to the specific anatomical and physiological context of each patient, rather than applied as uniform, protocol-driven interventions. A first anatomical consideration is about the saphenous compartment that acts as a biomechanical constraint limiting outward vein expansion. When reflux develops, chronic venous hypertension eventually overwhelms this containment, leading to compartmental dilation, vein elongation, and tortuosity. Segments that remain intrafascial may demonstrate better responsiveness to sclerotherapy due to more efficient vein wall apposition during spasm, whereas extrafascial segments often require higher sclerosant volumes and demonstrate higher recanalization rates [22]. The great saphenous vein receives multiple tributaries along its course, including anterior and posterior accessory saphenous veins. These accessory systems frequently serve as parallel reflux pathways and may be the dominant source of clinical symptoms despite a relatively preserved main trunk. Failure to recognize and treat these pathways can result in apparent procedural failure following otherwise technically successful catheter sclerotherapy [23]. Anatomical duplication of the great saphenous vein, present in a minority of patients, poses a unique challenge. In duplicated systems, catheterization of only one channel may leave the parallel trunk untreated, leading to persistent reflux and symptom recurrence. Comprehensive duplex mapping is therefore mandatory prior to catheter-based interventions [24]. The small saphenous vein arises from the lateral marginal vein of the foot and ascends posteriorly in the midline of the calf. Unlike the great saphenous vein, the small saphenous vein demonstrates marked variability in termination, draining into the popliteal vein at variable levels or continuing proximally as the vein of Giacomini. These anatomical variations have direct implications for catheter length selection, access site planning, and junctional safety margins [25]. The proximity of the small saphenous vein to the sural nerve further distinguishes it from the great saphenous vein. Although catheter-directed sclerotherapy avoids thermal nerve injury, aggressive sclerosant dosing in superficial or ectatic small saphenous vein segments may still result in inflammatory neuropathy, reinforcing the need for anatomical precision [26]. Venous valves are more densely distributed in the distal segments of the saphenous veins, with decreasing frequency proximally. Valve orientation and cusp morphology vary considerably, influencing local flow patterns and susceptibility to failure. For catheter-based sclerotherapy, this observation supports treatment strategies targeting entire pathological segments rather than isolated reflux points, even when duplex imaging suggests focal incompetence. Saphenous reflux may originate at junctional valves, isolated truncal valves or incompetent perforators. Once established, reflux leads to sustained venous hypertension, which drives progressive vein wall remodeling and further valvular dysfunction. Descending reflux from the SFJ is a frequently observed pattern in great saphenous vein disease, together also with the ascending reflux from calf perforators.

Catheter-directed sclerotherapy is uniquely suited to address both patterns by enabling treatment of continuous reflux segments irrespective of directionality.

Chronic reflux induces profound histopathological changes, including smooth muscle cell hypertrophy, collagen accumulation, elastin fragmentation, and inflammatory infiltration. These alterations reduce vein wall contractility and responsiveness, diminishing the efficacy of chemical ablation in advanced disease unless delivery is carefully optimized. Larger vein diameters correlate strongly with recanalization after sclerotherapy. Catheter-based techniques partially mitigate this risk by ensuring consistent sclerosant exposure, but vein wall degeneration remains a limiting factor in late-stage disease. Recurrent varicose veins often demonstrate complex reflux patterns involving neovascular channels, residual saphenous stumps or accessory veins. These anatomies are frequently unsuitable for thermal ablation but remain amenable to catheter-directed sclerotherapy, provided detailed duplex assessment is performed. Importantly, recurrent disease is often hemodynamically significant despite relatively small vein diameters, emphasizing the need for functional rather than purely anatomical treatment criteria [27]. The efficacy of sclerotherapy is fundamentally dependent on local hemodynamics. High venous flow rates promote sclerosant dilution, foam fragmentation and premature washout, reducing endothelial injury. Catheter-directed techniques seek to counteract these effects by enabling controlled, segmental delivery under low-flow conditions. Venous pressure varies significantly with patient position. Supine or Trendelenburg positioning reduces hydrostatic pressure and vein diameter, facilitating vein wall apposition and enhancing sclerosant contact. Failure to optimize positioning may result in incomplete ablation, particularly in large-diameter trunks. Foam sclerosants are rheologically complex, with behavior influenced by bubble size, gas composition, and shear forces. In high-flow environments, foam degradation accelerates, reducing effective sclerosant concentration. Catheter-based pullback techniques reduce turbulence and allow progressive luminal filling, improving foam stability. Controlled injection speed is critical. Rapid injection increases proximal migration and systemic exposure, whereas slow, steady delivery enhances endothelial interaction and reduces adverse events [28]. The hemodynamics at the sapheno-femoral junction and sapheno-popliteal junction represent a critical safety consideration. Direct sclerosant delivery into junctional segments increases the risk of deep venous propagation. Most catheter-based protocols intentionally terminate injection several centimeters distal to the junction, accepting short residual stumps with minimal clinical consequence. Compression applied during and immediately after catheter withdrawal further modulates junctional flow, promoting proximal vein collapse and reducing the risk of sclerosant escape.

3 Patient Selection and Indications

Patient selection is the single most critical determinant of success in catheter-directed sclerotherapy of the saphenous veins. Unlike thermal ablation, which relies on predictable circumferential heat injury, chemical ablation depends on a complex interplay of anatomical configuration, venous hemodynamics, vein wall biology, and patient-specific factors. As a result, identical procedural techniques may yield markedly different outcomes in different patients. Historically, suboptimal outcomes associated with truncal sclerotherapy were often attributable not to intrinsic limitations of the technique but to inappropriate patient selection, insufficient understanding of disease patterns, or inadequate procedural control. Contemporary catheter-based approaches have mitigated many technical limitations, shifting the emphasis decisively toward refined clinical judgment. In modern venous practice, catheter-directed sclerotherapy should be conceptualized as a precision tool, ideally suited for specific clinical and anatomical scenarios rather than a universal substitute for thermal ablation. Its optimal use requires systematic assessment of symptoms, duplex findings, disease stage, comorbidities, and patient priorities. The fundamental indication for catheter-directed sclerotherapy is symptomatic superficial venous reflux involving the great or small saphenous vein, confirmed by duplex ultrasound and correlated with clinical findings. Symptoms may include pain, heaviness, fatigue, edema, nocturnal cramps, skin changes, or ulceration attributable to superficial venous hypertension. Patients with continuous truncal reflux over long vein segments are particularly suitable candidates, as catheter-based delivery enables uniform sclerosant exposure along the entire pathological segment. This advantage is less pronounced in focal disease, where simpler injection techniques may suffice. Catheter-directed sclerotherapy is especially attractive in patients seeking minimally invasive treatment with rapid recovery, avoidance of tumescent anesthesia, and minimal post-procedural discomfort. These preferences increasingly influence treatment selection in contemporary venous care. Vein diameter plays a central role in patient selection. Moderate-diameter saphenous veins are generally more responsive to chemical ablation than severely dilated or aneurysmal trunks. However, catheter-directed techniques partially compensate for larger diameters by ensuring continuous sclerosant replenishment and prolonged endothelial contact. Hemodynamically, patients with isolated superficial reflux and preserved deep venous function derive the greatest benefit. In contrast, extensive deep venous incompetence may limit symptomatic improvement following superficial ablation alone, regardless of technical success.

Absolute contraindications include acute deep vein thrombosis, severe peripheral arterial disease compromising limb perfusion, known allergy to sclerosants, pregnancy, and active infection. In these settings, catheter-directed sclerotherapy poses unacceptable risk or limited benefit.

Relative contraindications are more nuanced and include extreme vein dilation, severe post-thrombotic changes, uncontrolled hypercoagulable states, and prior severe neurologic reactions to foam sclerosants. In such cases, alternative modalities or modified protocols may be preferable. Importantly, contraindications should be interpreted in context: experienced operators may safely perform catheter-directed sclerotherapy in borderline cases through appropriate sclerosant/foam selection, staged treatment, or adjunctive compression strategies. Care should be placed in venous trunks in proximity of the skin as the post-procedural inflammatory process could be more pronounced, therefore leading to discomfort and possible hyperpigmentation. Worthy of notice is the publication highlighting the feasibility and the good result of CDS also in venous ulcer treatment, presenting a healing rate of 65% at 1 year follow-up [29]. Thermal ablation remains the reference standard for many patients due to consistently high occlusion rates and extensive long-term data. However, catheter-directed sclerotherapy occupies a distinct niche within the treatment spectrum. Compared with thermal techniques, catheter-based sclerotherapy avoids nerve injury, skin burns, and the need for tumescent anesthesia. These advantages are particularly relevant for veins with superficial course, proximity to nerves, or complex anatomy. When compared with other non-thermal techniques, catheter-directed sclerotherapy offers greater flexibility, lower material costs, and applicability across a wider range of vein diameters, albeit with potentially higher retreatment rates. Recurrent disease following surgery or endovenous intervention often involves complex anatomies unsuitable for thermal ablation. Catheter-directed sclerotherapy allows targeted treatment of residual or neovascular channels with minimal additional tissue trauma. In elderly patients, treatment goals often prioritize symptom relief and functional improvement over perfect anatomical results. Catheter-directed sclerotherapy offers a low-stress, outpatient solution well suited to this population. Catheter-directed sclerotherapy can often be performed without interrupting anticoagulation, reducing thrombotic risk in high-risk patients. Careful technique and ultrasound surveillance are essential to ensure safety and efficacy. The choice between modalities should therefore be individualized, incorporating anatomical and hemodynamics feasibility, patient comorbidities, cost considerations, and patient preference.

4 Pre-procedural Evaluation

Duplex ultrasound is indispensable for both diagnosis and procedural planning in chronic venous disease. For catheter-directed sclerotherapy, duplex evaluation is not merely confirmatory but prescriptive, directly determining treatment feasibility, technique selection, and risk mitigation strategies. A comprehensive duplex examination must assess vein patency, valve competence, reflux duration, flow direction, vein diameter, and connectivity with deep and perforating systems. Incomplete duplex assessment leads to inappropriate truncal treatment and suboptimal clinical outcomes. Reflux is typically defined as retrograde flow exceeding 0.5 s in superficial veins. However, in catheter-based sclerotherapy, the extent, continuity, and hemodynamic significance of reflux are often more important than absolute duration thresholds. Pre-procedural mapping should trace the entire saphenous vein from distal calf to its junction with the deep system, documenting anatomical variants, accessory veins, large tributaries, perforators, and areas of compartmental exit (Fig. 10.4). These features influence sclerosant containment and foam propagation. Mapping should be performed with the patient standing or in reverse Trendelenburg position to maximize venous filling and reflux detection. Failure to assess veins under physiologic loading conditions may underestimate disease severity and lead to incomplete treatment planning. Precise documentation of reflux origin (junctional, truncal, perforator-related), direction (ascending vs. descending), and continuity allows tailored catheter pullback strategies and optimized sclerosant delivery. Duplex findings directly influence access site selection, catheter length, sclerosant concentration, total injected volume and compression planning. For example, reflux extending into distal calf segments may necessitate more distal access to ensure complete treatment. Identification of large tributaries or perforators adjacent to the planned treatment segment may prompt staged therapy or adjunctive compression to reduce sclerosant escape and systemic exposure. Vein diameter is one of the strongest predictors of sclerotherapy success. Larger saphenous veins demonstrate increased luminal volume, higher flow velocities and reduced wall contractility, all of which diminish sclerosant efficacy. Catheter-directed delivery improves outcomes in larger veins by maintaining continuous sclerosant replacement and prolonged endothelial contact. However, extreme dilation or aneurysmal degeneration remains a relative contraindication due to high recanalization risk,

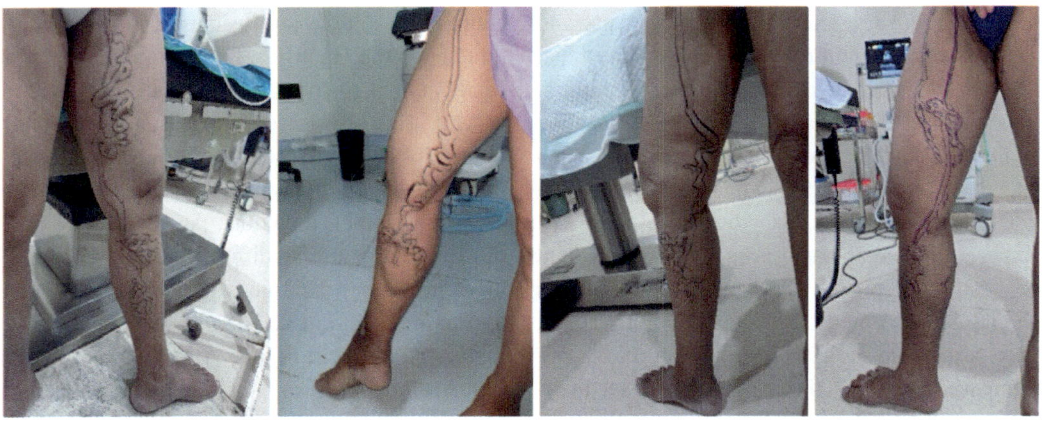

Fig. 10.4 Preprocedural mapping

despite successful treatment cases have been reported also following non CDS [30]. Diameter should be measured at multiple standardized points in the standing position, as focal dilation may not reflect overall trunk behavior. Reliance on supine measurements systematically underestimates treatment complexity. The longitudinal extent of reflux is particularly relevant for catheter-based techniques. Long, continuous reflux segments are ideal candidates, as catheter pullback ensures uniform treatment. Short, discontinuous reflux segments may be more appropriately treated with focal injection techniques or alternative modalities, avoiding unnecessary truncal ablation. Accurate assessment of reflux length also informs sclerosant dose calculation, minimizing systemic exposure while ensuring adequate endothelial injury. Vein tortuosity is a key technical consideration. While catheter-directed sclerotherapy can accommodate moderate curvature, severe tortuosity may prevent safe catheter advancement and result in uneven sclerosant distribution.

Pre-procedural recognition of tortuous segments allows modification of access strategy, use of shorter catheters, or adoption of hybrid approaches combining catheter-based and segmental injection techniques. Informed consent for catheter-directed sclerotherapy must explicitly address modality-specific benefits and limitations. Patients should understand that chemical ablation may involve higher retreatment rates than thermal ablation but offers advantages in terms of recovery, anesthesia requirements and nerve safety. Common risks include superficial thrombosis, skin hyperpigmentation, matting, local inflammation and transient neurologic symptoms. Rare but serious complications, such as deep vein thrombosis or paradoxical embolization, should also be discussed [31]. Expectation management is especially important in catheter-directed sclerotherapy. Patients should be informed that clinical improvement may occur even in the absence of complete anatomical closure and that staged or repeat treatments may be necessary. Informed consent also serves as a forum for aligning treatment goals with patient priorities, particularly in elderly or comorbid populations where symptom relief may outweigh anatomical perfection. Baseline assessment of thrombotic risk is mandatory prior to catheter-directed sclerotherapy. Risk factors include prior venous thromboembolism, inherited or acquired thrombophilia, malignancy, immobility, obesity, and advanced age. Although the overall risk of thrombotic complications is low, catheter-based sclerotherapy involves deliberate endothelial injury and intraluminal thrombosis, necessitating careful patient selection and surveillance [32]. One of the advantages of catheter-directed sclerotherapy is its feasibility without interruption of anticoagulation in many patients. This is particularly relevant for individuals with high thrombotic risk where anticoagulant cessation is undesirable. However, anticoagulation may reduce thrombotic occlusion and increase recanalization risk, requiring optimized sclerosant concentration, compression, and follow-up protocols. Early post-procedural duplex ultrasound thrombotic risk is performed naturally as after sclerotherapy, a follow-up visit should always performed in the few weeks later, in order to eventually also refine the sclerotherapy act.

In selected high-risk patients, short-term pharmacologic thromboprophylaxis may be considered, although evidence remains limited and decisions should be individualized [33, 34]. Last but not least, adapting the sclerosing drug concentration, volume and wetness to the catheter-directed rather than direct injection scenario is fundamental to preserve safety and efficacy. Indeed, the catheter is allowing delivery of the foam close to the junctions, without the blood-mediated inactivation and dilution happening following a direct injection. At the same time, different catheters and different speed and modality of injection (continuous vs pulsed) could alter the foam half-life: knowing the exact features of the sclerosant both in the syringe and at the exit of the catheter is of top importance for both clinical and research purposes.

5 Catheter Systems and Equipment

Catheter systems and ancillary equipment constitute the mechanical interface between pharmacologic intent and biological effect in catheter-directed sclerotherapy of the saphenous veins. Unlike thermal ablation, where energy delivery creates relatively predictable tissue effects once contact is established, chemical ablation depends on precise sclerosant dispersion, controlled flow dynamics, and sustained endothelial contact, all of which are profoundly influenced by catheter design and access strategy. Inadequate appreciation of catheter mechanics or access-related variables may negate the advantages of catheter-based sclerotherapy, resulting in heterogeneous sclerosant exposure, early recanalization or increased risk of systemic or local complications. Conversely, meticulous equipment selection and technique optimization allow catheter sclerotherapy to approach the reproducibility of thermal modalities in selected patients. Initial attempts at catheter-directed sclerotherapy relied on general-purpose angiographic catheters, which were ill-suited for superficial venous anatomy. These devices were often excessively stiff, poorly visualized on ultrasound, and optimized for liquid contrast injection rather than foam sclerosant delivery. As a result, early outcomes were inconsistent and operator-dependent [4]. The development of dedicated saphenous vein catheters represented a pivotal advance. Modern designs emphasize atraumatic tips, enhanced ultrasound visibility, controlled lumen geometry, and flexibility profiles tailored to the superficial venous system. These refinements have significantly improved the feasibility of treating long truncal segments with predictable sclerosant distribution. Most contemporary saphenous vein catheters range from approximately 4 to 6 French in outer diameter, balancing low access-site morbidity with adequate internal lumen diameter for foam delivery. Smaller lumens increase injection resistance and may destabilize foam structure, whereas excessively large lumens increase access trauma and venous spasm. Internal lumen geometry influences foam integrity during injection. Narrow or irregular lumens increase shear forces that may fragment foam bubbles, reducing sclerosant efficacy before endothelial contact is achieved. Purpose-designed catheters aim to preserve foam architecture during delivery. Flexibility gradients along the catheter shaft are critical. Distal segments must be soft enough to navigate curved or compliant vein segments without perforation, while proximal segments require sufficient stiffness to transmit push and torque. Poorly balanced flexibility profiles may result in catheter kinking or uncontrolled advancement. Trackability is particularly important, particularly where post-interventional scarring or neovascularization may distort normal anatomy. Catheter length should be selected based on duplex-defined reflux extent rather than generic anatomical assumptions. Insufficient catheter length may necessitate multiple access sites, increasing procedural complexity and risk. Centimeter markings along the catheter shaft facilitate precise correlation between ultrasound mapping and catheter position. These markings are especially valuable during controlled pullback techniques, allowing uniform sclerosant exposure along the treated segment. End-hole catheters deliver sclerosant through a single distal aperture, producing a concentrated sclerosant column immediately adjacent to the catheter tip. This configuration offers maximal control over sclerosant location and timing, which is advantageous in anatomically complex or junction-adjacent segments. During pullback, end-hole catheters require precise coordination between injection rate and withdrawal speed. Inconsistent technique may lead to segmental overexposure or untreated intervals, particularly in long reflux segments. Multi-hole catheters incorporate multiple lateral exit ports along the distal segment, allowing sclerosant to disperse over a broader longitudinal area. This design aims to reduce focal concentration peaks and promote circumferential endothelial exposure. In large-diameter or straight saphenous veins, multi-hole catheters may improve uniformity of foam distribution. However, the reduced localization may increase sclerosant escape into tributaries or perforators if flow is not adequately controlled. For the saphenous trunk, which is relatively smaller and more tortuous, the use of catheters made of polyethylene or polyurethane is preferred because they have low to moderate stiffness, good memory shape and are easy to negotiate through tortuous blood vessels. Authors usually use selective diagnostic catheters. The size of selective diagnostic catheters ranges from 4 to 6 Fr, with lengths ranging from 50 to 125 cm. Simple curve, Head Hunter (H1), Bernstein, multipurpose (MPA, MPB). No high-level evidence definitively favors one design over the other, and catheter selection remains largely operator-dependent. End-hole catheters are often preferred in tortuous veins or near junctions, whereas multi-hole catheters may be advantageous in long, straight trunks with uniform diameter. Expert operators frequently adapt technique rather than catheter choice, modifying pullback speed, foam density, and compression to achieve optimal endothelial exposure regardless of catheter design. Percutaneous access under ultrasound guidance is standard for catheter-directed sclerotherapy. Access site selection should prioritize straight vein segments with sufficient diameter to accommodate the introducer sheath while minimizing spasm and patient discomfort. Distal access allows treatment of the entire refluxing segment during proximal pullback, but proximal access may be required in cases of distal spasm, severe tortuosity or post-thrombotic changes. Accurate catheter tip positioning is critical near the saphenofemoral and saphenopopliteal junctions. Most protocols recommend maintaining a safety margin of several centimeters distal to the junction to reduce the risk of sclerosant migration into the deep venous system. During sclerosant injection, ultrasound enables visualization of foam filling, vein spasm, and immediate hemodynamic response. Absence of expected vein wall reaction may indicate dilution, extravasation or technical error requiring immediate correction. Continuous ultrasound monitoring during pullback allows detection of untreated segments, sclerosant escape or deep venous propagation, significantly enhancing procedural safety and treatment completeness.

6 Procedural Technique

An appropriate procedural technique begins with an appropriate patient positioning as it is a critical determinant of venous hemodynamics during catheter-directed sclerotherapy. Optimal positioning reduces venous diameter, lowers hydrostatic pressure, and minimizes antegrade flow, thereby enhancing sclerosant–endothelium contact and reducing washout. The best venous access is obtained with ultrasound guidance (Fig. 10.5). Blind puncture of veins that do not

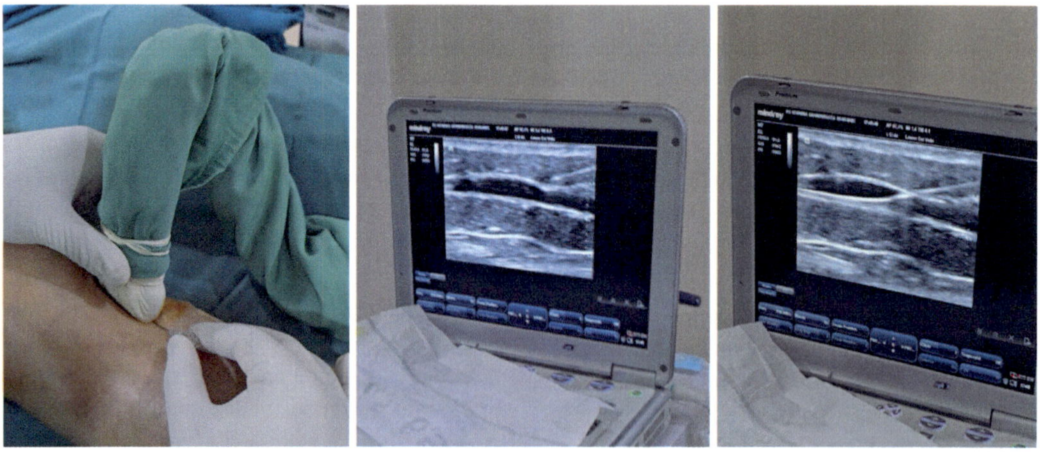

Fig. 10.5 Ultrasound-guided access puncture. Line up the needle parallel to the longitudinal vein wall, observe the vein wall being pushed by the needle, and position the needle precisely in the center of the blood vessel

have a pulse and have more flexible walls will make it difficult to place the needle in the lumen. Multiple puncture attempts may result in vasospasm, which reduces the chances of successful cannulation of the vein. If this happens, venous surgical access is required.

Elevation of the limb above the level of the heart reduces venous filling and promotes vein wall apposition, particularly in large-diameter saphenous trunks. Inadequate elevation may result in persistent venous flow, foam fragmentation, and increased risk of proximal sclerosant migration. Conversely, excessive elevation may collapse the vein lumen prematurely, complicating catheter advancement and sclerosant distribution. One of the principal advantages of catheter-directed sclerotherapy is the avoidance of tumescent anesthesia, unless the operator opt for a further mechanical vein compression by the same tumescence, eventually adding the biochemically induced spasm obtained by the use of adrenalin. Other experts prefer the absence of tumescent anesthesia so to preserve native vein anatomy and to avoid perivenous compression that might otherwise alter sclerosant distribution. In selected patients with anxiety, low pain tolerance, or prolonged procedures, conscious sedation may be used, though excessive sedation risks loss of patient feedback during catheter advancement and injection. Access is typically obtained distally to allow treatment of the entire refluxing segment during proximal catheter withdrawal. The access site should correspond to a straight, adequately sized vein segment identified during duplex mapping (Fig. 10.4). After access and sheath placement, the catheter is advanced proximally under continuous ultrasound guidance. Advancement should be gentle, avoiding forceful manipulation that may cause venous spasm, dissection, or perforation. Catheter tip position is critical. Most protocols recommend positioning the tip 2–5 cm distal to the saphenofemoral or saphenopopliteal junction, creating a safety buffer to reduce the risk of sclerosant migration into the deep venous system. The junction should be compressed during the injection to avoid displacement of the sclerosant into the deep venous system. Controlled pullback is the defining technical feature of catheter-directed sclerotherapy. Unlike single-site injection, pullback techniques ensure uniform sclerosant exposure along the entire treated segment, reducing untreated intervals and dilution effects. The objective is to synchronize injection rate, sclerosant volume, and catheter withdrawal speed to achieve continuous vein wall contact without overexposure or proximal escape. Pullback speed is typically slow and deliberate, adjusted based on vein diameter, sclerosant concentration, and foam stability. Larger veins generally require slower pullback to ensure adequate endothelial exposure. Inconsistent pullback speed is a common cause of segmental recanalization. Many expert operators rely on catheter depth markings and timed withdrawal to standardize exposure. The variable presence of saphenous tributaries flushing in or out can significantly alter the sclerosant dilution, therefore representing a factor altering the possible standardization among the different procedures in light of the sclerosant dilution and inactivation by the blood proteins. In very long or large-diameter veins, segmental pullback with brief pauses may be employed to allow vein spasm and sclerosant action before further withdrawal. Staged procedures, treating the vein in multiple sessions, may improve safety and durability in extensive disease while limiting total sclerosant volume. Continuous ultrasound monitoring during sclerosant injection is essential. Ultrasound allows real-time visualization of foam propagation, vein wall response, and immediate identification of complications. Effective sclerosant delivery is typically accompanied by vein spasm, wall thickening, and loss of compressibility, indicating adequate endothelial injury. Absence of expected ultrasound findings may indicate dilution, leakage into tributaries, or excessive venous flow. Immediate correction, such as adjusting position, compression, or injection rate, is required to avoid ineffective treatment. Compression during injection enhances vein wall apposition, reduces luminal volume, and limits sclerosant escape into tributaries or perforators. Manual compression may be applied proximally during injection to control flow dynamics. Care must be taken to avoid excessive compression that collapses the vein prematurely, preventing uniform sclerosant distribution. Following catheter removal, immediate application of compression bandaging or stockings is standard practice. Evidence suggests that appropriate compression reduces post-procedural pain, inflammation, and the risk of thrombosis, although optimal dosing and duration remains debated [34]. Compression regimens should be individualized based on vein size, disease severity, and patient tolerance. Extended compression may be particularly beneficial in large-diameter veins or advanced chronic venous disease [35, 36].

7 Post-procedural Care and Follow-Up

Post-procedural care and follow-up represent a continuation of treatment rather than a passive observation phase in catheter-directed sclerotherapy of the saphenous veins. Unlike thermal ablation, which produces immediate vein wall necrosis and mechanical collapse, chemical ablation initiates a time-dependent biologic cascade involving endothelial destruction, thrombus formation, inflammatory remodeling, and eventual fibrosis. The success or failure of this process is strongly influenced by post-procedural management. Failure to provide structured post-treatment protocols is a major contributor to avoidable complications such as thrombosis, hyperpigmentation, delayed recanalization and patient dissatisfaction. In expert venous practice, follow-up is an active, interventional phase, during which outcomes can be optimized and complications mitigated through timely ultrasound surveillance and targeted intervention. Immediately following catheter withdrawal and access site closure, a focused clinical and ultrasound assessment should be performed. This includes evaluation of the treated saphenous segment for luminal echogenicity, loss of compressibility and absence of continuous flow, which collectively suggest effective sclerosant action. Ultrasound assessment should also confirm that no significant sclerosant migration has occurred into the deep venous system, particularly at the saphenofemoral or saphenopopliteal junction. Early detection of junctional thrombus extension allows prompt intervention before progression. Access sites should be inspected for bleeding, hematoma, or localized sclerosant extravasation. Although access-related complications are uncommon with modern low-profile sheaths, their incidence is higher in anticoagulated patients and those with fragile skin. Early ambulation is a cornerstone of post-procedural care. Patients should be encouraged to walk immediately after treatment and to maintain regular ambulation during the first days following the procedure. Calf muscle pump activation reduces venous stasis and lowers the risk of deep vein thrombosis. Prolonged immobilization should be avoided, as it may promote thrombus propagation and exacerbate post-procedural pain and swelling. However, patients should be advised to avoid strenuous lower-limb exercise, heavy lifting, or prolonged standing during the first 24–48 h. Post-procedural discomfort after catheter-directed sclerotherapy is usually mild and self-limited. When required, analgesia is typically limited to a short course of non-steroidal anti-inflammatory drugs. Routine use of anti-inflammatory medication is not universally recommended, yet certified compression and validated venous active drugs can significantly improve the post-procedural symptoms. Micronized Purified Flavonoid Fraction and Sulodexide demonstrated also a possible effect in hyperpigmentation risk reduction [37, 38]. Compression therapy is particularly important following catheter-directed sclerotherapy because chemical ablation represents a controlled but prolonged inflammatory stimulus that is appropriately counteracted by adequate compression. The idea that compression actually "compresses" the treated vein is questioned by even magnetic resonance imaging studies showing how in the subcutaneous tissue the vein is simply pushed down deeper in the limb. The benefit of compression is to be found more in its anti-inflammatory and anti-edema action, eventually adding a hemodynamic effect in case of adequate stiffness of the material [39]. Elastic bandaging may be used immediately post-procedure to provide uniform compression, particularly when treating long truncal segments. This is often followed by transition to compression stockings once ambulation is established. The optimal duration of compression following sclerotherapy remains debated. Evidence suggests that compression for at least several days improves comfort and reduces inflammatory complications, while extended compression may provide incremental benefit in selected patients. In expert practice, compression regimens are individualized based on vein diameter, disease severity, patient tolerance, and ultrasound findings rather than applied uniformly [1]. Duplex ultrasound surveillance is essential following catheter-directed sclerotherapy. Initial follow-up is commonly performed within 7–14 days to assess early treatment response and detect complications. Subsequent examinations are scheduled based on disease severity, initial findings, and symptom evolution. Early imaging allows differentiation between expected post-sclerotherapy thrombosis and pathologic thrombus extension into the deep venous system. Unlike thermal ablation, where immediate vein non-patency is expected, sclerotherapy produces a dynamic ultrasound appearance. Early findings may include partial luminal filling, heterogeneous echogenic thrombus, and residual compressibility, all of which may evolve toward complete fibrosis over weeks. Progressive thrombus organization and loss of compressibility are favorable signs. Persistence of flow without thrombus progression suggests treatment failure and may prompt early intervention. Duplex ultrasound is the primary modality for detecting complications such as thrombus extension into the common femoral or popliteal vein, residual reflux or unexpected recanalization. Surveillance is particularly important in high-risk populations, including anticoagulated patients, those with prior venous thromboembolism and patients treated with large foam volumes. Treatment success after catheter-directed sclerotherapy should be defined using combined clinical, hemodynamic and anatomical criteria. Complete anatomical occlusion is desirable but not mandatory if symptoms have resolved and reflux is absent or minimal. Conversely, persistent symptoms, ongoing reflux or progressive disease constitute clinically meaningful failure, even if partial occlusion is present. Retreatment decisions should generally be deferred until the biologic effects of sclerotherapy have stabilized, typically several weeks to months after the initial procedure. Premature retreatment may disrupt evolving fibrosis and increase complication risk. Early retreatment may be appropriate in cases of clear technical failure, such as untreated long segments or immediate recanalization with persistent reflux. Retreatment options include repeat catheter-directed sclerotherapy, focal ultrasound-guided foam injection or alternative modalities such as thermal ablation, depending on anatomy and prior response (Table 10.1).

Table 10.1 Post-catheter directed sclerotherapy fundamental actions to properly complete the procedure

Post-cahtetered directed sclerotherapy fundamental actions	
Immediate ultrasound scanning	*To verify effective sclerosis:* (1) Luminal echogenicity (2) No compressibility (3) Absence of continuous flow (4) Exclude migration into the deep venous system and in not targeted areas
Monitor access site	*Exclude*: (1) Bleeding (2) Hematoma (3) Localized sclerosant extravasation
Early ambulation	*Minimize complications*: (1) After 20 min from the procedure, avoid sedentarism and promote deambulation to reduce the risk of venous stasis and related thrombosis (2) Avoid strenuous lower-limb exercise, heavy lifting, or prolonged standing during the first 24–48 h

(continued)

Table 10.1 (continued)

Post-cahtetered directed sclerotherapy fundamental actions	
Manage inflammation and hyperpigmentation risk	Consider certified compression and validated venous active drugs
Thromboprophylaxis	*Thrombotic risk assessment* (1) Patient thrombotic risk (2) Procedure extenesion and related thrombotic risk
Follow-up visit (about 2 weeks after)	*Finalize the treatment*: (1) Remove eventually trapped blood (2) Complete missing segments treatment (3) Promptly manage eventual complications

8 Outcomes

Assessment of outcomes following catheter-directed sclerotherapy of the saphenous veins requires a fundamentally different conceptual framework than that applied to thermal or adhesive-based endovenous interventions. Whereas thermal ablation is quite easily standardized in its energy delivery and device use, CDS is characterized by many variables in terms of both catheter and sclerosant use (liquid/foam, concentration, wetness, etc.), therefore making the latter extremely difficult to be assessed in homogenous settings. Indeed, reported anatomical occlusion rates for catheter-directed sclerotherapy vary widely due to heterogeneity in study design, sclerosant type, foam preparation, catheter systems, vein diameters, and follow-up duration. At 6–12 months, occlusion rates for the great saphenous vein commonly range from approximately 70% to 90% in contemporary series. A 2020 meta-analysis analyzed 62 studies, for a total of 3689 patients. A benefit compare to direct sclerotherapy was demonstrated thanks to a relative risk of 1.06 and 1.15 at short (up to 12 months) and mid-term (in between 12 and 36 months), respectively. Moreover, less major and minor complications were reported in the catheter-directed sclerotherapy group (Relative Risk 0.23, Relative Risk 0.43–0.76, $p < 0.05$). In particular, a complete ablation was reported in 82.4% of CDS cases vs direct foam sclerotherapy at 36 months of follow-up. Major complications were reported in 0.23% vs 0.97% of CDS and direct sclerotherapy, respectively. Comparing minor complications in the CDS and direct sclerotherapy groups, pain was present in 15.5% vs 19.9%, hyperpigmentation, hyperpigmentation in 9.92% vs 15.2%, superficial venous thrombosis in 5.93% vs 13.7%, respectively. All the above mentioned minor complications were significantly different in the two groups [20]. In 2020, same year of the above mentioned meta-analysis, Dos Santos et al. published a randomized trial comparing CDS with tumescence vs direct injection foam sclerotherapy. At 1 year follow-up the results were overlapping but less patients in the CDS group had needed adjunctive sclerotherapy injection [40]. Interestingly, a similar study compared high ligation and CDS vs direct foam sclerotherapy, reporting better occlusion rates for the CDS group, but no differences in post-procedural quality of life and venous clinical severity score [41]. Always in 2020, Kakraman et al. demonstrated the performance of CDS in elderly patients (over 65 yo), reporting an occlusion rate of 86.4% (over 65 yo) and 86.3% (under 65 yo) [42]. The authors of this chapter were able to identify only one study comparing CDS with Flebogriff™. The investigation was performed on 79 CDS and 25 Flebogriff™ cases. Complete occlusion rate was 54.43% in CDS and 88% in Flebogriff™ groups. Complications developed in 22 cases following CDS and in five cases after Flebogriff™. Patients were more satisfied after Flebogriff™. The discrepancy in the number of the two groups and the methodological limits of the investigation do not allow solid conclusions for which further investigations are needed on the topic [43]. A 2022 meta-analysis on Flebogriff™ highlighted the paucity of available data, extracting only five studies with a maximum follow up of 12 months, for which further investigations are needed [44]. The authors identified one publication only also in the comparison of Clarivein™ with CDS and specifically with the Sclerosafe™ catheter, characterized by the possibility of aspirating the residual sclerosant following the procedure. The investigation reported no significant differences in venous ulcer healing [45]. A 5 year follow-up study on Clarivein™ reported a freedom from anatomical failure of 78.7%, with no clear clinical predictors of failure [46]. A similar study with the same follow up on the same device demonstrated a similar anatomical success 76.3%, yet BMI was a predictor of failure [47]. Such heterogeneity is confirmed by another investigation on Clarivein™ identifying another predictor of failure in the saphenous diameter >7 mm, already at 3 years follow-up [48]. All these data questions the real benefit of mechano-chemical ablation over catheter-directed sclerotherapy and highlight a heterogeneity in the study designs demanding a proper data collection on the topic.

In conclusion, catheter-directed sclerotherapy appears to be a safe and effective option in specific anatomical and hemodynamic reflux patterns, yet proper scientific validation is still needed to determine this technique real positioning.

References

1. Gianesini S, Obi A, Onida S, et al. Global guidelines trends and controversies in lower limb venous and lymphatic disease: narrative literature revision and experts' opinions following the vWINter international meeting in Phlebology, Lymphology & Aesthetics, 23–25 January 2019. Phlebology. 2019;34(1 Suppl):4–66.
2. Gianesini S, Chi YW, Agüero C, et al. Fake-news-free evidence-based communication for proper vein-lymphatic disease management. Int Angiol. 2023;42(2):89–189.
3. Khan A, Sorour AA, E Anton G, et al. Venous insufficiency: endovascular and surgical treatment. Curr Cardiol Rep. 2025;27(1):67.
4. Parsi K. Catheter-directed sclerotherapy. Phlebology. 2009;24(3):98–107.
5. Gatto A. La Sclerose de La Saphene Interne Jusqua La Crosse avec Catheter (Video). In: Davy A, Stemmer R, editors. Phlebologie. John Libbey Eurotext Ltd; 1989. p. 797.
6. Grondin L, Soriano J. Duplex-echosclerotherapy, the quest for the safe technique. Phlebologie. Paris: John Libbey; 1992. p. 824–5.
7. Robert C, Robert JL. La sclerose par echo-catheterisme. Phlebologie. 1995;48:13–6.
8. Parsi K, Lim AC. Extended long line echosclerotherapy (ELLE)—review of technique. Aust NZ J Phlebol. 2000;4:6–10.
9. Navarro L, Min RJ, Boné C. Endovenous laser: a new minimally invasive method of treatment for varicose veins-preliminary observations using an 810 nm diode laser. Dermatologic Surg. 2001;27:117–22.
10. Brodersen JP, Geismar U. Catheter-assisted vein sclerotherapy: a new approach for sclerotherapy of the greater saphenous vein with a double-lumen balloon catheter. Dermatologic Surg. 2007;33:469–75.
11. Almeida JI, Raines JK. Catheter-directed sclerotherapy for saphenous vein incompetence. An update on the recent progress and current areas of clinical study and development using this therapeutic option. Endovasc Today. 2008;39:32–4.
12. Thibault P. Internal compression (peri-venous) following ultrasound guided sclerotherapy to the great and small saphenous veins. Aust NZ J Phleb. 2005;9:29–32.
13. Devereux N, Recke AL, Westermann L, et al. Catheter-directed foam sclerotherapy of great saphenous veins in combination with pre-treatment reduction of the diameter employing the principals of perivenous tumescent local anesthesia. Eur J Vasc Endovasc Surg. 2014;47(2):187–95.
14. Donnelly LF, Bissett GS III, Adams DM. Combined sonographic and fluoroscopic guidance: a modified technique for percutaneous sclerosis of low-flow vascular malformations. Am J Roentgenol. 1999;173:655–7.
15. Lcu AJ, Inderbitzi R. Balloon sclerotherapy: a new method for the treatment of truncal varicose veins. Vasa. 2008;37(2):165–73.
16. Salerno M, Bissacco D, Chi YW, Narayanan S, et al. Empty vein ablation innovative technique for chronic venous disease treatment: proof of concept and ex-vivo analysis. Int Angiol. 2023;42(5):420–6.
17. Elias S, Raines JK. Mechanochemical tumescentless endovenous ablation: final results of the initial clinical trial. Phlebology. 2012;27(2):67–72.
18. Zubilewicz T, Terlecki P, Terlecki K, et al. Application of endovenous mechanochemical ablation (MOCA) with Flebogrif™ to treat varicose veins of the lower extremities: a single center experience over 3 months of observation. Acta Angiologica. 2016;22(4):137–42. https://doi.org/10.5603/AA.2016.0012.
19. Camillo O. Is catheter-directed foam sclerotherapy more effective than the usual foam sclerotherapy for treatment of the great saphenous vein? Phlebology. 2018;33(9):646–52.
20. Lim SY, Tan JX, D'Cruz RT, Syn N, et al. Catheter-directed foam sclerotherapy, an alternative to ultrasound-guided foam sclerotherapy for varicose vein treatment: a systematic review and meta-analysis. Phlebology. 2020;35(6):369–83.
21. Gianesini S, Danese M, AlQedrah D, et al. Multi-specialty recommendations for the appropriate and

affordable lower limb vein-lymphatic disorders management. Int Angiol. 2026;45:1–64.
22. Molino Lova R, Cappelli M, Macchi C, et al. Macroscopic anatomy of the superficial veins of the lower limb: a systematic review based upon echography. Ital J Anat Embryol. 2001;106(3):215–20.
23. Shadid N, Nelemans P, Lawson J, et al. Predictors of recurrence of great saphenous vein reflux following treatment with ultrasound-guided foamsclerotherapy. Phlebology. 2015;30(3):194–9.
24. Kockaert M, de Roos KP, van Dijk L, et al. Duplication of the great saphenous vein: a definition problem and implications for therapy. Dermatologic Surg. 2012;38(1):77–82.
25. Corcos L, Macchi C, de Anna D, et al. The anatomical variables of the sapheno-popliteal junction visualization by radiological and echographic examinations. Ital J Anat Embryol. 1996;101(1):15–28.
26. Garagozlo C, Kadri O, Atalla M, et al. The anatomical relationship between the sural nerve and small saphenous vein: an ultrasound study of healthy participants. Clin Anat. 2019;32(2):277–81.
27. Szary C, Wilczko J, Plucinska D, et al. The analysis of selected morphological and hemodynamic parameters of the venous system and their presumable impact on the risk of recurrence after varicose vein treatment. J Clin Med. 2021;10(3):455.
28. Carugo D, Ankrett DN, O'Byrne V, et al. The role of clinically-relevant parameters on the cohesiveness of sclerosing foams in a biomimetic vein model. J Mater Sci Mater Med. 2015;26(11):258.
29. Williamsson C, Danielsson P, Smith L. Catheter-directed foam sclerotherapy for chronic venous leg ulcers. Phlebology. 2014;29(10):688–93.
30. Seo SH, Kim MB, Kwon KS, et al. Primary venous aneurysms of the superficial venous system. Angiology. 2008;59(5):593–8.
31. Wong M, Parsi K, Myers K, et al. Sclerotherapy of lower limb veins: indications, contraindications and treatment strategies to prevent complications—a consensus document of the International Union of Phlebology-2023. Phlebology. 2023;38(4):205–58.
32. Danneil O, Dörler M, Stockfleth E, et al. Factors influencing superficial and deep vein thrombosis after foam sclerotherapy in varicose veins. J Dtsch Dermatol Ges. 2022;20(7):929–38.
33. Watanabe S, Okamura A, Iwamoto M, et al. A randomized controlled trial to evaluate the safety and efficacy of transluminal injection of foam sclerotherapy compared with ultrasound-guided foam sclerotherapy during endovenous catheter ablation in patients with varicose veins. J Vasc Surg. 2021;10:10.
34. de Aguiar ET, Dos Santos JB, Carvalho DD. Venous thromboembolism after ultrasound guided foam sclerotherapy. Phlebology. 2021;36:233–9.
35. Cavezzi A, Mosti G, Colucci R, et al. Compression with 23 mmHg or 35 mmHg stockings after saphenous catheter foam sclerotherapy and phlebectomy of varicose veins: a randomized controlled study. Phlebology. 2019;34(2):98–106.
36. Belramman A, Bootun R, Lane TRA, et al. COmpressioN following endovenous TreatmenT of Incompetent varicose veins by sclerotherapy (CONFETTI). J Vasc Surg Venous Lymphat Disord. 2024;12(2):101729.
37. Bogachev VY, Boldin BV, Turkin PY. Administration of micronized purified flavonoid fraction during sclerotherapy of reticular veins and telangiectasias: results of the national, multicenter, observational program VEIN ACT PROLONGED-C1. Adv Ther. 2018;35(7):1001–8.
38. Gonzalez Ochoa AJ, Carrillo J, Manríquez D, et al. Reducing hyperpigmentation after sclerotherapy: a randomized clinical trial. J Vasc Surg Venous Lymphat Disord. 2021;9(1):154–62.
39. Partsch H, Mosti G, Mosti F. Narrowing of leg veins under compression demonstrated by magnetic resonance imaging (MRI). Int Angiol. 2010;29(5):408–10.
40. Dos Santos JB, Júnior WC, Porta RM, et al. Catheter-directed foam sclerotherapy with tumescence of the great saphenous vein versus ultrasound-guided foam sclerotherapy: a randomized controlled trial. Phlebology. 2020;35(2):84–91.
41. Yu S, Li R, Cheng J, et al. Is catheter-based foam sclerotherapy more effective than direct foam sclerotherapy when combined with high ligation for the treatment of primary great saphenous vein incompetence? Vascular. 2023;31(5):981–8.
42. Kahraman N, Özsin KK. Ultrasound-guided catheter-directed foam sclerotherapy can be safely applied for the treatment of great saphenous varicose veins in elderly patients. Vascular. 2020;28(5):597–603.
43. Hamed EA, Elwakeel HA, Eldin HA. Chemical and mechanochemical catheter-directed sclerotherapy in varicose vein ablation. Egypt J Surg. 2021;40:90–8.
44. Alozai T, Huizing E, Schreve M, et al. A systematic review and meta-analysis of mechanochemical endovenous ablation using Flebogrif for varicose veins. J Vasc Surg Venous Lymphat Disord. 2022;10(1):248–257.e2.
45. Avrahami M, Silverberg D, Elias S, et al. Inframalleolar access in endovenous treatment of venous ulcers and C5 disease with nonthermal nontumescent techniques. J Vasc Surg Venous Lymphat Disord. 2022;10(2):417–22.
46. Thierens N, Holewijn S, Vissers WH, et al. Five-year outcomes of mechano-chemical ablation of primary great saphenous vein incompetence. Phlebology. 2020;35(4):255–61.
47. Witte ME, Holewijn S, van der Veen D, et al. Long-term results and predictors of failure after mechanochemical endovenous ablation in the treatment of primary great saphenous vein incompetence. Phlebology. 2024;39(1):9–19.
48. Vähäaho S, Halmesmäki K, Mahmoud O, et al. Three-year results of a randomized controlled trial comparing mechanochemical and thermal ablation in the treatment of insufficient great saphenous veins. J Vasc Surg Venous Lymphat Disord. 2021;9(3):652–9.

Sclerotherapy for Lower Limb Telangiectasia Treatment

11

Nathalia Cardoso Oliveira and Sergio Gianesini

1 Background

Telangiectasias are intradermal dilated small vessels with a diameter of less than 1 mm. Popularly known as "spider veins" and fairly visible to the naked eye, they can usually be of red, blue, or purplish in color. They are classified as C1 in the Clinical, Etiological, Anatomical, Pathophysiological (CEAP) classification, along with reticular veins (1–3 mm), which often act as feeding veins [1]. With an unknown cause and a long historical perception as a merely aesthetic problem, they can also be associated with symptoms such as pain, burning, itching, and a sensation of heaviness in the limbs, representing an early stage of chronic venous disease (CVD) [2, 3]. Risk factors include family history, pregnancy, local trauma, obesity, and hormonal factors [4, 5]. The global prevalence is high: studies estimate that between 60% and 86% of the adult population has telangiectasias or reticular veins, with a higher frequency in females and a progressive increase with age [4, 6–9]. The aesthetic and psychosocial impact is important, leading many patients to seek treatment even in the absence of clinical symptoms. Multicenter programs, such as the Vein Consult Program, have demonstrated that 63.9% of the patients evaluated were between C1 and C6; the initial stages (C0s–C2) accounted for approximately 58% of the sample. C1–C3 were more frequent in women, regardless of the country [10]. Sclerotherapy has established itself as the standard treatment for telangiectasias. The therapeutic principle consists of injecting a sclerosing agent into the venous lumen, promoting endothelial damage, thrombosis, and subsequent fibrosis of the vascular wall, with the disappearance of the treated vessel [11]. The development of detergent agents such as polidocanol and sodium tetradecyl sulfate (STS) has allowed for efficacy and a lower complication rate when compared to solutions used in the past [11, 12]. More recently, the use of image-guided techniques, such as transillumination, augmented reality, and ultrasonography, has increased the accuracy in identifying and treating feeding veins, increasing the clinical success rate [13, 14].

N. C. Oliveira
Private Clinic Nathalia Cardoso Saúde Vascular, São Luís, Brazil
e-mail: atendimento@nathaliacardoso.com

S. Gianesini (✉)
Department of Translational Medicine, University of Ferrara, Ferrara, Italy

Department of Surgery, Uniformed Services University of Health Sciences, Bethesda, MD, USA
e-mail: gnssrg@unife.it

S. Gianesini, Y. W. Chi (eds.), *Sclerotherapy*, https://doi.org/10.1007/978-3-032-32794-9_11

2 Pathophysiology of Telangiectasias of the Lower Limbs

An understanding of the pathophysiology of these vessels is essential to ensure effective treatment. Telangiectasias are intradermal dilations of the subpapillary venous plexus. Histopathological studies demonstrate that these vessels have a thickened venous wall composed of collagen, muscle fibers, and, in some cases, elastic fibers, reflecting progressive structural remodeling [6]. Current evidence shows that these telangiectasias might share some mechanisms of advanced chronic venous disease (CVD), with different proposed theories including localized venous hypertension and microvascular inflammation [2, 4]. Engelhorn et al. found that up to 46% of patients with only telangiectasias have saphenous reflux on Duplex ultrasound [15]. On the other hand, Blin discovered communications between telangiectasias and the deep venous system through small perforators while performing the technique of micro-venography [16]. Besides that, several authors [17–20] described a relation between feeder veins or incompetent perforators and telangiectasias. Theses feeders veins can be often responsible for the persistence or recurrence of telangiectasias after superficial treatments [18]. In telangiectasias on the lateral side of the thigh, a feeding reticular vein (Fig. 11.1) connected to posterolateral perforators (lateral subdermal plexus described by Albanese) is common. This circuit may support "resistant vessels" and promote matting or recurrence when only the superficial network is treated [17]. This evidence reinforces the need to map and treat feeder veins, either with Doppler ultrasound (Fig. 11.2) or assisted visualization techniques, as an essential part of the therapeutic strategy [6].

The inflammatory and parietal theory suggests that a primary alteration of the venous wall, with initial dilation of the venules, leads to blood stasis, leukocyte adhesion, and additional wall damage, resulting in further dilation and progression of telangiectasias [21]. Complementarily, the connective and adipose tissue theory proposes that fat lobules may reduce venous return, generating localized venous hypertension and favoring the emergence of these lesions [22]. Thus, both hypotheses point to structural and hemodynamic mechanisms that, possibly interconnected, contribute to the development and worsening of telangiectasias, although further evidence is needed to confirm their clinical and therapeutic implications. Although rare, arteriovenous microshunts have been described in some studies [20] and may explain therapeutic failures and complications such as skin necrosis after sclerotherapy [6]. The presence of these shunts requires caution in injection, with small volumes and low pressure, to reduce the risk of inadvertent passage of sclerosant into the arterial circulation.

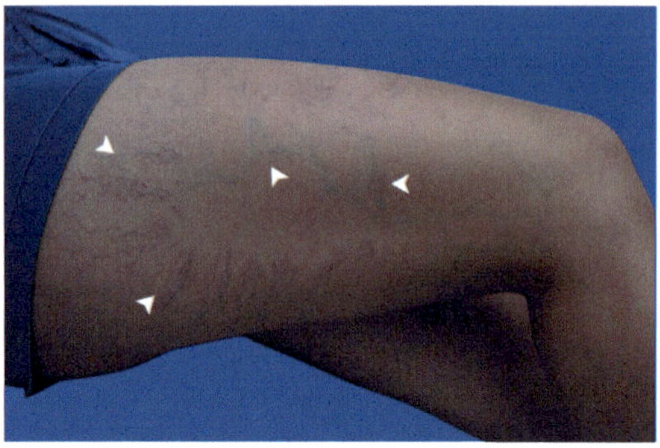

Fig. 11.1 Feeder veins underlying lateral-thigh telangiectasias. Clinical image of the lateral thigh showing a telangiectatic plexus with reticular "feeder" veins that communicate with the intradermal network—key targets to map and treat for durable results

Both types are venous, but present significant pathophysiological differences (Fig. 11.3):

- Red Telangiectasias: more superficial, reduced diameter, greater resistance to sclerosing treatment.
- Blue Telangiectasias: associated with deeper reticular veins, generally more responsive to treatment [6].

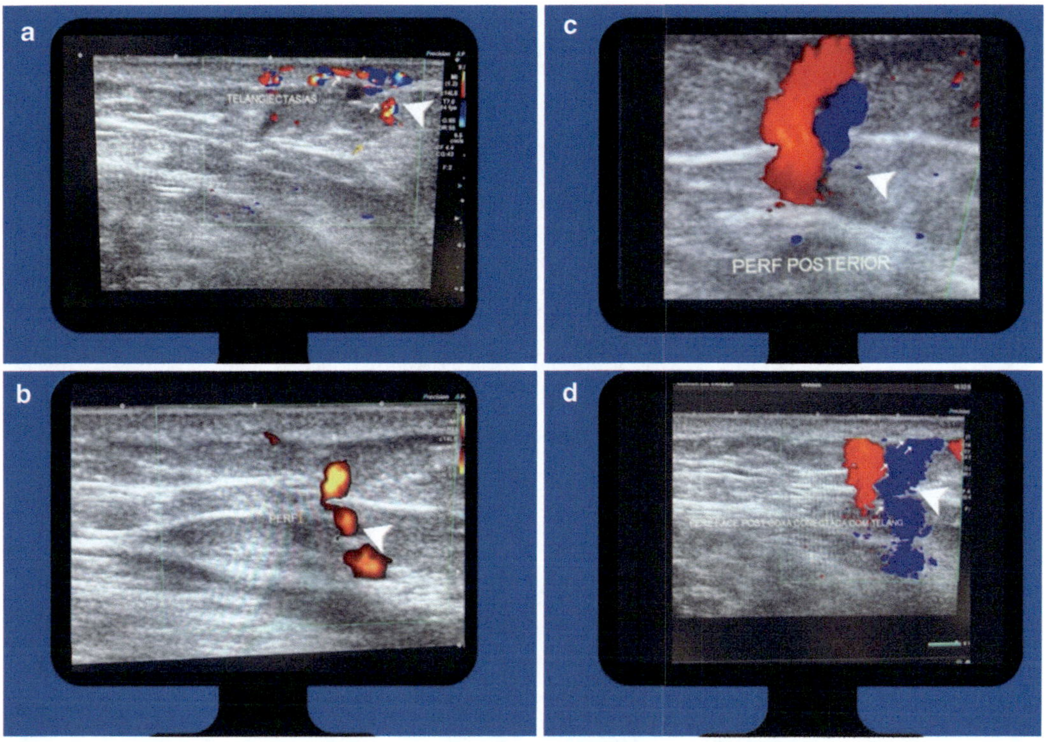

Fig. 11.2 Duplex ultrasound showing an incompetent perforator feeding the telangiectatic plexus. Longitudinal color Doppler view of the lateral thigh in the same patient demonstrates a subfascial perforator (**b**, **c**) with retrograde flow after distal compression release (**d**), connecting the deep system to a reticular feeder vein that supplies the intradermal telangiectasias (**a**)

Fig. 11.3 Red (**a**) and blue (**b**) telangiectasias

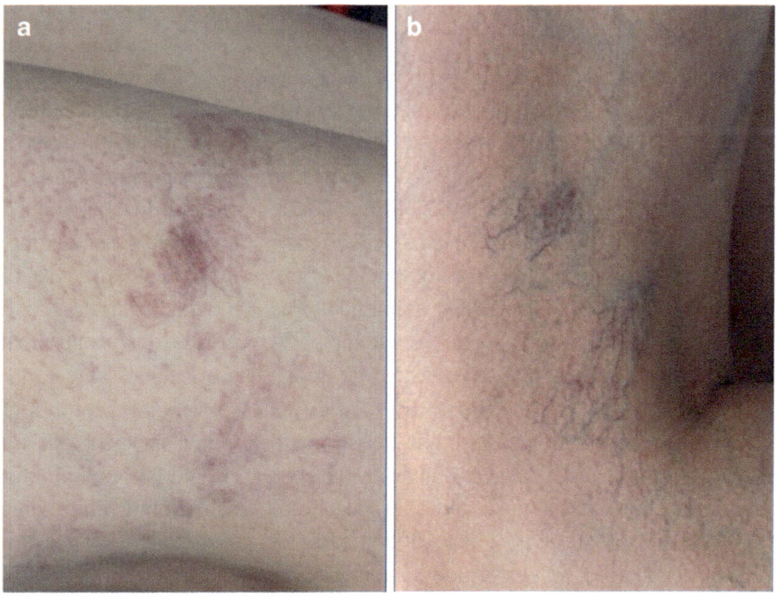

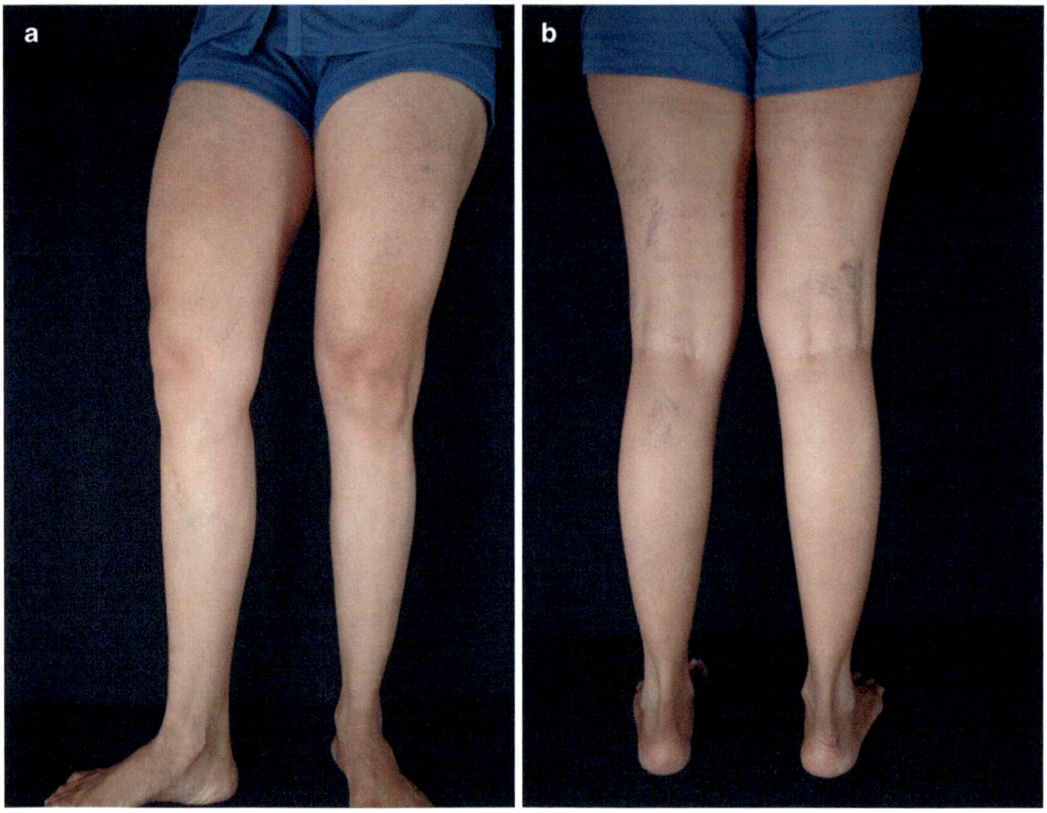

Fig. 11.4 Patient in upright position during physical examination

Patient evaluation should begin with a detailed personal and family history, addressing a history of venous disease, thrombosis, previous treatments, and risk factors such as pregnancy, hormone therapy, obesity, and prolonged standing. The Caprini Score is recommended for stratifying thromboembolic risk, providing a comprehensive view of the patient's profile [23, 24]. The physical examination should be performed in the upright position (Fig. 11.4), with special attention paid to differentiating telangiectasias (≤1 mm, intradermal) from reticular veins (1–3 mm, often feeding veins). During the examination, it is essential to assess the filling rate after compression, the color of the vessels, and the number of feeding veins. These findings guide not only the diagnosis but also the choice of therapeutic strategy. Photodocumentation (Fig. 11.5) should be performed systematically, enabling objective comparison during clinical and scientific follow-up.

The procedure includes multiple standardized photographs documenting all telangiectasias with the patient in both standing and supine positions. In the upright position, sequential images are taken of the anterior aspect of each leg, followed by the medial region (including the saphenous area), then the lateral and posterior aspects, with additional focused photographs of specific telangiectasias when required. In the supine position, the same sequence is repeated (anterior, medial, lateral, and posterior views), complemented by prone positioning to capture the full posterior surface.

Venous color Doppler ultrasound examination of the lower limbs is the diagnostic method of choice, allowing the physician to rule out deeper causes and map hidden connections (Fig. 11.6). The evaluation should include, in addition to the classic vein protocol [25], a detailed investigation with the following objectives:

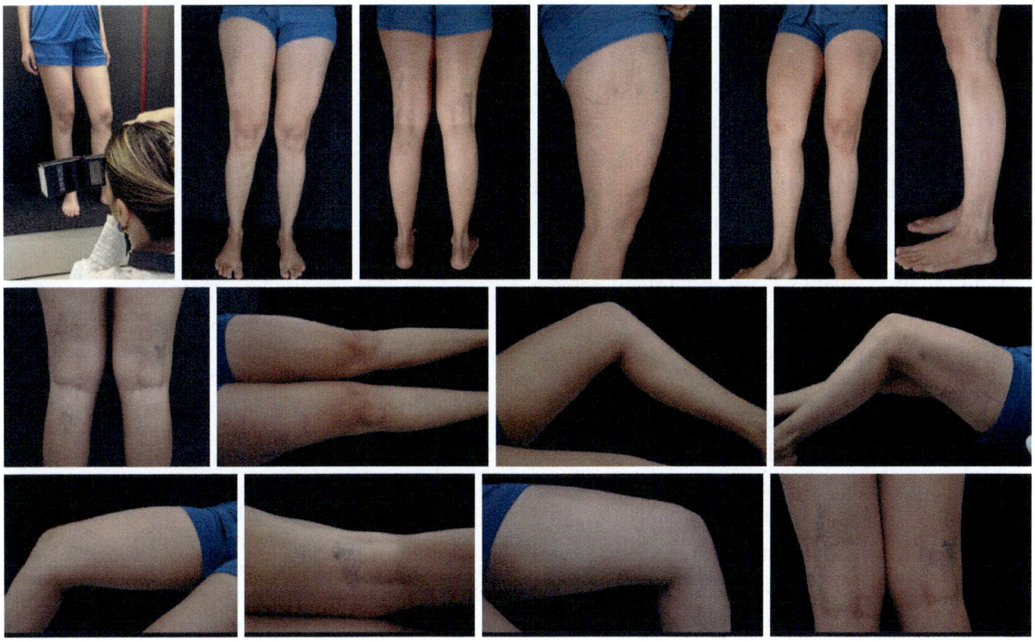

Fig. 11.5 Systematic photodocumentation for objective clinical and scientific follow-up

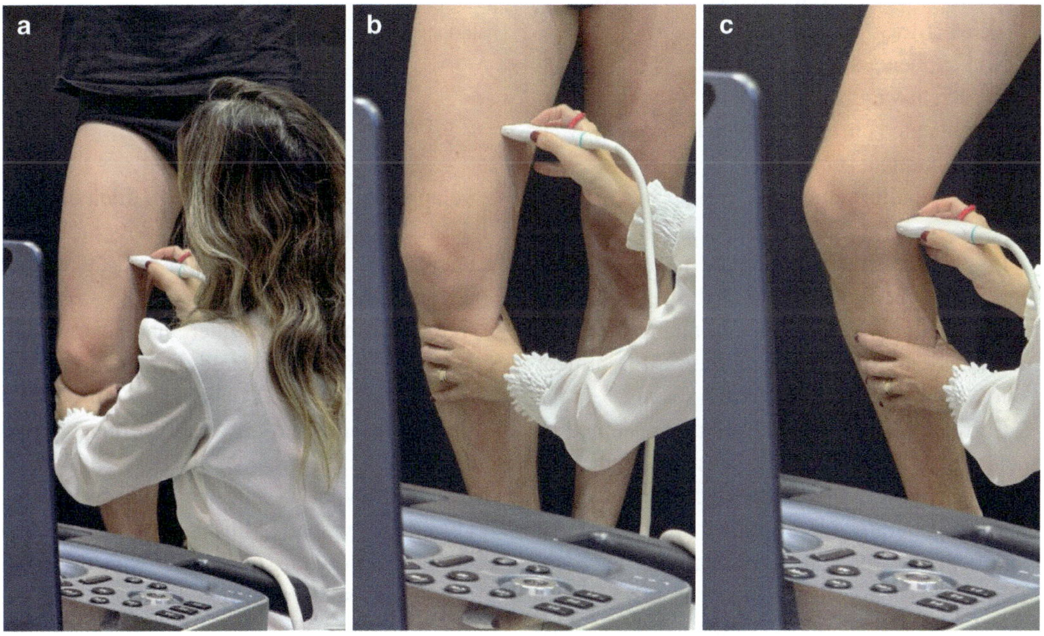

Fig. 11.6 Venous color Doppler ultrasound of the lower limbs with the patient in supine position. Images **a–c** show the same finding, highlighting the method's role in ruling out saphenous and perforator insufficiency, pelvic reflux, and mapping telangiectasia plexuses

- Rule out saphenous insufficiency (great and small saphenous veins).
- Identify perforating vein insufficiency, which may supply superficial plexuses.
- Rule out reflux originating from the pelvic region [26], which may manifest as atypical varicose veins associated with telangiectasias or recurrent veins.
- Individually evaluate each telangiectasia plexus, checking for connections with larger veins or deep pathways.

Although the use of ultrasound in all patients is debated, when seeking diagnostic accuracy and individualized treatment planning, its use should be strongly considered. According to the UIP Consensus Document on Duplex Ultrasound Investigation of the Veins in Chronic Venous Disease [27], the main formal indications include:

- Primary varicose veins in the great saphenous vein territory.
- Primary varicose veins in the small saphenous vein territory.
- Non-saphenous varicose veins.
- Recurrent varicose veins.
- Complicated chronic venous disease.
- Post-treatment surveillance.
- Venous malformations.

In all these situations, duplex ultrasound can locate and specify the origin of the venous problem, providing a true diagnostic map. This mapping is essential for selecting the best treatment option and objectively evaluating results.

Currently, there is no universally accepted or standardized classification system dedicated exclusively to telangiectasias. In clinical practice, they are generally incorporated into the CEAP classification of chronic venous disorders (Table 11.1), being categorized as C1 together with reticular veins. CEAP remains as the most internationally recognized, offering consistency in both clinical documentation and scientific communication.

However, there are some practical definitions to standardize documentation and planning of C1 subtypes such as:

Table 11.1 CEAP classification (Clinical Etiological Anatomical Pathophysiological)

Category	Subcategories/description
C—Clinical	*C0*: No visible or palpable signs of venous disease*C1*: Telangiectasias or reticular veins *C2*: Varicose veins (>3 mm) *C2r*: Recurrent varicose veins *C3*: Edema *C4a*: Pigmentation, eczema *C4b*: Lipodermatosclerosis, atrophie blanche *C4c*: Corona phlebectatica *C5*: Healed venous ulcer *C6*: Active venous ulcer *(add: "s" for symptomatic; "a" for asymptomatic)*
E—Etiological	*Ec*: Congenital *Ep*: Primary *Es*: Secondary (e.g., post-thrombotic) *En*: No venous cause identified
A—Anatomical	*As*: Superficial veins *Ap*: Perforator veins *Ad*: Deep veins *An*: No venous location identified
P—Pathophysiological	*Pr*: Reflux *Po*: Obstruction *Pro*: Reflux + obstruction *Pn*: No venous pathophysiology identifiable

- Telangiectasias: confluence of dilated intradermal venules <1 mm, lined by a single endothelial layer with thin muscular and adventitial layers.
- Venulectasias: veins wider than telangiectasias (1–2 mm) in the mid-dermis/subdermis, often slightly raised or arranged in "grape-like" clusters, and invariably connected to feeder veins.
- Reticular Veins: subdermal dilated veins (1–3 mm), typically bluish; correspond to normally visible veins in patients with thin skin or to larger subdermal vessels.

In the Edinburgh Vein Study, authors reported reticular veins in approximately 50% of subjects and a positive correlation between superficial venous incompetence and the presence of telangiectasias [28]. According to the European Society for Vascular Surgery (ESVS) 2022 guidelines for

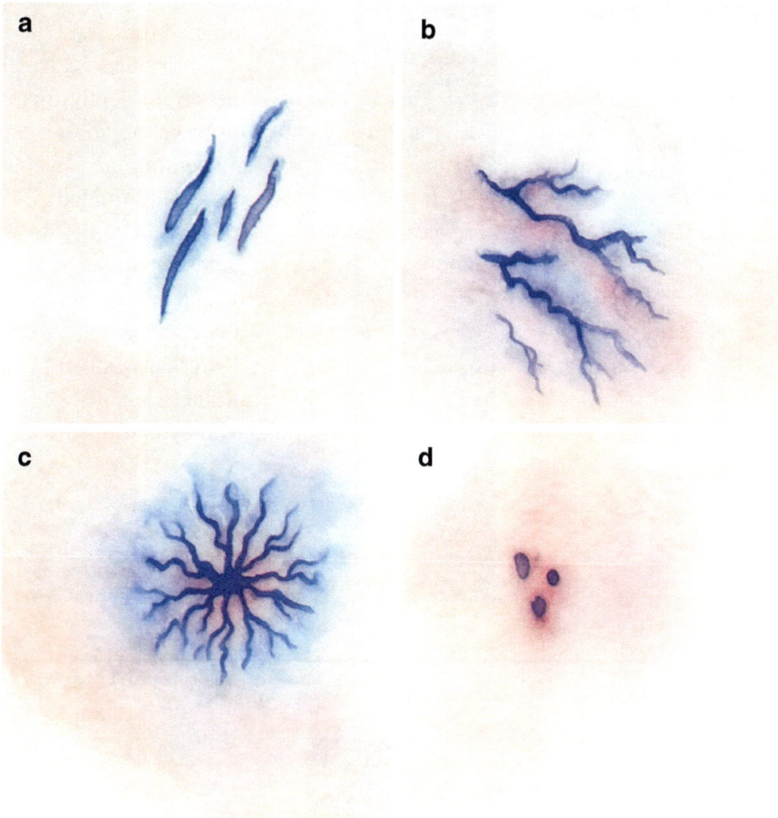

Fig. 11.7 Morphological patterns of telangiectasias. (After Redisch & Pelzer, 1949): (**a**) simple/linear; (**b**) arborizing; (**c**) spider (stellate); (**d**) papular. (Artwork © 2025 Joana Storino, MD)

chronic venous disease, recommendations for liquid sclerotherapy are: reticular veins—Grade IA; telangiectasias—Grade IIA [29].

In addition to CEAP, some morphological classifications have been proposed to describe telangiectasias. The pioneering work of Redisch and Pelzer (1949) identified four distinct clinical patterns (Fig. 11.7) of localized vascular dilatations [30]:

1. *Simple/Linear Telangiectasia*—a single red or blue vessel, flat and non-palpable, varying in length and diameter.
2. *Arborizing Telangiectasia*—a branching vessel pattern similar to tree limbs.
3. *Spider (Stellate) Telangiectasia*—a central point with multiple radiating branches in 360°, often raised, resembling a "spider."
4. *Papular Telangiectasia*—small, elevated red papules, usually ranging from pinpoint to 1 cm in diameter.

Histological and capillaroscopic analysis by the same authors demonstrated that these structures consist of dilated venous or capillary channels lined only by endothelium, without muscular or adventitial layers. This finding excluded a true arteriolar origin, even in spider telangiectasias where pulsation was sometimes observed. In such cases, the pulsation was interpreted as transmitted from adjacent arterioles, not as intrinsic arterial flow.

Later, Goldman and Bennett (1987) [31] complemented these observations by proposing a clinical distinction (Fig. 11.8) between:

- *Arteriolar-Type Telangiectasias*: small, bright red, superficial, frequently located on the face and upper trunk.
- *Venular-Type Telangiectasias*: larger, blue or violet, often located on the lower extremities and associated with venous hypertension.

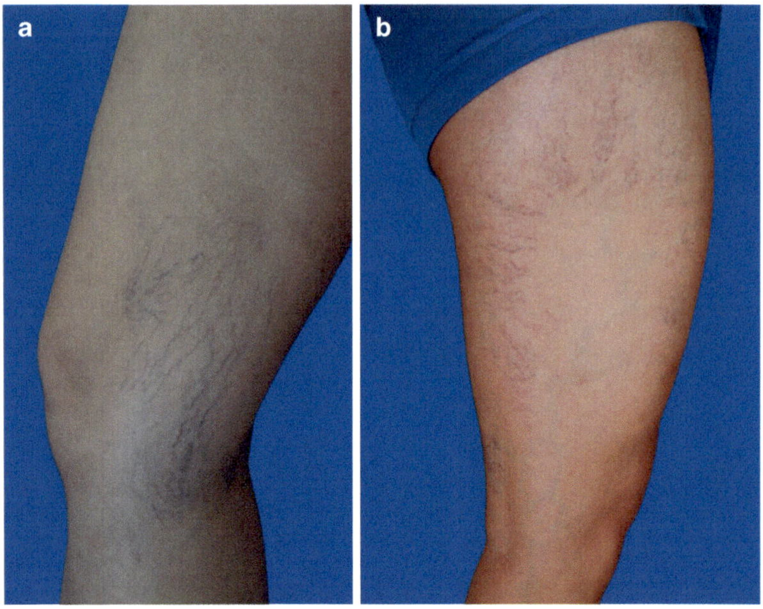

Fig. 11.8 Distribution patterns of lower-limb telangiectasias. (**a**) Parallel linear pattern along the medial thigh. (**b**) Arborizing or "sunburst" pattern on the lateral thigh

	absent	NO feeder vein	WITH feeder vein
	TELEANGECTASIA		
absent	1	2	3
NO saphenous, pelvic, perforating origin	4	5	6
WITH saphenous, pelvic, perforating origin	7	8	9

Fig. 11.9 Score 9–1. Diagram of the 9-cell matrix proposed by Kasuo Miyake detecting telangiectasias with feeder connections. Nine possible scenarios, supporting treatment decisions when clinical evaluation alone is ambiguous. Scheme created by the author, adapted from the original publication. (Source: Miyake K, Davidson JRP. *Augmented Reality and Duplex Ultrasound in Medical Treatment Decision: Score 9–1*. J Phlebol Lymphol. 2019;12(1):1–2)

They also described typical distribution patterns, such as the parallel linear pattern on the medial thigh and the arborizing or "sunburst" pattern on the lateral thigh.

Although these morphological systems are descriptive rather than universally standardized, they remain clinically useful for photographic documentation, patient communication, and treatment planning.

In 2005, Miyake and colleagues [14] proposed the Score 9–1 (Fig. 11.9), a 9-cell matrix combining duplex ultrasound (DU) and augmented reality (AR).

- *DU* defines whether there is reflux in saphenous or perforator veins.
- *AR* identifies whether telangiectasias are connected to feeder veins.

By crossing these two variables, the table generates nine possible scenarios, from absence of disease to combined reflux and feeder-associated telangiectasias.

This system does not replace CEAP or VCSS but offers a practical adjunct to refine treatment decisions, particularly when clinical evaluation alone is ambiguous.

3 Principles of Aesthetic Sclerotherapy

Produce controlled endothelial injury sufficient to achieve occlusion and lasting fibrosis of the unwanted vein; inadequate denaturation leads to persistence/recanalization, whereas extravascular diffusion risks tissue necrosis. One of the most important concepts in sclerotherapy is to destroy the most extension of vessel wall possible with the least amount of sclerosant necessary to do it (Fig. 11.10). Excessive doses increase the risk of adverse effects, while very low concentrations favor recanalization and therapeutic failure.

Endothelial destruction can be total or partial, depending on the concentration used. Irreversible endothelial damage promotes organized thrombosis and replacement of the vascular wall with fibrous tissue. Insufficient concentrations result in unstable thrombi and a greater likelihood of recanalization.

An important thing to notice is that, immediately after injection, the sclerosant mixes with the blood, and the concentration that truly matters is the one that reaches the endothelium, not the one in the vial. This gradient creates three effect zones (Fig. 11.11) around the injection site:

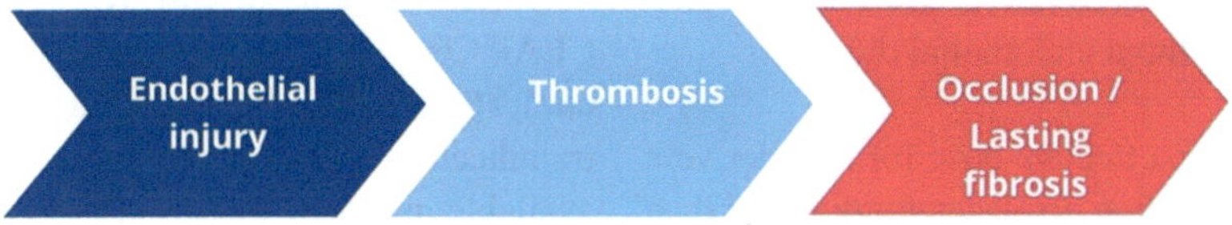

Fig. 11.10 Flowchart of the desired mechanism for sclerotherapy. Pathophysiological sequence: (1) endothelial injury (concentration/contact time-dependent wall denaturation) → (2) intraluminal thrombosis and spasm → (3) scar remodeling with fibrosis and definitive vessel occlusion (author's adaptation)

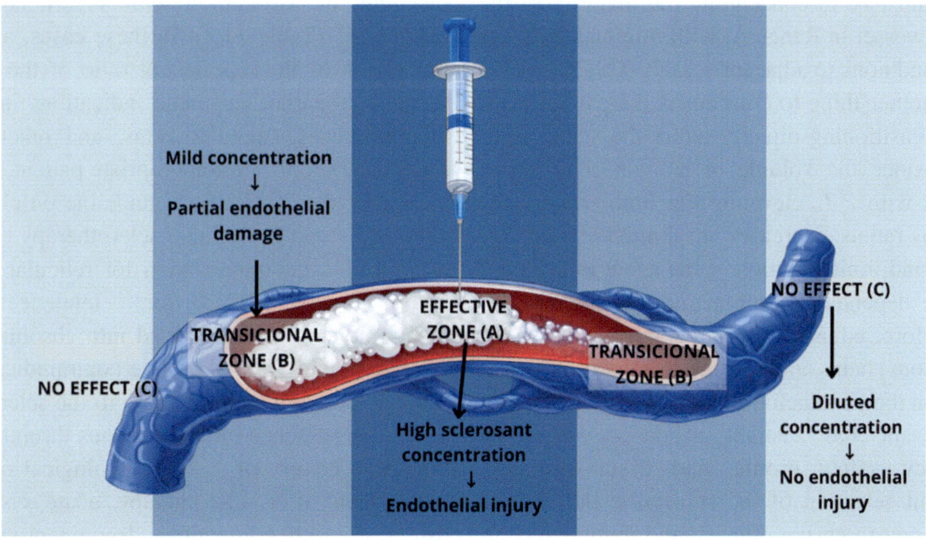

Fig. 11.11 Radial dilution of the sclerosant. Representation of the three action zones (A: irreversible injury and fibrosis; B: partial thrombosis with recanalization; C: no injury) formed by dilution of the agent from the injection site

Table 11.2 UIP Consensus 2023—Lower limb sclerotherapy: indications, contraindications and practical points (summary)

Topic	Practical summary
Indications	Chronic venous disease CEAP C0s–C6s with signs/symptoms; cosmetic for C1 after evaluation; selected situations even without complaints when DUS reveals relevant incompetence (e.g., extensive subdermal network, risk of bleeding)
Absolute contraindications	Allergy to the agent; acute VTE; recent history of severe neurological/cardiac events; infection/decompensated systemic disease; severe PAD
Relative contraindications/require selection	Pregnancy, postpartum period, lactation; increased risk of VTE (personal/family history, thrombophilia); PFO/neurological risk; poorly controlled comorbidities
Precautions (cutaneous/ aesthetic)	Avoid extravasation and local overdose (necrosis); reduce matting and hyperpigmentation with appropriate technique, concentration, and volumes; compression and photoprotection as appropriate

- Range A—concentration sufficient for irreversible wall damage, leading to occlusion and fibrosis of the target vessel.
- Range B—suboptimal damage with partial/temporary thrombosis, which tends toward recanalization.
- Range C—concentration below the damaging threshold, without endothelial damage.

In practice, an effective dose for a spider vein (where the fluid often displaces more blood than it mixes) may fail in a reticular/truncular vein due to intraluminal dilution. Moreover, very high doses expand the A/B zones beyond the target, increasing the risk of unwanted tissue injury. The goal must be to concentrate the majority of the target vessel in Range A, with minimal spillover to B and none to adjacent vessels (C) [32].

Another thing to consider is the patient position. Positioning directly alters the sclero dilution: since the volume of a cylindrical vessel varies with $r^2 \cdot L$, elevating the limb reduces the venous radius, decreases intraluminal blood volume, and limits dilution of the agent in the wall; in the dependent position, the opposite occurs. Therefore, adjusting posture (and manual compressions) helps optimize the effective concentration on the endothelial surface [32]. Each type of sclerosant has distinct properties regarding potency, safety profile, and tissue response. Careful selection of the substance and dose is important to ensure efficacy and minimize complications. Although there is no absolute consensus on universal dilution protocols, modern practice emphasizes individualized treatment, considering vessel caliber, local flow, and patient anatomy. According to the 2023 UIP Consensus, sclerotherapy may be indicated for clinical, preventive, or cosmetic reasons [33]. Clinical indications include patients with symptoms or signs of chronic venous disease (CVD), classified as CEAP C0s to C6s, or asymptomatic patients with clinical signs of CVD, provided there are no contraindications. Preventive indications are also available in selected cases of individuals without complaints, but where Doppler ultrasound reveals significant venous incompetence, such as an extensive network of incompetent veins, the presence of subdermal varicose veins with a risk of bleeding, or association with superficial vein thrombosis (Table 11.2). In these cases, a prior discussion of the risk-benefit ratio of the treatment is essential. Cosmetic indications include telangiectasias, reticular veins, and other aesthetic alterations, after appropriate patient evaluation. Per the 2022 ESVS guideline on chronic venous disease [34], liquid sclerotherapy carries a Grade IA recommendation for reticular veins and Grade IIA for telangiectasias. Contraindications are divided into absolute and relative (Table 11.2). Absolute contraindications include known hypersensitivity to the sclerosing agent, the presence of acute venous thromboembolism, a history of severe neurological or cardiac events after sclerotherapy, acute systemic diseases or active infections, decompensation of chronic diseases, and severe peripheral arterial disease. Relative contraindications include

Table 11.3 Classification of sclerosing agents according to mechanism of action

Class	Agents	Commercial examples	Main mechanism
Detergents	Sodium tetradecyl sulfate, Polidocanol, Sodium morrhuate, Ethanolamine oleate	Sotradecol®, Aethoxysklerol®, Scleromate®, Ethamolin®	Disruption of endothelial lipid membranes
Osmotic agents	Hypertonic saline, Saline/dextrose	Hypertonic saline 15–30%, Sclerodex®, Hipertonic glucose	Dehydration and cell lysis by osmotic gradient
Chemical irritants	Chromated glycerin, Polyiodinated iodine	Sclermo®, iodine-based solutions	Direct caustic injury to the venous wall

pregnancy, the postpartum period, and lactation, as well as conditions associated with an increased risk of venous thromboembolism, such as a personal or family history of thrombosis and hereditary or acquired thrombophilias. Patients with a patent foramen ovale or high neurological risk, increased cardiac risk, or poorly controlled systemic diseases should also be carefully evaluated. In cases where there is a risk of thrombosis, appropriate stratification and consideration of thromboprophylaxis measures before the intervention are recommended.

Sclerosing agents are classified into three main groups (Table 11.3): detergents (sodium tetradecyl sulfate, polidocanol, sodium morrhuate, and ethanolamine oleate), osmotic agents (hypertonic saline and hypertonic glucose), and chemical irritants (such as chromated glycerin and iodinated solutions). In Brazil, hypertonic glucose (commonly 75%) is widely used in daily practice, either alone or in combination with low concentrations of polidocanol, although scientific evidence supporting its efficacy is less robust compared to detergent agents. In the context of sclerotherapy for telangiectasias and reticular veins, the detergents polidocanol (Aethoxysklerol®) and sodium tetradecyl sulfate (Sotradecol®) are the most commonly used [31, 35]. The choice of sclerosant concentration depends on the vessel caliber. For telangiectasias (≤1 mm), the recommended concentration is polidocanol between 0.25 and 0.5% or STS between 0.1 and 0.2%. For reticular veins (1–3 mm), the ideal concentrations range from 0.5 to 1% for polidocanol and 0.2 to 0.5% for STS. In both situations, reduced volumes should be used per injection site, respecting the maximum limit of 10 mL of pure sclerosant per session, in order to minimize systemic complications [33]. As for some evidence on the use of sclerosants, the EASI trial [11] was a double-blind RCT in C1 comparing Polidocanil 0.5%, STS 1% and isotonic saline: both detergents superior to saline for efficacy; local adverse effects were more frequent with STS than Polidocanol. In the same line, a Brazilian triple-blind RCT [36] comparing POL 0.2% + Glucose 70% vs. Glucose 75%: greater clearance of telangiectasias and reticulars with the combination, no increase in complications. Examples: elimination of reticulars 95.2% vs. 85.4%; mean residual length 3.07 vs. 8.30 cm; all $p < 0.01$. Thus, sclerotherapy of telangiectasias and reticular veins, when performed with an appropriate technique, careful selection of the sclerosing agent and subsequent compression, presents high rates of efficacy and safety (Table 11.4).

Foam vs. Liquid in C1 For telangiectasias/reticular veins, liquid sclerotherapy is the standard; foam can be used selectively, especially when there are larger caliber reticular feeding veins [34].

Photodocumentation is considered a fundamental step in the monitoring of patients undergoing sclerotherapy (Fig. 11.12). Photographs should be taken in a standardized manner, always respecting the same lighting conditions, distance, and positioning, both pre- and post-treatment. In addition to allowing for an objective analysis of the results, this practice helps reduce disputes regarding the causality of complications and reliably document clinical progress. Studies show that photodocumentation, in addition to its medicolegal utility, increases the perception of patient

Table 11.4 Dose guardrails for liquid sclerotherapy in C1

Agent	C1 target	Typical liquid concentration	Session limits	Notes
Polidocanol (POL)	Telangiectasias (≤1 mm); reticular veins (1–3 mm)	Up to 0.5% for both	Max systemic dose: 2 mg/kg	Calculate mg = (% × mL × 10). Keep small aliquots; slow, low-pressure injections.
Sodium tetradecyl sulfate (STS)	Telangiectasias; reticular veins	Telangiectasias: up to 0.1% Reticulars: up to 0.5%	Max per session: ~10 mL at low concentrations	Higher local irritation than POL; prefer minimal volumes and careful extravasation avoidance

Adapted from Rabe et al., *Phlebology* 2014; and ESVS 2022

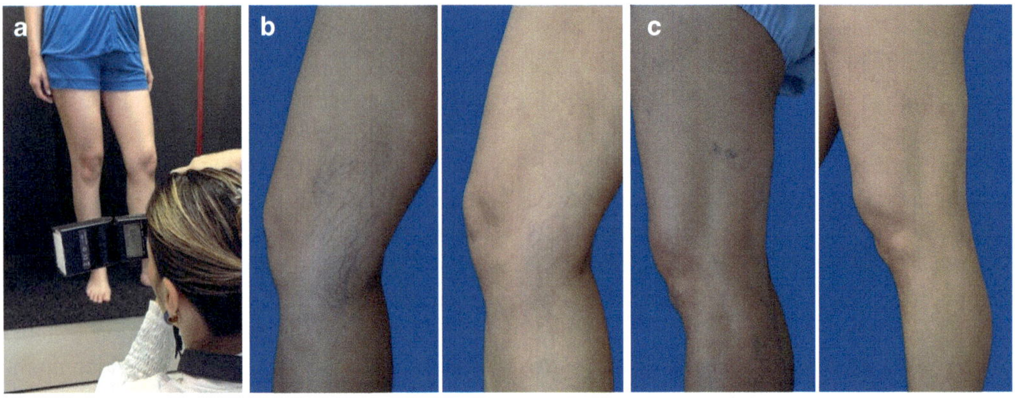

Fig. 11.12 Photodocumentation in sclerotherapy. (**a**) Standardized photodocumentation procedure, performed under controlled lighting and positioning conditions. (**b**) Pre- and post-treatment images of the medial thigh, showing significant reduction of telangiectasias after the therapeutic cycle. (**c**) Pre- and post-treatment images of the lateral thigh, demonstrating aesthetic improvement at the completion of treatment

satisfaction, as they can concretely visualize the improvement achieved, as highlighted by Santiago in his analysis of photographic recording practices in phlebology [37].

Written informed consent is equally essential. It should include a clear explanation of the sclerosing agent's mechanism of action, the procedural steps, available therapeutic alternatives, and potential adverse events. It is essential to detail both minor effects, such as local pain, hyperpigmentation, or matting, as well as serious, albeit rare, complications, such as skin necrosis, venous thrombosis, or anaphylactic reactions. The document, duly signed and filed in the patient's medical record, not only meets ethical and legal requirements but also strengthens the doctor-patient relationship, promoting transparency and safety. International literature reinforces that adequate communication of risks and benefits, combined with objective treatment records, is crucial for therapeutic success and patient satisfaction [33, 38]. Proper selection of equipment is essential for the safe and effective performance of sclerotherapy of telangiectasias and reticular veins. Needles should be thin, typically between 27 and 32G, suitable for small-caliber vessels. In the case of foam sclerotherapy, needle gauge and length directly influence product stability. Experimental studies have shown that 32G (~0.26 mm) needles are associated with rapid foam disintegration and should be avoided. A relevant finding was the greater stability of 0.5% polidocanol foam when injected through a 30G × 6 mm needle, a behavior considered atypi-

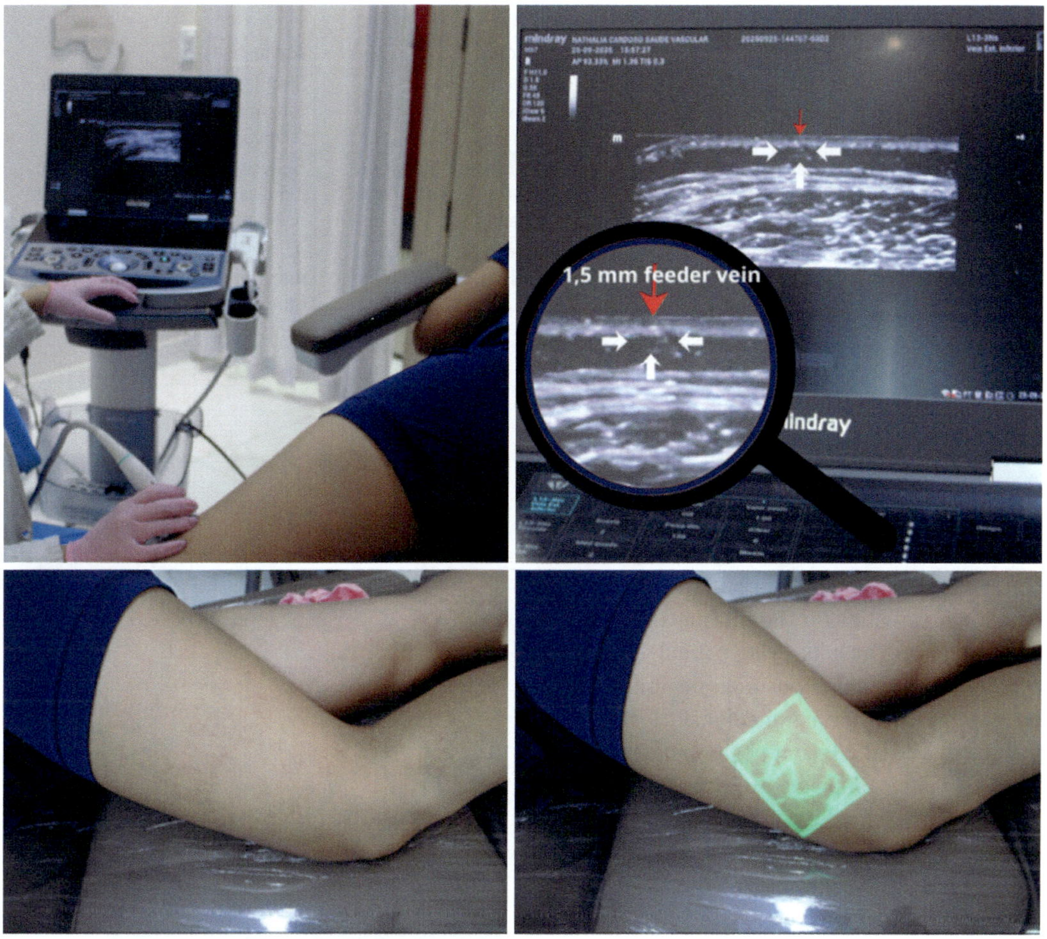

Fig. 11.13 Ultrasound-guided and image-guided puncture in a patient with resistant telangiectasias. A small 1.5 mm feeding vein was identified and punctured with the aid of duplex ultrasound and augmented reality, demonstrating how these tools enhance precision, safety, and selectivity in sclerotherapy

cal. For STS, better performance was observed with the use of longer needles, approximately 13 mm, which contributes to greater homogeneity and stability of the preparation [35]. Syringes and connections also influence foam quality. The use of low-silicone materials is recommended, as silicone accelerates the disintegration of microbubbles. Foam preparation should follow established methods, such as the Tessari method or the Double Syringe System (DSS), both based on the use of two syringes connected by a three-way stopcock, allowing adequate mixing of the sclerosant with air [31, 35]. Ultrasound should be available for situations requiring greater precision, such as guided punctures, assessment of the hemodynamic pattern, or mapping of associated feeding and perforating veins. This practice increases the safety of the procedure and allows for greater treatment selectivity [39]. Finally, elastic compression with stockings or bandages could be part of post-procedure care. This measure contributes to more comfort after procedure [40]. The sclerotherapy technique is relatively simple, but it requires meticulous attention to detail to ensure safety and adequate aesthetic results (Fig. 11.13). The different types are shown in Table 11.5.

Table 11.5 Comparative overview of sclerotherapy techniques

Technique	Indications	Devices/tools	Advantages
Direct	Isolated telangiectasias, superficial visible veins	30–32G needles, low sclerosant volumes	Simple, fast, low-cost; suitable for small, well-visualized telangiectasias
Image-guided	Telangiectasias with suspected feeder veins	*Veinlite*® (transillumination), *AccuVein*® (NIR), augmented reality systems	Better visualization of feeders; reduces recurrence; real-time mapping
Ultrasound-guided (UGS)	Recurrent telangiectasias; suspicion of reflux in hidden feeders or perforators	Duplex ultrasound, high-frequency linear probe, foam sclerosant	Allows precise puncture and injection; identifies hidden reflux; improves efficacy in complex cases

4 Technical Notes

The procedure should begin with the signing of a consent form and prior photodocumentation, which are essential for monitoring the progress and comparing results. The patient should be positioned in a supine position, beginning treatment on the anterior and medial sides. They can then be placed in a lateral position and finally in a prone position, allowing access to the entire circumference of the leg. This sequence avoids blind spots and ensures that all areas of concern are addressed. No prior vein dilation is necessary. Skin antisepsis is performed with 70% alcohol or alcoholic chlorhexidine, which, in addition to providing asepsis, increases the visibility of telangiectasias by altering the refraction of light on the skin. The use of magnifying lenses (2.5–5×) can aid visualization and puncture accuracy.

The choice of instruments should consider the caliber of the target vessel. Materials checklist (single-use) (See Fig. 11.14).

- Skin Prep: gauze/cotton, ethyl alcohol, 2% alcoholic chlorhexidine.
- Syringes: 1 to 3 ml, preferably with a threaded (luer lock) for greater precision and safety.
- Needles: between 27G 1/2 and 30G 1/2, up to 32G for thinner vessels.
- Post-puncture Tamponade: microporous tape with small cotton balls or pre-made dressings.
- Optional Optics: loupes with light to enhance accuracy.

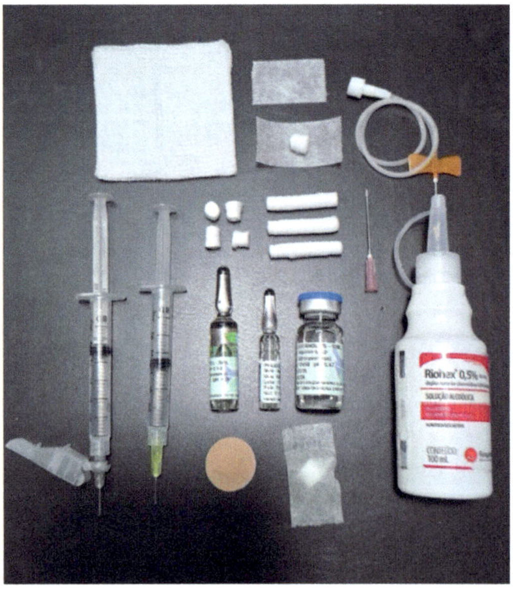

Fig. 11.14 Basic equipment required for sclerotherapy of telangiectasias and reticular veins. Including sterile gauze, cotton swabs, rolled cotton, micropore, hemostatic dressing (BloodStop), 27G ½ and 30G ½ needles, 3 mL syringes with sclerosants (e.g., polidocanol, glucose), and antiseptic solutions such as alcoholic chlorhexidine

The needle should be inserted parallel to the skin, at the smallest possible angle, with the bevel facing upward. It is recommended to use your non-dominant hand to pull the skin, facilitating the puncture.

When holding the syringe, we can use three points of support, increasing stability. The puncture should be precise and delicate, avoiding sudden movements that can increase pain and the risk of extravasation.

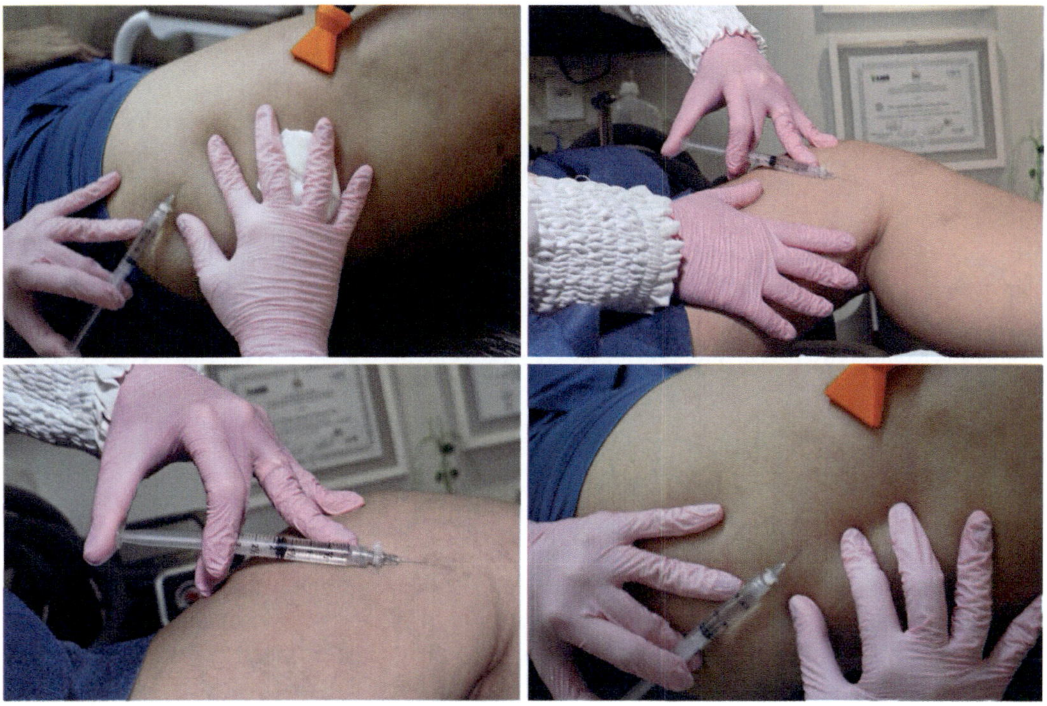

Fig. 11.15 Puncture technique for sclerotherapy with liquid sclerosant. The sequence of four images demonstrates the parallel introduction of the needle at the smallest possible angle, bevel facing upward, and the use of three-point support with the dominant hand for stability and precision

After confirming entry into the lumen, the sclerosant is slowly injected:

- Volume Per Point: ≤0.3 ml, to reduce the risk of necrosis, matting, and extravasation.
- Sequence: The treatment sequence should be in order from largest to smallest vessel, and sessions can be repeated every three to four weeks. Start with feeding and reticular veins, moving toward thinner telangiectasias.

In case of resistance or subcutaneous papule, stop immediately and reposition the needle.

Tips for Ergonomics and injection workflow:

- Dominant Hand Support: rest middle/ring/little fingers on the skin; thumb and index operate the plunger.
- Counter-Traction: with the non-dominant hand, stretch the skin using a thumb–index triangle to align vessel and needle (Fig. 11.15).
- Sequence: treat reticular feeder veins first, then the telangiectatic plexus from the root outward.
- Safety Rules: use multiple entry points, small aliquots, slow injection, low pressure.
- Before Microsclerotherapy: rule out and address significant truncal reflux per ESVS 2022 [34].

After the injection, digital compression should be applied to the treated area for a few seconds, followed by a dressing:

- A small square of cotton or a cotton ball secured with micropore tape.
- In complex or branched areas, the micropore tape can be reinforced for better fixation.
- Some professionals use small rollers adapted to apply greater local pressure.

It is recommended to keep the dressings in place for at least 3 h, and may be removed earlier if itching occurs.

After treating all the planned areas, the use of elastic compression stockings over the dressings may be recommended. According to the Society for Vascular Surgery (SVS) and American Venous Forum (AVF) guidelines, immediate compression after treatment should be preferred over no compression, as it is associated with improved clinical and cosmetic outcomes (GRADE 2; level of evidence C) [41]. Although there is no consensus on the ideal duration, the guidelines suggest that the decision should be guided by individual clinical judgment, as studies show heterogeneous results regarding compression timing, modality, and intensity.

In practice, most specialists use compression for at least 24 h after the procedure, in some cases extending its use for additional days or weeks. The physiology of compression—increased deep venous flow velocity, reduced superficial venous capacity, improved tissue oxygenation, and decreased stasis—justifies its use, even in the absence of definitive evidence regarding the optimal duration. In summary, although robust data defining compression timing and dose are lacking, the current clinical consensus is that immediate compression therapy after sclerotherapy improves venous wall apposition, reduces thrombus formation, and enhances the efficacy of the sclerosant, which is why it remains an essential component of the therapeutic protocol [42–45].

Early ambulation should be encouraged, as it reduces the risk of thrombosis. If thrombosis occurs in the treated vessel, the thrombus should be evacuated mechanically.

Auxiliary devices can be employed to improve patient tolerance and enhance outcomes during sclerotherapy. Skin coolers, which release jets of cold air, reduce the painful sensation associated with sclerosant injection and increase patient comfort throughout the procedure. Another adjunctive strategy is the use of tumescent anesthesia, consisting of perivenous infiltration of saline solution. Beyond its analgesic effect, this technique may also provide mechanical compression of the vein, helping to maintain sclerosant–endothelium contact for a longer period. Ramelet (2012) reported that this approach could improve results in resistant or larger reticular veins; however, the available evidence remains limited, and further studies are needed to confirm these findings [46, 47].

The efficacy of sclerotherapy relies on physical-chemical principles that promote endothelial damage and subsequent fibrosis. Wall contact time and sclerosant concentration determine the degree of mural denaturation, leading to vein occlusion and scarring [38]. Compared to liquid, foam (Fig. 11.16) displaces intraluminal blood, prolongs contact with the endothelium, and is ultrasound-visible, though its relative instability has been associated with rare transient neurological events, emphasizing the need for optimized preparation [38]. Foam stability is influenced by multiple variables, including sclerosant concentration, mixing pressure, syringe material (silicone content), needle caliber/length, and even solution temperature—with lower temperatures increasing viscosity and bubble stability [48–50]. Beyond the pharmacology of the sclerosant itself, the efficacy of sclerotherapy is ultimately governed by the interplay of physical factors, which must be taken into account to achieve consistent and safe clinical outcomes.

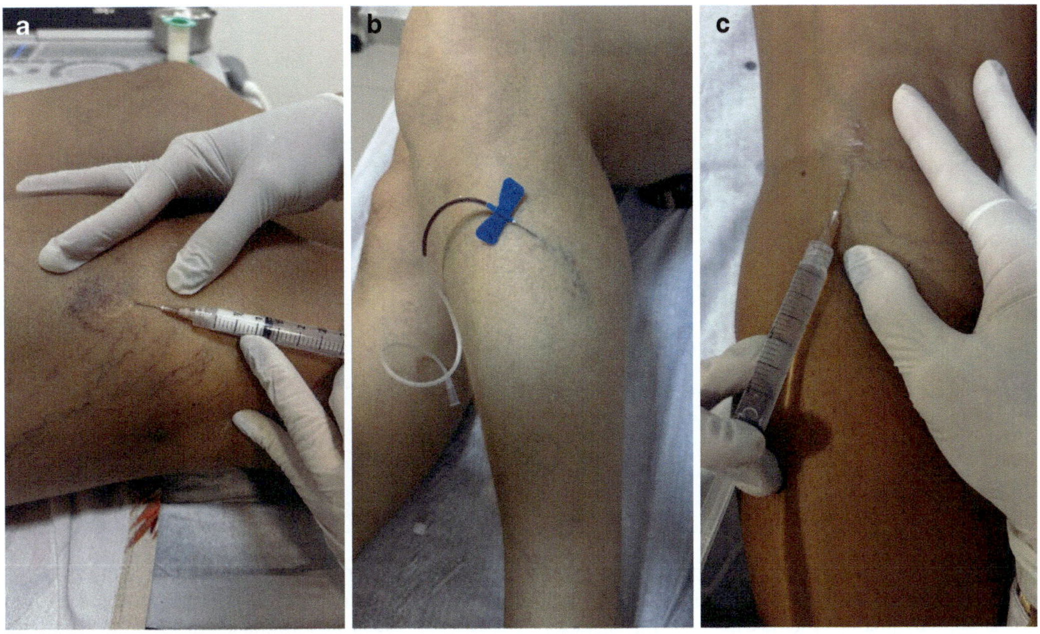

Fig. 11.16 Different sclerotherapy modalities: (**a**) foam sclerotherapy; (**b**) sclerosant injection with saline wash through a feeding vein; (**c**) liquid sclerotherapy of a vessel in the popliteal fossa. (Picture copyright: dr. Nathalia Cardoso)

5 Complications Management

Although sclerotherapy is considered a safe procedure, with an estimated incidence of complications (Fig. 11.17) of only 0.22% for liquid sclerosants and 0.58% for foam [51, 52].

It is essential to understand the most common adverse reactions and how to prevent them. Many of these situations arise not only from the drug itself, but also from the application technique, the volume injected, and post-procedure handling. Early recognition and the adoption of simple measures can prevent serious complications and reduce the aesthetic impact, ensuring better results.

- Residual Hyperpigmentation.

Hyperpigmentation occurs due to hemosiderin deposition resulting from superficial thrombosis and incomplete blood reabsorption. It can be avoided by using microvolumes, taking care not to overflow the solution, and, most importantly, by early evacuation of retained blood when indicated. Studies show that up to 90% of cases resolve spontaneously within one year.

- Trapped Blood.

The accumulation of a clot within the treated vein increases the risk of pigmentation. The recommended approach is puncture and early evacuation. This simple measure significantly reduces subsequent hyperpigmentation [51, 52].

- Pigmentation Care.

Evacuate trapped blood; avoid UV exposure for 2 weeks after treatment (Grade 1C).

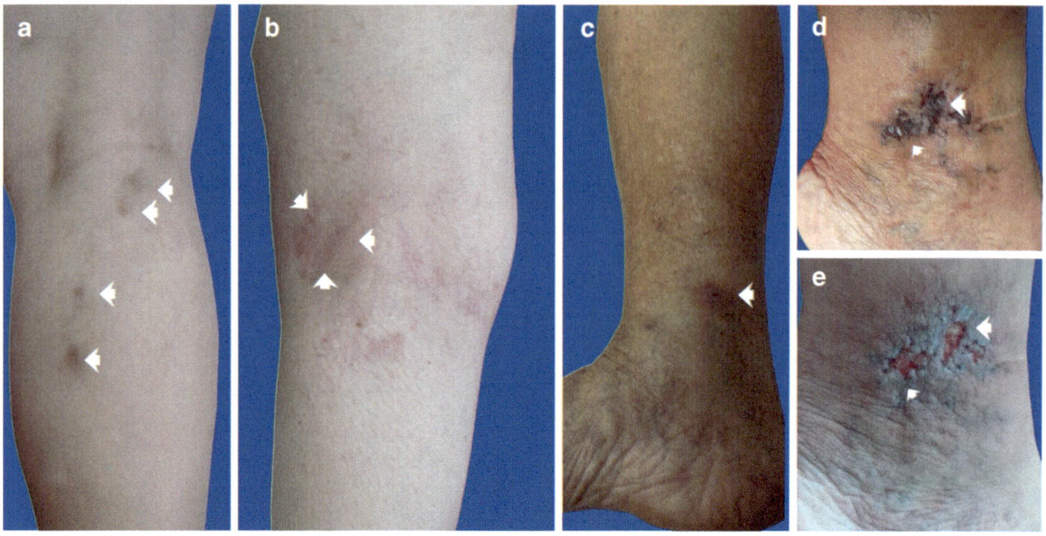

Fig. 11.17 Complications of sclerotherapy. (**a**) Post-sclerotherapy hyperpigmentation due to hemosiderin deposition. (**b**) Matting (neovascularization), characterized by the appearance of fine telangiectasias in the treated area. (**c**) Cutaneous ulcer following sclerotherapy. (**d**) Skin necrosis caused by extravasation of the sclerosing agent. (**e**) Established ulcerated wound on the foot after sclerotherapy complication

- Matting (Neovascularization).

Two types: inflammatory (individual, unpredictable; can also follow thermal/surgical ablation) and hemodynamic (due to untreated reflux).

Characterized by the appearance of fine reddish vessels near the treated area, usually associated with excess volume, concentration, or injection pressure. Local trauma should be minimized, overtreatment avoided, and, in cases of rapid recurrence, ultrasound evaluation should be performed to identify incompetent feeders or perforators. Treat reflux sources and tailor concentration/volume; avoid high-pressure injections [51].

- Ulceration and Necrosis.

These are rare but serious events, often related to sclerosant extravasation, inadvertent intra-arterial injection, or the use of high volumes/concentrations. Necrosis should be immediately recognized: interruption of the procedure, attempts at local neutralization when possible, and wound management according to advanced care protocols are recommended. The use of ultrasound during puncture and the avoidance of small-bore syringes (which generate greater injection pressure) are additional preventive strategies [53].

- Venous Thrombosis.

Deep venous thrombosis is uncommon after sclerotherapy, <1% [54] overall; meta-analysis [55] distal 0.6%. As measures to decrease the risk, we recommend the use of Caprini's score for risk; consider prophylaxis in high-risk patients; encourage mobilization and finally, use small volumes/inject with low pressure.

- Superficial Thrombophlebitis.

Incidence reports 0–45.8% (mean ~ 4.7%). Differentiate local inflammatory response at the injected site from true superficial vein thrombosis at a non-injected vein.

- Neurological/Visual Symptoms.

Migraine-like symptoms can occur after any sclerotherapy; PFO approximately 30% may allow foam microbubbles to reach arterial circulation. Endothelin-1 release has been shown after injections. Mitigate with multiple small-volume punctures.

- Anaphylaxis (Rare).

This is a very rare but drastic and life-threatening complication. The recommendation is to Stop the procedure immediately; give the patient hemodynamic/ventilatory support and epinephrine as needed (Grade 1A) [56].

Liquid sclerotherapy is highly effective in the treatment of telangiectasias and reticular veins, promoting 70 to 90% lightening after 2 to 4 sessions in different clinical series and controlled trials [51, 57, 58]. The result is not immediate: progressive lightening occurs over weeks, with continuous improvement after each session. The use of foam on reticular veins increases therapeutic efficacy, as it promotes greater contact of the sclerosant with the venous wall and less intraluminal dilution [57, 59].

The final result can take up to 12 weeks, the period necessary for complete reabsorption of the sclerosed segments. Among the transient effects, residual hyperpigmentation resolves spontaneously within 6 months in approximately 90% of cases.

Aesthetic satisfaction among patients undergoing the procedure is high, often exceeding 80%, with a positive impact not only on appearance but also on self-esteem and overall well-being. This benefit has been documented by validated quality of life instruments, confirming significant improvement after sclerotherapy [51, 53, 59].

6 Future Perspectives

Even though its widespread use and proven efficacy, sclerotherapy still lacks global standardization in technical protocols, success criteria, and post-treatment follow-up. High-quality comparative clinical trials that integrate not only occlusion rates but also clinical and quality-of-life outcomes, using validated instruments, are needed. Furthermore, the standardization of ultrasound protocols is considered essential to better define recurrences, residual incompetence, and complications [60]. In this scenario, the creation of international multicenter clinical registries emerges as a strategic tool to strengthen the evidence base. These registries allow us to capture "real-world" data, identification of practice patterns, regional variations, and long-term outcomes, complementing clinical trials. Combined with the development of new sclerosing agent formulations, automated systems [61] and the use of digital monitoring platforms, they represent a promising path to consolidate more robust global recommendations and maintain sclerotherapy as a safe and effective reference treatment.

References

1. Eklof B, Perrin M, Delis KT, et al. Updated terminology of chronic venous disorders: the VEIN-TERM transatlantic interdisciplinary consensus document. J Vasc Surg [Internet]. 2009. [cited 2024 Oct 18];49:498–501. https://doi.org/10.1016/J.JVS.2008.09.014.
2. Bergan JJ, Schmid-Schönbein GW, Coleridge Smith PD, et al. Chronic venous disease from the Departments of Surgery [Internet]. www.nejm.org.
3. Krizanova O, Penesova A, Hokynkova A, Pokorna A, et al. Chronic venous insufficiency and venous leg ulcers: aetiology, on the pathophysiology-based treatment. Int Wound J. 2024;21. https://doi.org/10.1111/iwj.14405.
4. Eberhardt RT, Raffetto JD. Chronic venous insufficiency. Circulation. Lippincott Williams and Wilkins. 2014:333–46. https://doi.org/10.1161/CIRCULATIONAHA.113.006898.
5. Fowkes FGR, Lee AJ, Evans CJ, et al. Lifestyle risk factors for lower limb venous reflux in the general population: Edinburgh vein study. Int J Epidemiol. 2001;30. https://doi.org/10.1093/ije/30.4.846.
6. Kern P. Pathophysiology of telangiectasias of the lower legs and its therapeutic implication: a systematic review. Phlebology. SAGE Publications Ltd. 2018:225–33. https://doi.org/10.1177/0268355518756480.
7. Salim S, Machin M, Patterson BO, et al. Global epidemiology of chronic venous disease: a systematic review with pooled prevalence analysis. Ann Surg. 2021; https://doi.org/10.1097/SLA.0000000000004631.
8. Lacroix P, Aboyans V, Preux PM, Houlès MB, Laskar M. Epidemiology of venous insufficiency in an occupational population. Int Angiol. 2003;22.

9. Jawien A. The influence of environmental factors in chronic venous insufficiency. Angiology. 2003; https://doi.org/10.1177/000331970305400 1s04.
10. Rabe E, Guex JJ, Puskas A, et al. Epidemiology of chronic venous disorders in geographically diverse populations: results from the vein consult program. Int Angiol. 2012;31.
11. Rabe E, Schliephake D, Otto J, et al. Sclerotherapy of telangiectases and reticular veins: a double-blind, randomized, comparative clinical trial of polidocanol, sodium tetradecyl sulphate and isotonic saline (EASI study). Phlebology [Internet]. 2010;25:124–31. https://doi.org/10.1258/phleb.2009.009043.
12. Bush R, Bush P. Evaluation of sodium tetradecyl sulfate and polidocanol as sclerosants for leg telangiectasia based on histological evaluation with clinical correlation. Phlebology [Internet]. 2017;32:496–500. https://doi.org/10.1177/0268355516673768.
13. Breu FX, Guggenbichler S, Wollmann JC. Duplex ultrasound and efficacy criteria in foam sclerotherapy from the 2nd European Consensus Meeting on Foam Sclerotherapy 2006, Tegernsee, Germany. Vasa J Vasc Dis. 2008; https://doi.org/10.1024/0301-1526.37.1.90.
14. Miyake K, Pires Davidson JR. Augmented reality and duplex ultrasound in medical treatment decision: score 9-1. J Phlebol Lymphol. 2019;12.
15. Engelhorn CA, Engelhorn ALV, Cassou MF, Salles-Cunha S. Patterns of saphenous venous reflux in women presenting with lower extremity telangiectasias. Dermatologic Surg. 2007;33. https://doi.org/10.1111/j.1524-4725.2007.33063.x.
16. Blin E. Techniques to study telangiectasias and reticular veins. Phlebologie Annales Vasculaires. 2011;64:35–9.
17. Albanese AR, Albanese AM, Albanese EF. Lateral subdermic varicose vein system of the legs: its surgical treatment by the chiseling tube method. Vasc Endovasc Surg. 1969;3. https://doi.org/10.1177/153857446900300205.
18. Schuller-Petrović S, Pavlović MD, Schuller S, Schuller-Lukic B, Adamič M. Telangiectasias resistant to sclerotherapy are commonly connected to a perforating vessel. Phlebology. 2013;28. https://doi.org/10.1258/phleb.2012.012019.
19. Engelhorn CA, Engelhorn ALDV, et al. Initial patterns of unilateral great saphenous vein reflux in women with telangiectasias and varicose veins. Veins Lymphat. 2017;6. https://doi.org/10.4081/vl.2017.6757.
20. Böhler-Sommeregger K, Karnel F, Schuller-Petrovič S, et al. Phlebology: do telangiectases communicate with the deep venous system? J Dermatol Surg Oncol. 1992;18. https://doi.org/10.1111/j.1524-4725.1992.tb03693.x.
21. Schmid-Schönbein GW, Granger DN, Coleridge-Smith P, et al. Inflammation in venous disease. Molecular basis for microcirculatory disorders. Springer Paris; 2003;489–500.
22. Curri SB. Anatomie microvasculaire de la peau et de ses annexes. Phlebologie. 1990;43:407–30.
23. Wilson S, Chen X, Cronin MA, et al. Thrombosis prophylaxis in surgical patients using the Caprini Risk Score. Curr Probl Surg. 2022;59. https://doi.org/10.1016/j.cpsurg.2022.101221.
24. Braet DJ, Loi K, Stabler C, et al. Thromboembolic outcomes are decreased with the use of a standardized venous thromboembolism risk assessment and prophylaxis protocol for patients undergoing superficial venous procedures. J Vasc Surg Venous Lymphat Disord. 2023; https://doi.org/10.1016/j.jvsv.2023.04.008.
25. De Maeseneer M, Pichot O, Cavezzi A, et al. Duplex ultrasound investigation of the veins of the lower limbs after treatment for varicose veins – UIP consensus document. Eur J Vasc Endovasc Surg. 2011;42. https://doi.org/10.1016/j.ejvs.2011.03.013.
26. Barros FS, Storino J, Cardoso da Silva NA, et al. A comprehensive ultrasound approach to lower limb varicose veins and abdominal-pelvic connections. J Vasc Surg Venous Lymphat Disord. Elsevier Inc. 2024;12. https://doi.org/10.1016/j.jvsv.2024.101851.
27. Coleridge-Smith P, Labropoulos N, et al. Duplex ultrasound investigation of the veins in chronic venous disease of the lower limbs – UIP consensus document. Part I. Basic principles. Eur J Vasc Endovasc Surg. 2006;31. https://doi.org/10.1016/j.ejvs.2005.07.019.
28. Lee AJ, Evans CJ, Allan PL, et al. Lifestyle factors and the risk of varicose veins: Edinburgh Vein Study. J Clin Epidemiol. 2003;56. https://doi.org/10.1016/S0895-4356(02)00518-8.
29. Nyamekye IK. European Society for Vascular Surgery (ESVS) 2022 clinical practice guidelines on the management of chronic venous disease of the lower limbs. JMV Journal de Medecine Vasculaire. Elsevier Masson srl. 2022;47:53–5. https://doi.org/10.1016/j.jdmv.2022.04.003.
30. Redisch W, Pelzer RH. Localized vascular dilatations of the human skin: capillary microscopy and related studies. Am Heart J. 1949;37. https://doi.org/10.1016/0002-8703(49)91433-7.
31. Goldman MP, Bennett RG. Treatment of telangiectasia: a review. J Am Acad Dermatol [Internet]. Mosby. 1987. [cited 2025 Sep 20];17:167–82. https://doi.org/10.1016/S0190-9622(87)70187-X.
32. Feied C. Sclerosing. Solutions. 2006; https://doi.org/10.1016/B978-0-12-369515-4.50016-8.
33. Wong M, Parsi K, Myers K, et al. Sclerotherapy of lower limb veins: indications, contraindications and treatment strategies to prevent complications – a consensus document of the International Union of Phlebology-2023. Phlebology. SAGE Publications Ltd. 2023:205–58. https://doi.org/10.1177/02683555231151350.
34. De Maeseneer MG, Kakkos SK, Aherne T, et al. Editor's choice – European Society for Vascular Surgery (ESVS) 2022 clinical practice guidelines on the management of chronic venous disease of the lower limbs. Eur J Vasc Endovasc Surg [Internet]. 2022. [cited 2024 Oct 18];63:184–267. https://doi.org/10.1016/J.EJVS.2021.12.024.

35. Wollmann JCGR, Goldman M. The history of sclerosing foams. Dermatologic Surg. 2004; https://doi.org/10.1111/j.1524-4725.2004.30208.x.
36. Bertanha M, Jaldin RG, Moura R, et al. Sclerotherapy for reticular veins in the lower limbs. JAMA Dermatol. 2017;153. https://doi.org/10.1001/jamadermatol.2017.3426.
37. Santiago FR, Piscoya M, Chi YW. Change in perception of sclerotherapy results after exposure to pre–post intervention photographs. Phlebology. SAGE Publications Ltd. 2018;33:282–7. https://doi.org/10.1177/0268355517736178.
38. Green D. Sclerotherapy treatment insights. Dermatol Clin [Internet]. Elsevier. 1998. [cited 2025 Sep 20];16:195–211. https://doi.org/10.1016/S0733-8635(05)70495-2.
39. Cartee TV, Wirth P, Greene A, et al. Ultrasound-guided foam sclerotherapy is safe and effective in the management of superficial venous insufficiency of the lower extremity. J Vasc Surg Venous Lymphat Disord. 2021;9. https://doi.org/10.1016/j.jvsv.2021.03.020.
40. Mohamed AH, Thadani S, Mohamed SH, et al. Compression following treatment of superficial venous incompetence: systematic review. Br J Surg. 2022; https://doi.org/10.1093/bjs/znac116.
41. Lurie F, Lal BK, Antignani PL, et al. Compression therapy after invasive treatment of superficial veins of the lower extremities: clinical practice guidelines of the American Venous Forum, Society for Vascular Surgery, American College of Phlebology, Society for Vascular Medicine, and International Union of Phlebology. J Vasc Surg Venous Lymphat Disord. 2019;7. https://doi.org/10.1016/j.jvsv.2018.10.002.
42. Weiss MA, Hsu JTS, Neuhaus I, et al. Consensus for sclerotherapy. Dermatologic Surg. 2014;40. https://doi.org/10.1097/DSS.0000000000000225.
43. El-Sheikha J, Carradice D, Nandhra S, et al. Systematic review of compression following treatment for varicose veins. Br J Surg. 2015; https://doi.org/10.1002/bjs.9788.
44. Khunger N, Sacchidanand S. Standard guidelines for care: sclerotherapy in dermatology. Indian J Dermatol Venereol Leprol. 2011;77. https://doi.org/10.4103/0378-6323.77478.
45. Nicolaides A, Kakkos S, Baekgaard N, et al. Management of chronic venous disorders of the lower limbs. Guidelines According to Scientific Evidence. Part I. Int Angiol. 2018 Jun; 37(3):181–254.
46. Ramelet AA. The START technique: sclerotherapy of reticular veins and telangiectasias under tumescent anesthesia. Haut. 2012.
47. Ramelet AA. Sclerotherapy in tumescent anesthesia of reticular veins and telangiectasias. Dermatologic Surg. 2012;38. https://doi.org/10.1111/j.1524-4725.2011.02287.x.
48. Skuła M, Hobot J, Czaja J, et al. The effect of the calibre and length of needle on the stability of sclerosing foam. Phlebology. SAGE Publications Ltd. 2021;36:322–8. https://doi.org/10.1177/0268355520953317.
49. Serkan M, Gokay D. Low temperature offers better foam stability. J Cosmet Dermatol. John Wiley and Sons Inc. 2024;23:3366–71. https://doi.org/10.1111/jocd.16398.
50. Patel SB, Ostler AE, Dos Santos SJ, et al. The effects of environmental and compositional manipulations on the longevity of Tessari-made foam for sclerotherapy. J Vasc Surg Venous Lymphat Disord. 2015;3. https://doi.org/10.1016/j.jvsv.2014.07.010.
51. Guex JJ. Complications of sclerotherapy: an update. Dermatologic Surg. 2010. https://doi.org/10.1111/j.1524-4725.2009.01409.x.
52. Scultetus AH, Villavicencio JL, Kao TC, et al. Microthrombectomy reduces postsclerotherapy pigmentation: multicenter randomized trial. J Vasc Surg. 2003. https://doi.org/10.1016/S0741-5214(03)00920-0.
53. Guex JJ, Allaert FA, Gillet JL, et al. Immediate and midterm complications of sclerotherapy: report of a prospective multicenter registry of 12,173 sclerotherapy sessions. Dermatologic Surg. 2005;31. https://doi.org/10.1097/00042728-200502000-00001.
54. Gillet J, Lausecker M, Sica M, et al. Is the treatment of the small saphenous veins with foam sclerotherapy at risk of deep vein thrombosis? Phlebology. 2014;29. https://doi.org/10.1177/0268355513497362.
55. Jia X, Mowatt G, Burr JM, et al. Systematic review of foam sclerotherapy for varicose veins. Br J Surg. 2007. https://doi.org/10.1002/bjs.5891.
56. Rabe E, Breu FX, Cavezzi A, et al. European guidelines for sclerotherapy in chronic venous disorders. Phlebology. 2014;29. https://doi.org/10.1177/0268355513483280.
57. Alòs Villacrosa J, Carreño P, López JA, et al. Efficacy and safety of sclerotherapy using polidocanol foam: a controlled clinical trial. Eur J Vasc Endovasc Surg. 2006;31. https://doi.org/10.1016/j.ejvs.2005.08.018.
58. Kern P, Ramelet AA, Wutschert R, et al. Single-blind, randomized study comparing chromated glycerin, polidocanol solution, and polidocanol foam for treatment of telangiectatic leg veins. Dermatologic Surg. 2004;30. https://doi.org/10.1111/j.1524-4725.2004.30102.x.
59. Rabe E, Otto J, Schliephake D, et al. Efficacy and safety of great saphenous vein sclerotherapy using standardised polidocanol foam (ESAF): a randomised controlled multicentre clinical trial. Eur J Vasc Endovasc Surg. 2008;35. https://doi.org/10.1016/j.ejvs.2007.09.006.
60. Gianesini S, Obi A, Onida S, et al. Global guidelines trends and controversies in lower limb venous and lymphatic disease: Narrative literature revision and experts' opinions following the vWINter international meeting in Phlebology, Lymphology & Aesthetics, 23–25 January 2019. Phlebology. SAGE Publications Ltd. 2019:4–66. https://doi.org/10.1177/0268355519870690.
61. Roche E, Pons R, Roche O, et al. A new automated system for the preparation of sclerosant foam: a study of the physical characteristics produced and the device settings required. Phlebology. 2020;35. https://doi.org/10.1177/0268355520937615.

Cryo-Laser and Cryo-Sclerotherapy (CLaCS)

12

Gisele Peron, Kasuo Miyake, and Sergio Gianesini

1 Introduction

Telangiectasias and reticular veins represent the most common visible expressions of chronic venous disease and are classified as CEAP 1. Although traditionally perceived as a predominantly cosmetic condition, a growing body of evidence demonstrates that C1 disease frequently carries clinically relevant symptomatology, including burning, aching, heaviness, localized pain, nocturnal discomfort, restless legs, and impaired quality of life. These symptoms may occur independently of overt reflux in axial veins and should not be dismissed as trivial manifestations of venous pathology [1]. From a public health and practice-management perspective, C1 disease constitutes a major proportion of venous consultations worldwide, particularly in ambulatory phlebology practices. Patient demand is driven not only by symptom relief but also by high expectations for aesthetic outcomes, minimal downtime, low pain, and avoidance of adverse sequelae such as hyperpigmentation or matting. These expectations place unique constraints on treatment strategies and have directly influenced the evolution of techniques targeting telangiectatic and reticular venous networks. Historically, injection sclerotherapy has been the cornerstone of C1 treatment, while transcutaneous laser therapy has developed as both an alternative, yet only for the most superficial branches, and an adjunct. Each modality in isolation exhibits its intrinsic limitations related to vessel size, depth, network architecture, pain, inflammatory response, and recurrence. The persistence of these limitations, despite decades of technical refinement, has driven interest in combined-modality approaches designed to exploit synergistic mechanisms while mitigating individual weaknesses. Within this context, Cryo-Laser and Cryo-Sclerotherapy (CLaCS) has emerged as a structured, same-session technique integrating transdermal laser photothermolysis, immediate microsclerotherapy, and continuous cutaneous cooling. CLaCS represents not merely a juxtaposition of two established modalities, but a reconceptualization of how C1 venous networks may be approached as dynamic, interconnected microvascular systems rather than isolated visible vessels [2, 3].

G. Peron
Department of Vascular Surgery, Sinop, Brazil

K. Miyake
Vascular Surgery Department, Centro de Estudos Hiroshi Miyake, Sao Paulo, Brazil

S. Gianesini (✉)
Department of Translational Medicine, University of Ferrara, Ferrara, Italy

Department of Surgery, Uniformed Services University of Health Sciences, Bethesda, MD, USA
e-mail: gnssrg@unife.it

S. Gianesini, Y. W. Chi (eds.), *Sclerotherapy*, https://doi.org/10.1007/978-3-032-32794-9_12

2 CLaCS Rationale

The therapeutic obliteration of superficial veins predates modern vascular medicine. Early forms of sclerotherapy, using corrosive or irritant substances, were empirically developed long before a coherent understanding of venous histology or hemodynamics. The modern era of sclerotherapy began with the recognition that controlled endothelial injury, rather than nonspecific tissue destruction, was sufficient to induce vein fibrosis and disappearance. By the late twentieth century, detergent sclerosants such as polidocanol and sodium tetradecyl sulfate became widely adopted due to their more predictable dose–response behavior and lower necrosis risk compared with earlier agents. This period also saw the rise of microsclerotherapy, emphasizing small needles, low injection pressures, precise targeting, and meticulous post-treatment compression [4, 5]. Despite technical refinement, long-term clinical experience revealed persistent challenges:

- Incomplete clearance in complex networks,
- Recurrence due to untreated feeder veins,
- Post-sclerotherapy hyperpigmentation, and,
- Telangiectatic matting.

These limitations were increasingly recognized as biological and architectural, rather than purely technical, problems [6]. The development and standardization of foam sclerotherapy represented a conceptual shift, particularly for larger superficial veins. Foam allowed improved endothelial contact and reduced sclerosant volume. However, in C1 disease, foam offered limited advantages over liquid for very small or intradermal vessels and introduced its own risks (e.g., inflammation, pigmentation, microthrombi). As a result, liquid microsclerotherapy remained dominant for telangiectasias [7]. Laser therapy entered the treatment landscape as an entirely different paradigm: selective photothermolysis, targeting hemoglobin within blood vessels while sparing surrounding tissue. Initial enthusiasm was tempered by pain, variable efficacy in leg veins (compared with facial vessels), and a narrow therapeutic window between efficacy and epidermal injury [8]. The introduction of long-pulsed 1064-nm Nd:YAG lasers improved penetration depth and made treatment of reticular veins and deeper telangiectasias feasible. Nevertheless, laser therapy alone often failed to address feeder networks adequately and was associated with procedure-related discomfort, necessitating cooling strategies [9, 10]. As clinical experience accumulated, it became evident that C1 venous disease behaves as a network pathology, not a collection of isolated vessels. Treating visible telangiectasias without addressing subdermal reticular veins frequently led to suboptimal results or early recurrence. This recognition laid the conceptual groundwork for combined approaches, culminating in CLaCS, which formalized the integration of laser, sclerotherapy, and cryoprotection into a reproducible procedural framework [2]. The rationale for CLaCS is rooted in the fundamentally different, but complementary, mechanisms of laser and sclerotherapy (Fig. 12.1):

- Laser photothermolysis induces thermal injury to blood-filled vessels, leading to endothelial denudation, collagen contraction, and partial or complete lumen collapse.
- Sclerotherapy produces chemical endothelial damage, triggering inflammation, thrombosis, and fibrosis.

When laser is applied first, the treated vessel often becomes narrowed, partially thrombosed, or hemodynamically altered, rendering it more susceptible to subsequent sclerosant action at lower volumes and concentrations [11]. Continuous cold-air cooling is not ancillary in CLaCS: it is structural to the technique. Cooling reduces nociceptor activation, improving patient tolerance, protects the epidermis from thermal injury, attenuates inflammatory cascades implicated in post-treatment pigmentation. This enables the operator to apply laser energy more effectively while maintaining safety margins, particularly in darker phototypes or extensive treatment fields [12]. CLaCS was explicitly designed to address common failure patterns such as residual patent feeders after laser alone, incomplete sclerosant penetration after sclero-

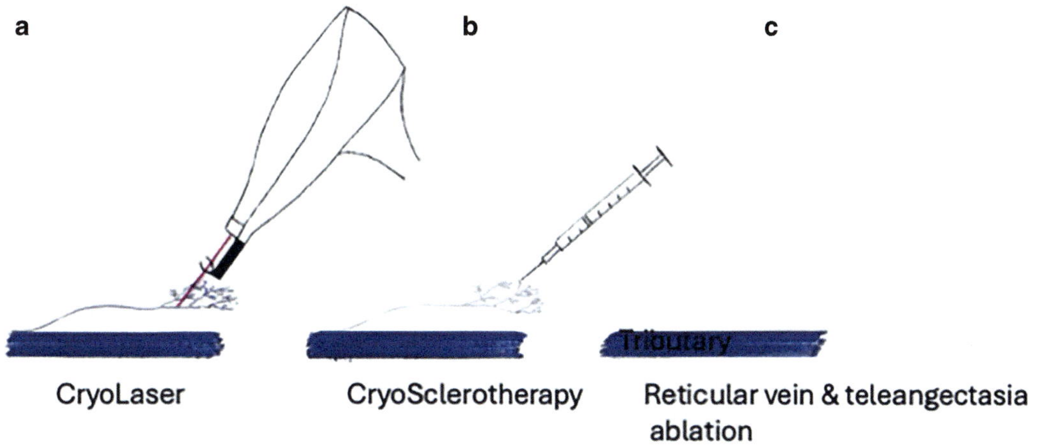

Fig. 12.1 CLaCS principle: laser-induced reduction of the targeted vein by means of low energy level use, completed by gentle sclerosant completion of the vessel occlusion. Figure copyright: dr. Celine Eggen (Centrum Oosterwal, Alkmaar (NETHERLANDS))

therapy alone, excessive inflammation leading to pigmentation and pin-limited treatment density. Clinical reports suggest that CLaCS can reduce pigmentation rates and improve clearance in selected patients when compared with conventional microsclerotherapy. CLaCS is defined as a same-session, integrated treatment protocol combining transcutaneous laser treatment of telangiectatic and reticular veins, immediate injection sclerotherapy of residual or feeder vessels with continuous cold-air skin cooling throughout the procedure. In its original conception, CLaCS uses Dextrose 75% (osmotic sclerosant) rather than detergents (polidocanol, sodium tetra decyl sulphate). It is critical to emphasize that CLaCS is not simply sequential laser and sclerotherapy performed coincidentally. Its defining feature is intentional integration, guided by vein architecture, hemodynamic logic, and procedural timing The scope of CLaCS primarily includes lower-limb telangiectasias, reticular veins serving as feeders, mixed networks resistant to single-modality therapy. Adjunctive technologies such as near-infrared vein visualization must be incorporated to enhance feeder identification [13]. In contemporary phlebology, CLaCS occupies an advanced, network-oriented niche rather than replacing established first-line therapies. It is particularly well suited for patients with complex telangiectatic–reticular networks, prior failure of laser or sclerotherapy alone, high concern for pigmentation or downtime, and low tolerance for pain or multiple sessions. From an expert standpoint, CLaCS should be viewed as a technique for experienced practitioners, requiring proficiency in duplex assessment, laser physics, microsclerotherapy, and complication management. When properly applied, it represents a logical evolution toward precision-based treatment of venous microvascular networks, aligning therapeutic intensity with biological complexity rather than vessel size alone.

3 Pertinent Anatomy and Pathophysiology

The effective treatment of telangiectasias and reticular veins requires an understanding that extends well beyond vessel diameter. These lesions arise from a complex interaction between dermal microvascular anatomy, subdermal venous networks, local hemodynamics, neurovascular regulation, and inflammatory biology. Unlike truncal venous disease, where pathology is often dominated by valve failure and axial reflux, C1 disease operates at the microcirculatory and mesovascular interface, where structure–function relationships are subtle, dynamic, and highly patient-specific. Historically, many therapeutic failures in C1 disease have stemmed from a reductionist view of spider veins as isolated cosmetic defects. Contemporary evidence instead supports a network-based pathophysiologic model, in which telangiectasias represent the visible terminal branches of deeper venous systems influenced by regional pressure gradients, microvalvular dysfunction, hormonal signaling, and cutaneous neurovascular control [14, 15]. This conceptual shift is foundational to CLaCS, which is explicitly designed to address the anatomic continuity and biological interdependence of superficial and subdermal venous structures. Telangiectasias are dilated intradermal venules, most commonly measuring 0.1–1.0 mm, located within the papillary and superficial reticular dermis. From a histological standpoint, they are characterized by a single layer of endothelial cells, a discontinuous or absent smooth muscle layer, a poorly developed adventitia, close proximity to collagen bundles and dermal fibroblasts. This minimal structural support explains both their high distensibility and their vulnerability to mechanical rupture, thermal injury, and chemical irritation. Clinically, telangiectasias are often subclassified by color (red, blue, violet) and morphology (linear, arborizing, spider-like). These visual patterns correlate imperfectly but meaningfully with depth, oxygenation, and venous versus capillary dominance, which in turn influence treatment response [9]. The dermis is not a homogeneous layer. The papillary dermis contains vertically oriented capillary loops supplying the epidermis, while the reticular dermis contains horizontally oriented venous plexuses. Telangiectasias may arise from either compartment or represent oblique connections between them [16]. Superficial red telangiectasias are often capillary-dominant and located closer to the epidermis. Blue or purple telangiectasias typically originate from venular structures deeper in the reticular dermis. This distinction is crucial for laser therapy, as wavelength penetration, spot size, and fluence must be adapted to vessel depth to avoid epidermal injury while achieving sufficient intravascular heating. The lack of smooth muscle in telangiectasias renders them incapable of active vasomotor control, highly sensitive to pressure fluctuations and prone to inflammation-mediated dilation. As a result, even mild inflammatory stimuli, such as extravasated sclerosant, thermal diffusion or post-procedure hyperemia, can result in persistent dilation or the appearance of new vessels. This explains why overly aggressive treatment often paradoxically worsens cosmetic outcomes. Reticular veins are subdermal veins, typically 1–3 mm in diameter, located at the dermo-hypodermal junction. They form a horizontal plexus that collects blood from intradermal venules and drains toward larger superficial veins. Structurally, reticular veins differ fundamentally from telangiectasias because they possess a recognizable smooth muscle layer, they exhibit greater compliance, and they demonstrate active vasomotor responsiveness. These features make reticular veins more resistant to laser-only treatment and more suitable for sclerotherapy, particularly when targeted accurately [17]. Although reticular veins operate at lower pressures than truncal veins, they are subjected to chronic hydrostatic loading in the lower extremities. Importantly, localized reflux or flow persistence in reticular veins can occur independently of saphenous reflux, sustained by microvalvular incompetence, gravitational pooling, and regional venous hypertension. This localized hemodynamic abnormality is sufficient to maintain telangiectasias even when duplex ultrasound of major trunks is normal. Reticular veins act as functional feeders, supplying pressure and flow to intradermal telangiectasias. Failure to recognize and treat these feeders is one of the most common reasons for incomplete clearance, early recurrence, and post-treatment telangiectatic matting [18, 19]. Network-based imaging and clinical observation confirm that effective C1 treatment must disrupt both visible endpoints and their subdermal supply lines. The skin contains a dense network of A-delta and C nociceptive fibers, closely associated with superficial blood vessels. These fibers respond to thermal stimuli, chemical irritation, and mechanical stretch. Both laser energy and sclerosant injection activate these pathways, explaining the historically significant pain possibly associated with C1 treatments [20, 21]. Cutaneous veins are under sympathetic autonomic control, which regulates venous capacitance through vasoconstriction and vasodilation. Temperature is a powerful modulator of this system: heat induces vasodilation and increased blood volume, cold induces vasoconstriction and reduced flow. Continuous cold-air cooling therefore stabilizes vessel diameter, reduces intravascular blood volume, and diminishes pain perception, all of which are essential to CLaCS efficacy and safety. Neuropeptides released from activated sensory fibers (e.g., substance P, CGRP) contribute to vasodilation, plasma extravasation, and inflammatory amplification. Excessive neurogenic inflammation increases the risk of pigmentation and matting. Cryoprotection attenuates these responses, providing a biological rationale for cooling beyond patient comfort. The most common cause of apparent treatment failure is incomplete network disruption. Treating telangiectasias without addressing reticular feeders allows rapid re-expansion of superficial vessels due to persistent pressure gradients. Aggressive or poorly controlled treatment can provoke a robust inflammatory response, leading to angiogenic signaling, recruitment of endothelial progenitor cells, and formation of fine neovessels (telangiectatic matting). This process is particularly common in hormonally sensitive patients and those with prior inflammatory skin conditions [22]. Pigmentation results from erythrocyte extravasation and subsequent hemosiderin deposition within dermal macrophages. Factors increasing this risk include incomplete vessel collapse, persistent intravascular thrombus, and excessive endothelial injury. Strategies that promote rapid and complete vessel closure, such as combined laser and sclerotherapy, may reduce pigmentary complications. Moreover, the use of low energy laser in combination with a mild sclerosant agent such as dextrose minimizes pigmentation risk in CLaCS [23, 24]. Outcomes are strongly influenced by dermal thickness and collagen density, inflammatory responsiveness, hormonal milieu, and genetic predisposition. CLaCS does not eliminate these variables but seeks to minimize their clinical impact by reducing procedural trauma while improving network-level efficacy. Moreover, the laser causes a focal and precise lesion, and the following sclerotherapy is performed with multiple low-volume injections to focus on treating the targeted vessels and not damaging adjacent normal veins. From an expert perspective, telangiectasias and reticular veins should be understood as elements of a multilevel, neurovascular, and hemodynamic system. CLaCS aligns with this model by targeting intradermal and subdermal compartments, structural and functional abnormalities, vascular and neural contributors to symptoms and recurrence. This integrative understanding represents a maturation of C1 disease management, moving beyond vessel diameter toward biologically informed, network-oriented therapy.

4 Patient Selection and Clinical Evaluation

In the treatment of telangiectasias and reticular veins, technical sophistication alone does not determine success. Nowhere in venous medicine is this more evident than in CEAP C1 disease, where outcomes are shaped less by the availability of tools than by the appropriateness of their application. CLaCS, as a synergy and relatively intensive intervention for superficial venous networks, magnifies this principle. Its potential benefits are substantial, but only when deployed in patients whose anatomy, skin biology, hemodynamics, and expectations align with the method's strengths. Unlike truncal venous disease, where patient selection is often dictated by objective findings such as reflux duration or vein diameter, C1 disease exists in a space where subjective symptoms, aesthetic priorities, and biological variability intersect. The clinician must therefore adopt a broader evaluative lens, integrating traditional vascular assessment with dermatologic, neurovascular, and psychosocial considerations. Failure to do so risks overtreatment, dissatisfaction, or avoidable complications, even when the technical execution is flawless. CLaCS should thus be understood not as a "better" treatment for spider veins, but as a more specific one. The most compelling indication for CLaCS arises in patients whose venous anatomy cannot be adequately addressed by a single modality without compromise. These patients frequently present with mixed telangiectatic–reticular networks, in which fine intradermal vessels are sustained by subdermal reticular veins. In such cases, isolated sclerotherapy may fail due to technical difficulty in cannulating the smallest vessels, while isolated laser treatment may inadequately address deeper feeders or provoke excessive discomfort. CLaCS, by design, addresses both compartments within a single session. Another common indication is prior treatment failure. Patients who present after multiple sessions of microsclerotherapy or laser therapy often do not lack treatable anatomy, rather they suffer from incomplete network disruption or biologically driven recurrence. In this population, CLaCS functions as a problem-solving strategy, allowing the clinician to modify both the physical and chemical injury patterns delivered to the venous network. CLaCS also finds a role in patients for whom procedural tolerance is a limiting factor. Laser energy is kept at very low levels, as well as the sclerotherapy aggressiveness, therefore limiting periprocedural pain. Finally, there is a growing body of interest in CLaCS for patients at high risk of post-treatment pigmentation, whether due to darker phototype, prior pigmentary complication, or heightened cosmetic sensitivity. While no intervention eliminates pigmentation risk entirely, combined approaches that reduce inflammation and promote rapid vessel closure may mitigate this outcome in selected patients. Contraindications to CLaCS must be considered additively, as the procedure combines laser energy, chemical injury, and mechanical manipulation. Sclerosant allergy is interestingly not present in the case of dextrose use, making CLaCS a great indication for the patients who cannot be candidates for detergent sclerosants or want to have a longer session with no sclerosing agent volume limitations, and therefore a faster result. Absolute contraindications include active venous thrombosis, pregnancy (in aesthetic practice), active skin infection, or severely compromised arterial perfusion. Relative contraindications are more nuanced and demand clinical judgment. These include autoimmune disease, connective tissue disorders, marked skin atrophy, photosensitivity syndromes, and a history of hypertrophic scarring. In such patients, CLaCS is not automatically excluded, but the threshold for proceeding should be higher, and the technique modified conservatively. Perhaps the most underappreciated contraindication is psychological or expectation-related unsuitability. Patients seeking absolute perfection, immediate results, or guarantees of permanence are poor candidates for any C1 intervention, particularly a combined technique that requires biological healing and time (Table. 12.1).

CLaCS experts usually refer to the so-called "Score 9–1." It represents a practical classification approach for lower-limb venous disease, specifically designed to account for the various presentations of varicose veins and telangiectasia. The scoring framework addresses two fundamental diagnostic considerations:

1. the presence of telangiectasia and reticular veins and, when present, whether these are associated with identifiable feeder veins.

Table 12.1 Indications and contraindications to CLaCS

Indications
Anatomic/hemodynamic patterns not suitable for a technique only.
Other techniques prior treatment failure
Intolerance to pain
Hyperpigmentation risk
High aesthetic demand
Relative contraindications
Autoimmune disease, Connective tissue, Disorders marked skin, Atrophy photosensitivity, Syndromes and a history of hypertrophic scarring, Psychological/expectation.
Absolute contraindications
Active thrombosis
Pregnancy
Severe peripheral arterial disese
Severe infections
Severe systemic disease

2. the presence of venous reflux originating from the saphenous, pelvic, or perforator venous systems. Within this classification, a feeder vein is defined as any reticular vein that demonstrates an anatomical connection to a telangiectasia.

The classification is visually structured as a grid. Along the horizontal axis, cases are differentiated based on the absence or presence of telangiectasia and reticular veins and, in cases of presence, on whether a feeding vessel can be identified. The vertical axis delineates three distinct conditions: absence of varicose veins, varicose veins not supplied by saphenous, pelvic, or perforator venous sources, and varicose veins supplied by saphenous, pelvic, or perforator venous systems. The final Score 9–1 is determined by the intersection of the venous dilation category on the vertical axis with the telangiectasia/reticular vein characteristics on the horizontal axis (Table. 12.2). Scores located below the red horizontal reference line (scores 7, 8, and 9) necessitate comprehensive duplex ultrasound evaluation to determine the most appropriate therapeutic strategy and treatment technique for the associated varicosities. Similarly, scores positioned to the right of the green vertical reference line (scores 3, 6, and 9) require detailed ultrasound assessment to accurately identify the veins supplying the telangiectasia and reticular veins targeted for treatment. At present, the Score 9–1 system has not been validated or published in an indexed scientific journal. It is intended as a descriptive classification tool only and is not designed to function as a grading system for disease severity.

Table 12.2 Score 9/1 for CLaCS indication

		Absent	NO feeder vein	WITH feeder vein
		Teleangectasia		
Absent	Varices	1	2	3
NO saphenous, pelvic, perforating origin		4	5	6
WITH saphenous, pelvic, perforating origin		7	8	9

Duplex ultrasound occupies a paradoxical position in C1 disease. Historically considered unnecessary for "cosmetic" veins, it is now recognized as a risk-reduction and outcome-optimization tool, particularly before advanced interventions. A recent clinical governance document lodged in the Italian Superior Institute of Health highlights its importance by suggesting it before whatever even just aesthetic phlebology procedure [25, 26]. In the context of CLaCS, duplex ultrasound is not primarily used to identify axial reflux, although this remains essential. Its greater value lies in mapping reticular feeders, localized reflux zones, and venous connectivity that may not be apparent on inspection alone. By visualizing subdermal venous anatomy, duplex allows the clinician to avoid treating superficial endpoints sustained by untreated deeper pathology, plan procedural sequencing, and document baseline anatomy for medicolegal protection. This mapping reinforces the conceptual shift from treating "what is visible" to treating what sustains visibility. Reticular veins can also be painful and an aesthetic concern, mostly on the lateral and posterior sides of women's thighs. As CLaCS treatment is focal, the treatment can have a better control and long-lasting results of more than a decade [27]. Duplex findings should be integrated with clinical examination and, whenever possible, with vein visualization technologies. Photodocumentation is also considered of pivotal importance in CLaCS practice, both for medicolegal and patient satisfaction purposes. Indeed, at this high level of aesthetics, patients might tend to forget the original appearance of their legs, therefore being comforted by the pre- and post-iconography. Moreover, the recommended number of photographs is 50–100 (with and without the VeinViewer), and this procedure helps to show the patient that the doctor is committed to the aesthetic result as well [28]. No evaluation for CLaCS is complete without a careful assessment of the skin itself. Laser energy interacts not only with blood but with melanin, collagen, and epidermal architecture, making skin biology a central determinant of risk. Patients with higher Fitzpatrick phototypes face increased risk of epidermal injury and post-inflammatory hyperpigmentation. Continuous cold-air cooling reduces this risk but does not eliminate it, necessitating conservative parameter selection and explicit counseling [29, 30]. Beyond phototype, dermal thickness and collagen density vary widely and influence both laser penetration and sclerosant diffusion. Thin, atrophic skin, often seen in older patients or those with chronic sun exposure, is particularly vulnerable to ulceration and pigmentation. Hormonal factors further complicate risk assessment. Patients using hormonal therapies or with a history of hormonally driven telangiectatic proliferation exhibit higher rates of matting and recurrence, regardless of technique [22]. CLaCS does not negate these risks, but when thoughtfully applied, it may reduce their clinical expression by limiting excessive inflammation and promoting more uniform vessel closure. The total energy used for CLaCS is much lower than the factory settings. The technique is based on lower energy and multiple passes ("slow cooking"), which has its effect amplified by the sclerotherapy synergy. In C1 disease, expectation management is inseparable from clinical care. Many patients arrive with unrealistic beliefs shaped by marketing, social media, or prior experiences. The role of the clinician is not merely to inform, but to reframe expectations within biological reality. Patients must understand that complete clearance is not guaranteed, multiple sessions may be required, pigmentation can persist for months, recurrence is possible even after technically successful treatment. Informed consent for CLaCS should explicitly address the combined nature of the procedure, its rationale, its potential advantages, and its unique risks. Ethically, the clinician must also recognize when not to treat. Declining CLaCS in patients with disproportionate expectations, poor adherence potential, or unfavorable biology is not a failure of care, but an affirmation of professional responsibility. Patient selection and clinical evaluation for CLaCS represent a philosophical stance as much as a technical one. They require the clinician to think in networks rather than vessels, in probabilities rather than guarantees, and in partnership rather than procedure. When these principles are respected, CLaCS becomes a powerful extension of modern phlebology, precise, restrained, and biologically informed.

5 Principles of Cryo-Laser Technology

The use of laser energy in the treatment of telangiectasias and reticular veins represents one of the most intellectually demanding aspects of aesthetic phlebology. Unlike sclerotherapy, where endothelial injury is direct and largely independent of surrounding tissues, laser therapy operates through complex, indirect interactions between light, blood, vessel walls, and skin. The introduction of cryogenic skin cooling into this equation further modifies these interactions, transforming laser treatment from a purely thermal intervention into a thermodynamically modulated procedure. Cryo-laser technology, as employed in CLaCS, is not simply a means of reducing discomfort. It fundamentally alters the safety margins, biological effects, and clinical usability of vascular laser therapy. Understanding these principles is essential for any practitioner seeking to apply CLaCS with precision rather than empiricism. Laser–tissue interaction in vascular applications is governed by the principle of selective photothermolysis, first articulated to describe how light of a specific wavelength can selectively damage a target chromophore while sparing surrounding tissue. In venous applications, the primary chromophore is hemoglobin, contained within intravascular blood. When laser energy is delivered to the skin, photons undergo reflection at the skin surface, scattering within the dermis, absorption by chromophores such as hemoglobin and melanin. Only absorbed photons contribute to therapeutic effect. Absorption by hemoglobin converts optical energy into heat, raising intravascular temperature and inducing endothelial injury, coagulation, and eventual vessel collapse [9]. However, this process is neither uniform nor predictable without careful parameter selection. Vessel diameter, blood volume, flow velocity, and wall thickness all influence heat accumulation. Small telangiectasias may heat rapidly but cool just as quickly, while larger reticular veins require deeper penetration and longer pulse durations to achieve meaningful thermal injury.

Pulse duration is particularly critical. To confine heat to the vessel, pulse duration must approximate or be shorter than the Thermal Relaxation Time (TRT) of the target vessel. Exceeding TRT allows heat to diffuse into surrounding tissue, increasing the risk of epidermal injury without improving vascular efficacy. In practice, this means that laser treatment of leg veins operates within a narrow therapeutic window, narrower than that for facial telangiectasias due to deeper vessel location, thicker dermis, and higher hydrostatic pressures [31]. Wavelength selection is the most consequential decision in vascular laser therapy. It determines not only which chromophores are targeted, but also how deeply laser energy penetrates the skin. Shorter wavelengths (e.g., 532 nm) are strongly absorbed by hemoglobin but also by melanin, limiting their safe use on the lower extremities and in darker skin types. These wavelengths are effective for very superficial red telangiectasias but carry a higher risk of epidermal injury and pigmentation when used on leg veins. Longer wavelengths, particularly 1064 nm (Nd:YAG), exhibit lower melanin absorption and deeper penetration, making them more suitable for blue telangiectasias and reticular veins. However, hemoglobin absorption is lower at this wavelength, necessitating higher fluence and careful pulse-duration selection to achieve adequate intravascular heating [10]. This trade-off reduced epidermal risk at the expense of higher energy requirements, defining the challenge of leg vein laser therapy. Cryo-laser technology was developed precisely to expand this therapeutic window, allowing effective fluence delivery while maintaining epidermal safety. Importantly, wavelength selection in CLaCS is not made in isolation. It is informed by vessel depth and color, skin phototype, and anticipated integration with sclerotherapy. Laser treatment in CLaCS is often used not to achieve complete vessel obliteration, but to modify vessel physiology, narrowing the lumen, slowing flow, and rendering the vessel more responsive to subsequent sclerosant injection, which can then be of the mildest and less prone to develop possible complications. Cryogenic skin cooling is frequently described in clinical terms as pain reduction and patient comfort, but its biological effects extend far deeper. Cooling influences thermal conduction, vascular tone, neural signaling, inflammatory response, making it a central component of cryo-laser technology rather than a mere adjunct. Cold-air cooling reduces epidermal temperature prior to laser exposure, increasing the temperature gradient between the epidermis and the intravascular space. This allows a greater proportion of laser-generated heat to be confined within the vessel, protecting the epidermis even when higher fluences are used [32]. Cooling also induces vasoconstriction in superficial vessels, reducing blood volume and stabilizing vessel diameter. This has two important consequences: reduced competing heat sink effect from flowing blood, more predictable laser–vessel interaction. From a neurophysiological perspective, cooling decreases nerve conduction velocity and dampens nociceptor activation. This not only improves patient tolerance but also reduces involuntary movement, enhancing procedural precision. Finally, cooling attenuates inflammatory mediator release, which is increasingly recognized as a contributor to post-laser hyperpigmentation and telangiectatic matting [33]. The defining feature of cryo-laser technology is the dynamic interaction between delivered laser energy and active epidermal cooling. Rather than acting independently, these forces shape each other's biological effects. By lowering epidermal temperature, cryoprotection allows higher fluence delivery, longer pulse durations, and larger spot sizes, without exceeding epidermal injury thresholds. This is particularly important for deeper or larger-caliber vessels, where insufficient energy delivery is a common cause of laser failure. At the same time, cooling modifies intravascular thermodynamics. Reduced baseline temperature means that a greater temperature rise is required to achieve endothelial damage. However, this is offset by reduced blood flow and increased thermal confinement, resulting in more controlled and uniform vessel injury rather than explosive coagulation. In CLaCS, this controlled injury is intentional. The goal is not maximal laser-induced destruction, but predictable vessel modification that synergizes with immediate sclerotherapy. The timing of cooling, before, during, and after laser exposure, is therefore critical. Inconsistent or delayed cooling undermines both safety and efficacy, collapsing the therapeutic window back to that of conventional laser therapy. When compared with conventional transcutaneous laser therapy, cryo-laser technology offers several clinically meaningful advantages that justify its role in CLaCS. First, cryo-laser expands the safety margin, particularly in darker phototypes and on the lower extremities, where epidermal injury risk is inherently higher. Second, improved pain control allows for more comprehensive treatment in a single session, reducing the need for multiple incomplete treatments driven by patient intolerance. Third, cryo-laser facilitates a strategic rather than destructive use of laser energy, enabling vessel modification that enhances sclerosant efficacy rather than competing with it. This represents a conceptual departure from laser-only paradigms. Finally, by reducing inflammation and epidermal injury, cryo-laser may contribute to lower rates of post-treatment pigmentation and matting, outcomes that are disproportionately important in aesthetic venous practice. Cryo-laser technology transforms vascular laser therapy from a narrow, pain-limited intervention into a modulated, biologically informed tool. Within CLaCS, it serves not as an isolated treatment, but as a physiologic primer, reshaping vessel behavior, improving tolerability, and expanding safety margins so that combined therapy can be delivered with precision and restraint. For the expert phlebologist, mastery of cryo-laser principles is not optional. It is the difference between applying CLaCS as a protocol and practicing it as a conceptual extension of modern venous science.

6 Principles of Cryo-Sclerotherapy

Sclerotherapy occupies a paradoxical position in modern phlebology. It is simultaneously the oldest therapeutic intervention in the field and one of the most biologically sophisticated. While the technical act of injecting a sclerosant appears deceptively simple, the cascade of events it initiates, spanning endothelial injury, thrombosis, inflammation, remodeling, and resorption, is exquisitely sensitive to context. Temperature, flow, vessel architecture, and host response all shape the final clinical outcome. Cryo-sclerotherapy, as integrated within Cryo-Laser and Cryo-Sclerotherapy (CLaCS), does not seek to replace conventional sclerotherapy. Instead, it redefines the environment in which sclerotherapy occurs. By deliberately altering tissue temperature before, during, and after sclerosant exposure, cryo-sclerotherapy transforms the pharmacodynamics of endothelial injury. The result is not weaker sclerotherapy, but more selective, confined, and predictable biological damage. To appreciate this evolution, one must abandon the notion that sclerotherapy success is proportional to sclerosant concentration or inflammatory intensity. In CLaCS, success is measured by precision of injury, not magnitude. Within CLaCS, sclerosant aggressiveness is intentionally reduced. Laser pretreatment alters vessel caliber and flow, while cryogenic cooling modifies endothelial susceptibility. Together, these changes allow effective sclerosis at lower chemical intensity, shifting the balance from destructive to biologically efficient therapy. Rather than traditionally used detergents, such as polidocanol and sodium tetradecyl sulphate, CLaCS relies on the osmotic sclerosing agent Dectrose 75%. The treatment of telangiectasias and reticular veins occupies a unique position within the broader field of chronic venous disease management. Although classified as CEAP C1 pathology, these lesions frequently represent the most visible manifestation of complex micro-hemodynamic dysfunction. Their treatment, therefore, has historically straddled the boundary between cosmetic intervention and legitimate medical therapy. Hypertonic glucose solutions, particularly at concentrations of 50–75%, represent the most widely used osmotic sclerosants in contemporary practice. Telangiectasia and reticular vein characteristics make them highly susceptible to chemical endothelial injury, but also prone to incomplete closure, recanalization, and post-treatment pigmentary change. The choice of sclerosant, therefore, must balance sufficient endothelial destruction with controlled inflammatory response. Hypertonic glucose exerts its sclerosant effect through osmotic stress rather than direct chemical toxicity. When injected intraluminally at high concentration, the glucose solution creates a steep osmotic gradient across the endothelial cell membrane. Water rapidly exits the endothelial cytoplasm, leading to cellular dehydration, membrane contraction and deformation, disruption of intercellular junctions, secondary exposure of the subendothelial matrix. The injury induced is nonspecific and concentration-dependent, relying heavily on contact time and intravascular retention. Thrombus formation follows endothelial compromise, and vein obliteration ultimately occurs through organization and fibrosis of the thrombotic material, rather than immediate wall destruction. This indirect mechanism explains both the relative safety and variable efficacy of hypertonic glucose, as well as its dependence on precise injection technique and adequate compression. Detergent sclerosants operate through a fundamentally different pathway. Polidocanol and sodium tetradecyl sulphate are amphiphilic molecules that integrate into lipid bilayers, forming micelles that solubilize membrane lipids and denature endothelial surface proteins. The result is immediate endothelial lysis, uniform circumferential injury, rapid exposure of collagen and elastin, intense platelet activation and inflammation. Polidocanol's additional local anesthetic effect reduces nociceptive signaling, making it subjectively less painful despite equivalent endothelial toxicity. The direct nature of detergent-induced injury accounts for the greater predictability and consistency observed clinically, particularly in reticular veins with thicker walls [34]. Histologic studies of treated veins reveal distinct patterns of injury. Detergent sclerosants produce complete endothelial denudation with extension into the superficial media, whereas osmotic agents often leave patches of intact endothelium, particularly when contact time is brief. These differences translate clinically into higher rates of immediate occlusion with detergents, greater reliance on thrombosis and fibrosis with glucose, increased recanalization risk with osmotic agents in larger-caliber vessels [6]. One of the most informative contemporary trials compared 75% hypertonic glucose with 0.2% STS for leg telangiectasias. This prospective randomized study demonstrated that glucose achieved equal or superior vessel disappearance scores, significantly lower post-treatment hyperpigmentation, comparable patient satisfaction. These findings challenge the assumption that detergents are universally superior in very small-caliber vessels [35]. Despite isolated advantages of glucose, detergent sclerosants remain the most extensively studied agents. Systematic reviews, including Cochrane analyses, emphasize that no sclerosing agent demonstrates universal superiority and that study heterogeneity limits definitive ranking. This reinforces the need for individualized agent selection rather than dogmatic preference [21]. Post-sclerotherapy hyperpigmentation is a major determinant of patient dissatisfaction. Evidence suggests higher pigmentation rates with detergents compared to dextrose. The reduced inflammatory response associated with osmotic injury likely contributes to this difference. Both sclerosant classes can cause skin necrosis following extravasation, ulceration, telangiectatic matting. Detergent sclerosants, particularly when used as foam, carry rare risks of systemic neurologic events, whereas hypertonic glucose may cause transient hyperglycemia without long-term consequence [36]. Across all studies, technique consistently emerges as the dominant determinant of outcome. Factors such as injection pressure, volume per injection, needle gauge, and immediate compression often outweigh the intrinsic properties of the sclerosant itself. The experienced practitioner tailors agent selection dynamically, based on vessel morphology, patient risk factors, and prior response. Temperature profoundly influences cellular biology, yet it has historically received little attention in sclerotherapy literature. Endothelial cells are metabolically active and possess intrinsic repair mechanisms that respond dynamically to injury. Cooling alters these processes at multiple levels. At reduced temperatures, cellular metabolism slows, membrane fluidity decreases, enzymatic repair pathways are suppressed, and inflammatory signaling is dampened. When a sclerosant is introduced into this environment, endothelial injury becomes less diffuse but more durable. Rather than provoking explosive inflammation and widespread endothelial sloughing, cooling favors localized membrane disruption with delayed repair, allowing thrombosis and fibrosis to proceed without excessive perivascular spillover [37]. This phenomenon helps explain why cryosclerotherapy may achieve effective vein closure with less pain, less inflammation, and fewer pigmentary sequelae than conventional approaches using identical agents. Importantly, cooling does not render endothelial cells resistant to injury. Instead, it alters the kinetics of injury and healing, favoring controlled luminal obliteration over inflammatory excess. Modifying CLaCS original technique substituting dextrose with detergents, even more if in foam formulation, demands maximum caution as a too aggressive endothelial damage and extravasation could happen following the laser and cold effect previously expressed on the vessel. These effects are magnified in superficial dermal vessels, where even modest inflammation becomes clinically visible. Within CLaCS, the biological environment is already optimized through laser-induced vessel modification and cryogenic vasoconstriction. Under these conditions, liquid sclerotherapy often provides superior control, allowing precise dosing and limited dispersion. Foam retains a role in selected reticular veins, particularly those with larger lumens or persistent flow, but its use must be selective and informed by anatomical depth, vessel size, and patient-specific inflammatory risk. In this case, a valuable alternative can be found in a pin-hole mini-phlebectomy [38]. Perhaps the most underappreciated effect of cooling in sclerotherapy is its influence on sclerosant diffusion. In warm tissue, vasodilation and increased capillary permeability facilitate sclerosant spread beyond the target vessel, exposing surrounding dermis to chemical injury. Cooling counteracts these processes by inducing vasoconstriction, reducing interstitial diffusion, and limiting capillary leakage. As a result, a greater proportion of sclerosant action is confined to the intraluminal space, increasing the efficiency ratio of desired to undesired injury. This confinement has downstream consequences. Reduced perivascular inflammation lowers the likelihood of hemosiderin deposition, prolonged induration, angiogenic signaling and matting. Clinical observations and emerging comparative data suggest that this refined injury pattern contributes to improved cosmetic outcomes in cryo-based combined approaches [24].

7 Technical Notes

The technical execution of CLaCS cannot be meaningfully separated from its conceptual foundations. To describe CLaCS merely as a sequence of laser application followed by sclerotherapy is to misunderstand its essence. CLaCS is not a hybrid procedure in the conventional sense: it is a single physiological intervention delivered through multiple modalities, each deliberately timed to exploit the transient vulnerabilities of the venous microcirculation. In conventional venous aesthetics, treatment steps are often compartmentalized. Laser is performed on 1 day, sclerotherapy on another. Cooling is applied intermittently, usually as an afterthought, primarily for comfort. CLaCS rejects this fragmentation. It proceeds from the premise that vascular biology is dynamic and that the window during which a vessel is most susceptible to intervention may be measured in minutes rather than days. The integrated protocol is therefore less about efficiency and more about biological opportunism, acting precisely when endothelial defenses are weakest and inflammatory escalation can still be restrained From this perspective, CLaCS is best understood as a continuum. At the heart of CLaCS lies a conceptual inversion. Traditional approaches aim for maximal immediate vessel destruction. CLaCS, by contrast, values instability over annihilation. The laser component is intentionally restrained. Its role is to destabilize the vessel biologically, not to close it definitively.

Under continuous cryogenic cooling, laser energy induces a state of controlled endothelial distress. The vessel wall experiences thermal stress sufficient to disrupt endothelial function and alter smooth muscle tone, yet insufficient to provoke uncontrolled coagulation or epidermal injury. Flow slows. The lumen narrows. Repair mechanisms are activated but not yet effective. The vessel enters a transiently compromised state. This state is fleeting. If nothing further is done, reactive vasodilation, endothelial repair, and flow restoration will follow. CLaCS intervenes precisely at this juncture. Sclerotherapy is administered immediately, before recovery can occur. The sclerosant encounters a vessel that is no longer physiologically intact, yet not so damaged that inflammation dominates the response. The chemical injury therefore completes what the laser initiated, producing a more predictable and confined endothelial collapse. This is the fundamental logic of CLaCS: laser creates vulnerability; sclerotherapy exploits it; cooling governs the entire process. Because CLaCS depends on uninterrupted physiological modulation, the procedural environment assumes outsized importance. The treatment room is not merely a setting; it is an active participant in the intervention. Patient positioning in CLaCS is a deliberate hemodynamic intervention. Venous filling, vessel diameter, and flow velocity vary dramatically with posture, and these variables directly influence both laser and sclerosant behavior. Complete limb dependency maximizes visibility but at the cost of increased intravascular pressure and flow, which oppose vessel collapse and promote sclerosant washout. Full elevation, on the other hand, collapses veins excessively, impairing visualization and cannulation. CLaCS therefore typically employs moderate dependency, most often with the patient supine and the limb slightly lowered. This positioning preserves enough venous filling for accurate targeting while maintaining a physiologic environment conducive to controlled injury. Importantly, cryogenic cooling and posture act synergistically: cooling induces vasoconstriction, while moderate dependency prevents excessive collapse. Together, they create a stable, predictable vascular field. Skin preparation follows the same philosophy of restraint. The objective is cleanliness without provocation. Overzealous antisepsis, aggressive scrubbing, or repeated alcohol application may prime the skin for inflammation and pigmentation, undermining the very outcomes CLaCS seeks to improve The procedural sequence begins with pre-cooling. Cold air is applied for sufficient time to establish analgesia and vasoconstriction before the first laser pulse. This step is not optional; it defines the safety and tolerability of everything that follows. Laser application then proceeds deliberately. The operator targets not only visible telangiectasias, but also strategic points within the network, junctions, convergences, and segments that will most influence downstream hemodynamics. The clinical endpoint is subtle transformation, not disappearance. Transient darkening, delayed blanching, or gradual narrowing are signs of effective conditioning. Excessive pursuit of immediate clearance is one of the most common errors among clinicians new to CLaCS. Aggressive laser application produces dramatic short-term results at the cost of inflammation, pigmentation, and prolonged recovery. CLaCS favors delayed success over immediate gratification. A neodymium:yttrium-aluminiumgarnet 1064 nm is used typically at an energy fluence ranging between 50 and 70 J/cm^2, combined with a 6 mm spot diameter and a pulse duration of 15 milliseconds at 1 Hz (1 shot per second)(Fig. 12.2). These settings are optimized for treating veins with an internal diameter of up to 1.5 mm. Using this protocol, one to three laser pulses are delivered to the same area after the entire vein pathway has been treated. Given the relatively low fluence applied in the CLaCS technique, it is recommended that laser shots overlap by approximately 10% to 20%. After completing

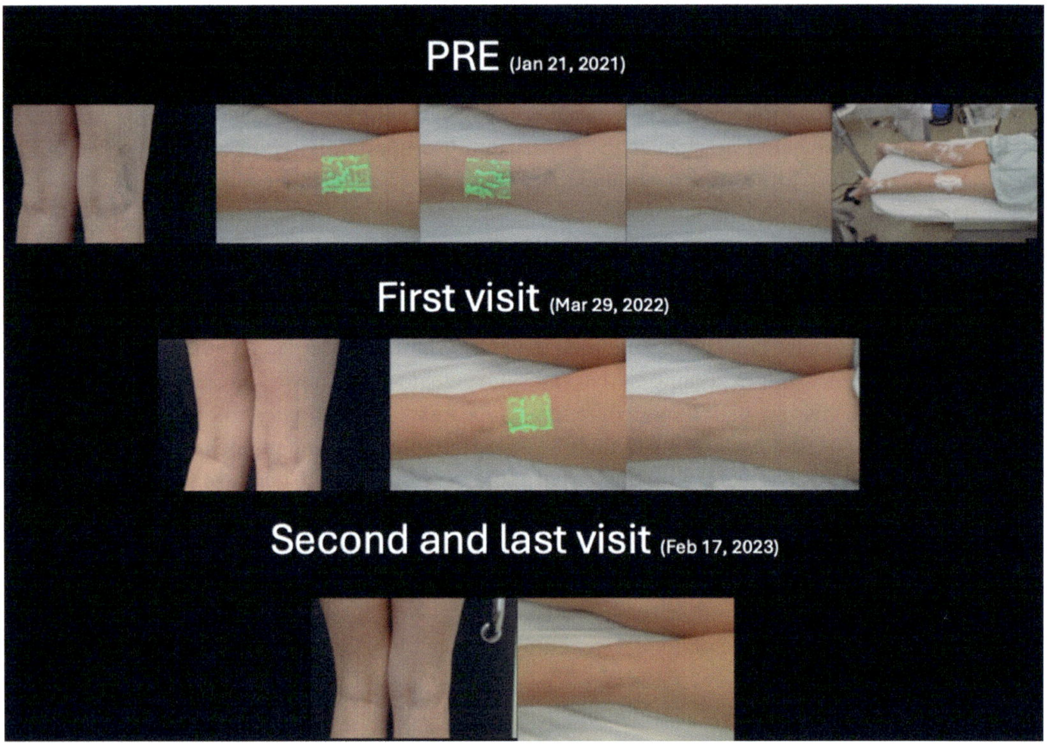

Fig. 12.2 CLaCS patient clinical case example. Laser parameters: 70 J/cm², 15 msec, 6 mm

laser treatment over an area of about 10 × 10 cm, the procedure proceeds with the sclerotherapy phase. Newer dedicated laser platforms are considerably more powerful and the 1064 nm laser is shot with 50–80 J/cm², combined with a 8 mm spot diameter and 15 millisecond fractioned consecutive pulse of 1.3 milliseconds. The rate of repetition is also faster and can reach 3 Hz. These advancements are particularly useful when the patient is sensitive and CLaCS is performed under endovenous sedation.

Both laser therapy and sclerotherapy are carried out with the assistance of visualization devices that emit infrared light, allowing the target vessels to be detected and displayed on the skin as a bright green image, thereby enhancing visibility. These visualizers do not provide hemodynamic information and cannot distinguish between normal and pathological venous drainage. Their primary function is to improve the detection of telangiectasias and associated feeder veins that are not visible to the naked eye. In accordance with the CLaCS approach, treatment is selectively applied only to vessels supplying the target telangiectasias and reticular veins, rather than to all visualized veins [13]. Without pausing cooling, sclerotherapy follows. The vessels encountered at this stage behave differently from untreated veins. They are less distended, less reactive, and more amenable to precise injection. Smaller volumes suffice. Lower pressures are effective. The sclerosant remains intraluminal longer due to reduced flow and vasoconstriction. The operator's mindset must shift accordingly. This is not conventional sclerotherapy. The aim is not to fill the vessel, but to touch the endothelium at a moment of maximum susceptibility. Over-injection negates the benefit of priming and reintroduces the risks of inflammation and diffusion. Compared with commonly used detergent sclerosants, a 75% dextrose solution is more viscous. This difference becomes apparent during injection, as greater force is required to depress the syringe plunger, particularly when very fine needles are used. Consequently, the use of 27-gauge needles paired with 3-mL syringes is advised, since 30-gauge needles tend to generate excessive resistance. Among the advantages of using dextrose are zero anaphylaxis risk, a lower pigmentation rate, and also zero chance of skin ulcer due to sclerotherapy. The laser damage added by the dextrose high viscosity impedes the sclerosing agent from being forced backwards into the arterio-capillary system and therefore cause an ischemic skin ulcer that heals slowly under second intention. This physiopathology was described in an experimental study in rabbit ears in 1972, but it was only accepted for publication in 2012 and therefore not spread out in the phlebology community [39]. Comprehensive photographic documentation is regarded as essential. Common pitfalls include escalating laser fluence in pursuit of instant results, injecting sclerosant volumes appropriate for untreated vessels, allowing cooling to lapse during transitions, treating visible telangiectasias while ignoring feeder dynamics. The greatest justification for CLaCS lies in its ability to manage heterogeneous venous networks, fields where telangiectasias, reticular veins, and transitional vessels coexist. Traditional single-modality approaches force compromise: laser struggles with depth, while sclerotherapy provokes inflammation in superficial vessels. CLaCS allows the clinician to speak multiple biological languages simultaneously. Laser addresses vessels too small or superficial for safe injection. Sclerotherapy treats larger feeders efficiently, eventually aided by mini-phlebectomies. Cooling moderates. The network is treated as a system rather than a collection of independent targets. In these cases, restraint is again paramount. It is neither necessary nor desirable to eliminate every vessel in a single session. CLaCS supports staged clearance without penalizing patience, preserving skin integrity and long-term aesthetics.

8 Safety Considerations and Complication Prevention

Complications in CLaCS is rarely idiosyncratic, particularly considering the low laser energy and the mild sclerosant utilization. They arise when the cumulative burden of injury exceeds the adaptive capacity of skin and microvasculature. Laser-induced thermal injury becomes hazardous when heat diffusion exceeds vascular confinement and spreads into surrounding dermis. This risk is heightened in superficial telangiectasias, thin or photoaged skin, and in patients with higher melanin content, where epidermal absorption competes with hemoglobin targeting. New dedicated laser platforms should be used with care because the stacking laser pulses may lead to complete destruction of the skin. To avoid that, new lasers have integrated infrared thermometers that shut down the laser if a set maximum temperature is reached [32]. Cryogenic cooling expands the therapeutic window by lowering epidermal temperature and increasing the margin between effective intravascular heating and epidermal damage. However, cooling does not nullify physics. Excessive fluence, inappropriate pulse duration, or repeated passes over the same area can overwhelm even well-cooled tissue. A common novice error is to interpret the absence of pain as evidence of safety. In reality, analgesia can mask impending injury. Cryogenic injury itself is theoretically possible but exceedingly rare when cold-air cooling is used appropriately. More relevant is the subtle ischemic stress imposed by prolonged vasoconstriction, particularly in patients with compromised microcirculation. Continuous visual monitoring of skin color, capillary refill, and texture is therefore essential throughout the procedure. Skin necrosis is the most feared complication in superficial venous treatment, not because it is common, but because it represents a catastrophic failure of biological balance. In CLaCS, necrosis almost never results from a single misstep. It is the endpoint of cumulative insult (thermal, chemical, mechanical, and ischemic) applied to tissue with limited reserve [32]. Early recognition of impending necrosis is critical. Persistent severe pain, non-blanching pallor, livedoid discoloration, or delayed capillary refill should prompt immediate cessation of treatment in the affected area. Early supportive care (local wound management, anti-inflammatory measures, and avoidance of further insult) can significantly limit tissue loss and long-term scarring. Post-treatment hyperpigmentation is the most common delayed complication of C1 treatment and one of the most emotionally charged. Although medically benign, pigmentation carries disproportionate weight in patient satisfaction and perception of success. The dominant mechanism is hemosiderin deposition, resulting from erythrocyte extravasation and hemoglobin breakdown within the dermis. Factors that increase pigmentation risk include: incomplete vessel collapse, prolonged intravascular thrombus, excessive endothelial inflammation, darker phototypes, sun exposure during the healing phase [40]. CLaCS mitigates pigmentation risk by using non-aggressive osmotic sclerosants and low laser energy. However, no technique abolishes pigmentation risk entirely. Overly aggressive treatment, particularly the pursuit of immediate clearance, remains the most common precipitant. Management of pigmentation begins with anticipatory counseling. Patients must understand that pigmentation is often transient and may persist for months before fading. Premature intervention—such as aggressive topical bleaching or repeated laser exposure—frequently worsens inflammation. Patience, sun avoidance, and gentle supportive care remain the cornerstone of management. Telangiectatic matting represents one of the most vexing phenomena in aesthetic phlebology. Characterized by the emergence of fine, reddish neovessels after treatment, matting is often perceived by patients as treatment failure. CLaCS offers theoretical advantages in matting prevention by addressing feeder networks more comprehensively, limiting the need for repeated high-intensity treatments and allowing a progressive adaptation of the circulation in a staged approach. Nevertheless, matting cannot be eliminated by technique alone. Prevention requires moderation, staging, and respect for biological variability, particularly in hormonally sensitive patients. When matting occurs, restraint remains essential. Further aggressive intervention often exacerbates angiogenesis. Observation, time, and delayed gentle laser therapy may allow gradual resolution. Pain and vasovagal reactions are often dismissed as minor or inevitable, yet they exert a profound influence on procedural safety and precision. In CLaCS, pain control is not merely a comfort issue: it is a safety mechanism. Cryogenic cooling provides analgesia by reducing nerve conduction velocity, dampening nociceptor activation, suppressing neurogenic inflammation. Effective analgesia stabilizes the patient, reduces movement, and improves injection accuracy, particularly in very superficial or fine vessels where precision is paramount. Despite this, vasovagal reactions may still occur, particularly in anxious or needle-sensitive patients, during prolonged procedures or in dehydrated individuals. Early warning signs (lightheadedness, nausea, diaphoresis) should prompt immediate intervention. Supine positioning, limb elevation, reassurance, and observation are usually sufficient. Importantly, vasovagal events should be normalized rather than minimized. Transparent communication preserves trust and reinforces the clinician–patient alliance.

9 Clinical Outcomes and Evidence

The evaluation of outcomes in the treatment of telangiectasias and reticular veins has always occupied an uneasy space between science and perception. Unlike truncal venous disease, where duplex-derived hemodynamic endpoints dominate, C1 disease is judged primarily by what is seen, what is felt, and what persists over time. CLaCS, as a deliberately integrated and physiologically nuanced intervention, demands an equally nuanced framework for outcome assessment. To ask whether CLaCS "works" is therefore an incomplete question. The more relevant inquiry is how, for whom, for how long, and at what biological and experiential cost it works. The existing evidence base, while still maturing, allows meaningful conclusions when interpreted with humility and contextual awareness rather than absolutism. The historical reliance on visual clearance as the primary outcome measure in C1 disease reflects both necessity and limitation. Telangiectasias are visible by definition, and photographic documentation provides a tangible metric. Yet, visibility is a poor proxy for vascular biology. Lighting conditions, skin tone, observer bias, and patient positioning can all exaggerate or minimize perceived change. In response, contemporary studies increasingly employ graded clearance scales, which quantify percentage improvement rather than binary success or failure. This approach aligns more closely with biological reality, acknowledging that partial vessel regression may represent optimal healing rather than incomplete treatment. CLaCS further complicates assessment by shifting the target from isolated vessels to networks. A telangiectasia that fades slowly over weeks after feeder modification may represent a superior biological outcome compared with one that disappears immediately after aggressive ablation but recurs months later. Traditional efficacy metrics often fail to capture this distinction. Objective adjuncts, such as duplex ultrasound or near-infrared vein visualization, have been proposed to document network disruption, but their role in routine outcome reporting remains limited. As a result, most CLaCS studies continue to rely on clinical and photographic endpoints, underscoring the need for interpretive sophistication when reviewing results. Comparative effectiveness research in C1 disease is inherently challenging. Patient populations are heterogeneous, disease patterns vary widely, and operator technique strongly influences outcomes. CLaCS studies often enroll patients with greater network complexity, prior treatment failure, or higher cosmetic expectations: factors that bias comparisons against it if not acknowledged. Despite these limitations, available comparative data suggest that CLaCS achieves equal or superior clearance in selected populations compared with laser-only or sclerotherapy-only approaches, particularly in mixed telangiectatic–reticular networks [2]. Comparative studies suggest that this integration can reduce the need for aggressive parameter escalation in either modality. A modified CLaCS using dextrose 67% + polidocanol 0.3% demonstrated overlapping result at 30 days in the comparison with the traditional CLaCS using dextrose 75%. A possible superiority in vein clearance was perceived in the dextrose 67% + polidocanol 0.3% group, yet more data in a homogeneous settings are needed to formulate a reliable conclusion [41]. Importantly, several studies report lower rates of post-treatment pigmentation with CLaCS compared with conventional microsclerotherapy, particularly when conservative sclerosant dosing is employed. These findings, while promising, are technique-dependent and should not be generalized indiscriminately. A Brazilian randomized comparative trial used a 2 months follow up, comparing CLaCS and polidocanol 0.5% foam on the contralateral leg. Fourty four patients were analyzed. No significant difference was reported in vein caliber reduction. Both groups improved in patients' satisfaction. Although the incidence of post-treatment hyperpigmentation in limbs treated for reticular veins did not differ statistically, the CLaCS technique was associated with reduced severity of skin discoloration, decreased formation and drainage of microthrombi, less bruising and a smaller volume of sclerosant required. The small population, the single sclerosing concentration option for the polidocanol 0.5%, and other confounding factors do not allow generalizations in the CLaCS performance. While extremely useful as starting point, this publication paves the way for further data collection [24]. Interestingly, the year before a quite similar investigation was performed in a totally different Egyptian population, therefore offering data from two different continents and ethnicities. The study population was about 4 times larger than the similar Brazilian investigation in number of patients and doubled in terms of follow up (8 weeks). The comparison arm was still with polidocanol 0.5% foam. The outcome reported a significant superiority for CLaCS in complete elimination rate and a lower incidence of postprocedural pigmentation and other complications. The different outcome compared to the Brazialian investigation highlights the importance of real-world data, homogeneous trials, and multi-ethnicity inclusion [23]. The clinical outcomes and evidence surrounding CLaCS support its role as a probability-shifting intervention rather than a categorical solution. It increases the likelihood of favorable outcomes in selected patients, particularly those with complex networks, pigmentary risk, or limited tolerance for conventional approaches. It does not abolish recurrence, nor does it override biological variability. For the expert clinician, the value of CLaCS lies in its alignment with vascular biology. By integrating physical, chemical, and thermal modulation, it allows treatment intensity to be distributed rather than concentrated, reducing collateral damage while preserving efficacy. When interpreted with appropriate humility, the evidence positions CLaCS not as a disruptive replacement for established therapies, but as a logical, evidence-informed evolution in the management of C1 disease, one that prioritizes durability, patient experience, and biological cooperation over immediate visual triumph.

10 Training and Learning Curve

The successful adoption of CLaCS depends far less on technology than on professional maturity. Unlike single-modality interventions, CLaCS cannot be reduced to a set of parameters that reliably produce acceptable outcomes in inexperienced hands. It is an integrative technique that demands fluency across disciplines: vascular medicine, laser physics, microsclerotherapy, dermatologic biology, and patient communication. As such, CLaCS exposes gaps in training more readily than it conceals them. This reality has important implications. CLaCS is not a shortcut to better outcomes, nor a substitute for foundational competence. Instead, it functions as a capstone technique, best introduced after mastery of its component parts. Understanding how clinicians acquire this competence, how errors arise during the learning curve, and how CLaCS can be responsibly integrated into a venous practice is therefore essential to its safe and sustainable use. The defining requirement for CLaCS proficiency is conceptual integration. The operator must understand not only how to perform laser therapy and sclerotherapy independently, but how these modalities interact biologically when combined under cryogenic modulation. This level of understanding cannot be achieved through device training alone. Equally important is training in clinical judgment. CLaCS is unforgiving of rigid protocol adherence divorced from biological feedback. Operators must learn to read subtle cues, changes in vessel color, skin temperature, patient response, and adjust dynamically. This skill is experiential and cannot be simulated fully through didactic instruction. The learning curve in CLaCS is not linear. Early adopters might report an initial phase of enthusiasm followed by frustration, as outcomes fail to match expectations despite apparent technical correctness. This phenomenon reflects the cognitive recalibration required to abandon maximalist habits acquired in single-modality practice. One of the most common beginner errors is overuse of laser energy. Clinicians accustomed to judging success by immediate vessel disappearance may escalate fluence when confronted with subtle CLaCS endpoints. Cryogenic analgesia masks pain, reinforcing the false impression that higher energy is safe. The result is increased inflammation, pigmentation, or delayed healing. A second frequent error is over-injection of sclerosant. Laser pretreatment reduces vessel caliber and flow, yet beginners often inject volumes appropriate for untreated veins. This negates the biological advantage of priming and increases the risk of necrosis, pigmentation, and matting.

Another pitfall is procedural fragmentation. Interrupting cooling to adjust equipment, prepare syringes, or reposition the patient allows vasodilation and recovery of endothelial function. The loss of continuity erodes CLaCS efficacy and safety, reducing the technique to a less effective hybrid. Finally, many beginners struggle with patient selection. Applying CLaCS indiscriminately rather than reserving it for complex networks or specific risk profiles leads to disappointment and unnecessary risk. CLaCS rewards selectivity: it punishes indiscriminate enthusiasm. Experienced operators consistently report that outcomes improve dramatically once these habits are unlearned. The learning curve therefore reflects not only skill acquisition, but conceptual restraint. The economic implications of CLaCS extend beyond the purchase price of equipment. While the capital investment in a vascular laser and cryogenic cooling system is substantial, the more meaningful cost lies in time, training, and opportunity. Laser systems suitable for lower-limb venous work represent a major capital expense, as does high-quality cold-air cooling equipment. These costs must be amortized over sufficient procedural volume to remain economically viable. Practices with low C1 caseloads or predominantly truncal disease may struggle to justify the investment. However, CLaCS also alters practice efficiency. By addressing complex networks more effectively, it may reduce the total number of sessions required for selected patients. Improved tolerability can enhance patient retention and satisfaction, indirectly supporting practice growth. From an economic standpoint, CLaCS integrates best into practices that already manage a high volume of C1 disease, emphasize aesthetic outcomes alongside vascular health, invest in longitudinal patient relationships rather than episodic procedures. The ultimate test of CLaCS is not technical success, but practice coherence. CLaCS should not exist as an isolated service line or marketing tool. It belongs within a comprehensive venous practice that values diagnostic rigor, patient education, and long-term disease management. Integration requires cultural as well as technical alignment. Staff must understand the rationale for CLaCS, support procedural continuity, and reinforce post-treatment care. Scheduling must allow sufficient time for unhurried execution. Follow-up protocols must be standardized to monitor outcomes and complications. Equally important is ethical integration. CLaCS should never be used to justify treatment of patients with unrealistic expectations or minimal clinical need. Training in CLaCS is less about learning a new procedure than about becoming a different kind of practitioner. The learning curve is therefore not merely technical: it is philosophical and deontological. Those who approach CLaCS as a shortcut or a marketing differentiator are likely to encounter frustration and complications. Those who adopt it as a capstone expression of vascular expertise often find that it reshapes their entire approach to C1 disease. In this sense, CLaCS does not simply integrate into a practice. It integrates the practitioner, aligning skill, judgment, economics, and ethics into a coherent whole.

References

1. Gianesini S, Chi YW, Agüero C, et al. Fake-news-free evidence-based communication for proper vein-lymphatic disease management. Int Angiol. 2023;42(2):89–189.
2. Miyake RK, Chi YW, Franklin IJ, Gianesini S. State of the art on cryo-laser cryo-sclerotherapy in lower limb venous aesthetic treatment. J Vasc Surg Venous Lymphat Disord. 2020;8(5):893–5.
3. Miyake RK, Ramacciotti E. Cryo-laser and cryosclerotherapy guided by augmented reality for telangiectasias, feeder, and small varicose vein treatment e the CLaCS technique white paper report. J Phlebol Lymphol. 2019;12(1):1–7.
4. Goldman PM. Sclerotherapy for superficial venules and telangiectasias of the lower extremities. Dermatol Clin. 1987;5(2):369–79.
5. Myers K. A history of injection treatments – II sclerotherapy. Phlebology. 2019;34(5):303–10.
6. Schwartz L, Maxwell H. Sclerotherapy for lower limb telangiectasias. Cochrane Database Syst Rev. 2011;2011(12):CD008826.
7. Wollmann JC. The history of sclerosing foams. Dermatol Surg. 2004;30(5):694–703; discussion 703. https://doi.org/10.1111/j.1524-4725.2004.30208.x. Erratum in: Dermatol Surg. 2005 Feb;31(2):249.
8. Anderson RR, Parrish JA. Selective photothermolysis: precise microsurgery by selective absorption of pulsed radiation. Science. 1983;220(4596):524–7.
9. Major A, Brazzini B, Campolmi P, et al. Nd:YAG 1064 nm laser in the treatment of facial and leg telangiectasias. J Eur Acad Dermatol Venereol. 2001;15(6):559–65.
10. Ozyurt K, Colgecen E, Baykan H, et al. Treatment of superficial cutaneous vascular lesions: experience with the long-pulsed 1064 nm Nd:YAG laser. ScientificWorldJournal. 2012;2012:197139.
11. Kikuchi R, Grill MH, Caffaro RA, et al. Effects of long-pulsed 1064-nm Nd:YAG laser on telangiectasias and reticular veins: a human in-vivo histological study. Int Angiol. 2023;42(6):457–64.

12. Zenzie HH, Altshuler GB, Smirnov MZ, et al. Evaluation of cooling methods for laser dermatology. Lasers Surg Med. 2000;26(2):130–44.
13. Miyake RK, Zeman HD, Duarte FH, et al. Vein imaging: a new method of near infrared imaging, where a processed image is projected onto the skin for the enhancement of vein treatment. Dermatologic Surg. 2006;32(8):1031–8.
14. Puruhito. Pathophysiology of microcirculation in venous disease. Clin Hemorheol Microcirc. 2000;23(2–4):239–42.
15. Miyake RK, Kikuchi R, Duarte FH, Davidson J, Miyake H. Digital vein mapping guiding laser and injection sclerotherapy to treat telangiectasias and feeder veins: report of 140 cases. Flebologia y Linfologia/Lecturas Vasculares. 2009;4:569–76.
16. Wang Y, Xu R, He W, et al. Three-dimensional histological structures of the human dermis. Tissue Eng Part C Methods. 2015;21(9):932–44.
17. Smith PC. Management of reticular veins and telangiectases. Phlebology. 2015;30(2 Suppl):46–52.
18. Miyake H, Miyake K. Tratamento das microvarizes e telangiectasias. In: Doenças vasculares periféricas, vol. 15. Rio de Janeiro: Medsi; 2002. p. 63–80.
19. Pascarella L, Schmid Schönbein GW. Causes of telengiectasias, reticular veins, and varicose veins. Semin Vasc Surg. 2005;18(1):2–4.
20. Bajerski JC, Giordani CB, Borges LB, et al. Treatment of lower limb telangiectasias with Nd: Yag 1064 nm laser with and without tumescent anesthesia – TTL technique. Phlebology. 2025;40(1):15–20.
21. Nakano LC, Cacione DG, Baptista-Silva JC, et al. Treatment for telangiectasias and reticular veins. Cochrane Database Syst Rev. 2021;10(10):CD012723.
22. Davis LT, Duffy DM. Determination of incidence and risk factors for postsclerotherapy telangiectatic matting of the lower extremity: a retrospective analysis. J Dermatol Surg Oncol. 1990;16(4):327–30.
23. Nasser MM, Ghoneim BM, Eldaly W, et al. A comparative study between cryo-laser cryo-sclerotherapy and sclerotherapy in the treatment of telangiectasia and reticular veins: a randomized controlled trial. J Vasc Surg Venous Lymphat Disord. 2024;12(4):101874.
24. Rodrigues A, Puggina J, da Silva VS, et al. Pigmentation after foam or cryo-laser cryo-sclerotherapy for lower limb reticular veins: a within-patient randomized trial. J Vasc Surg Venous Lymphat Disord. 2025;13(6):102285.
25. Miyake K, Pires Davidson JR. Augmented reality and duplex ultrasound in medical treatment decision: score 9-1. J Phlebol Lymphol. 2019;12(1):500–1.
26. Gianesini S, Danese M, AlQedrah D, et al. Multi-specialty recommendations for the appropriate and affordable lower limb vein-lymphatic disorders management. Int Angiol. 2026;45(1):1–64.
27. Miyake K, Grill MH, Feitoza HSN. Case report: novel leg vein treatment CLaCS guided by augmented reality 11 years follow-up. J Cosmet Dermatol. 2023;22:16–20.
28. Santiago FR, Piscoya M, Chi Y-W. Change in perception of sclerotherapy results after exposure to pre-post intervention photographs. Phlebology. 2018;33(4):282–7.
29. Husain Z, Alster TS. The role of lasers and intense pulsed light technology in dermatology. Clin Cosmet Investig Dermatol. 2016;9:29–40.
30. Soares I, Amaral IP, Correia MP, et al. Complications of dermatologic lasers in high Fitzpatrick phototypes and management: an updated narrative review. Lasers Med Sci. 2024;39(1):149.
31. Wall TL. Current concepts: laser treatment of adult vascular lesions. Semin Plast Surg. 2007;21(3):147–58.
32. Miyake RK, Miyake H, Kauffman P. Skin temperature measurements during intense pulsed light emission. Dermatologic Surg. 2001;27(6):549–54.
33. Das A, Sarda A, De A. Cooling devices in laser therapy. J Cutan Aesthet Surg. 2016;9(4):215–9. https://doi.org/10.4103/0974-2077.197028.
34. Rabe E, Schliephake D, Otto J, et al. Sclerotherapy of telangiectases and reticular veins: a double-blind, randomized, comparative clinical trial of polidocanol, sodium tetradecyl sulphate and isotonic saline (EASI study). Phlebology. 2010;25(3):124–31.
35. Bukina OV, Sinitsyn AA, Pelevin AV. Sclerotherapy of telangiectasias: a prospective, randomized, comparative clinical trial of hypertonic glucose versus sodium tetradecyl sulfate. Vasc Med. 2021;26(3):297–301.
36. Wong M, Parsi K, Myers K, et al. Sclerotherapy of lower limb veins: indications, contraindications and treatment strategies to prevent complications – a consensus document of the International Union of Phlebology-2023. Phlebology. 2023 May;38(4):205–58.
37. Hansen TN, Dawson PE, Brockbank KG. Effects of hypothermia upon endothelial cells: mechanisms and clinical importance. Cryobiology. 1994 Feb;31(1):101–6.
38. Weiss RA, Weiss MA. Ambulatory phlebectomy compared to sclerotherapy for varicose and telangiectatic veins: indications and complications. Adv Dermatol. 1996;11:3–16.
39. Miyake RK, King JT, Kikuchi R, Duarte FH, Davidson JRP, Oba C. Role of injection pressure, flow and sclerosant viscosity in causing cutaneous ulceration during sclerotherapy. Phlebology. 2012;27(8):383–9.
40. Bossart S, Ramelet AA, Seyed Jafari SM, et al. Revealing the origin of postsclerotherapy hyperpigmentation: identification of melanin and hemosiderin as causative pigments in a histopathological study. Phlebology. 2025:2683555251357095.
41. Fonseca MM, Mocelin FJ, Grill MH, et al. Nd:Yag laser combined with injection sclerotherapy in the treatment of reticular veins and telangiectasias (CLaCS method): A triple-blind randomized clinical trial comparing two sclerosing agents associated with same laser patterns. Phlebology. 2023;38(3):165–71.

13 Foam Sclerotherapy for Pelvic Venous Disorders Treatment

Zaza Lazarashvili, Yung Wei Chi, and Sergio Gianesini

1 Prevalence and Quality of Life of Chronic Pelvic Pain

CPP affects about 4% to 16% of women overall. In the United States, 1 in 7 women are affected by this condition [2]. In community samples, some studies find a higher prevalence—for example, one study reported a 24% three-month prevalence of CPP in women of reproductive age [3]. Quality of life (QoL) in women with chronic pelvic pain (CPP) is substantially and consistently reduced across physical, psychological, social, and sexual domains: Persistent pain leads to limitations in daily activities, work, and exercise, fatigue and sleep disturbance are common, high rates of work absenteeism, and reduced productivity [4]. Depression and anxiety are significantly more prevalent in women with CPP, pain unpredictability contributes to catastrophizing, stress, and reduced coping capacity, central sensitization, and pain amplification further worsen emotional burden. Dyspareunia and post-coital pain are common, reduced libido, avoidance of intimacy, and relationship strain—sexual dysfunction is a major independent driver of poor QoL. All this factors are causing social withdrawal and reduced participation in family or community activities. Between the factors affecting the QoL in women with CPP, following management flaws are important: long diagnostic delays, multiple overlapping pain conditions (endometriosis, IBS, bladder pain syndrome, pelvic venous disorders), inadequate pain control or fragmented care, lack of validation or understanding from healthcare providers. The impact is often comparable to or worse than other chronic pain conditions such as low back pain or rheumatoid arthritis.

Z. Lazarashvili
Department of Vascular Surgery, Chapidze Heart Center, Tblisi State University, Tbilisi, Georgia
e-mail: zaza.lazarashvili@ecc.ge

Y. W. Chi
Department of Cardiovascular Medicine, University of California, Davis Vascular Center, Sacramento, CA, USA
e-mail: ywchi@ucdavis.edu

S. Gianesini (✉)
Department of Translational Medicine, University of Ferrara, Ferrara, Italy

Department of Surgery, Uniformed Services University of Health Sciences, Bethesda, MD, USA
e-mail: gnssrg@unife.it

2 Nomenclature of Pelvic Venous Disorders

One of the main causes of the development of CPP is PeVD which accounts for 16% to 31% of all cases—it is second only to endometriosis in prevalence [5]. Pelvic venous disorder (PeVD) is a term that encompasses all the interrelated causes of chronic pelvic pain (CPP) and perineal/lower-extremity varicose veins of pelvic venous origin historically known as nutcracker syn-

S. Gianesini, Y. W. Chi (eds.), *Sclerotherapy*, https://doi.org/10.1007/978-3-032-32794-9_13

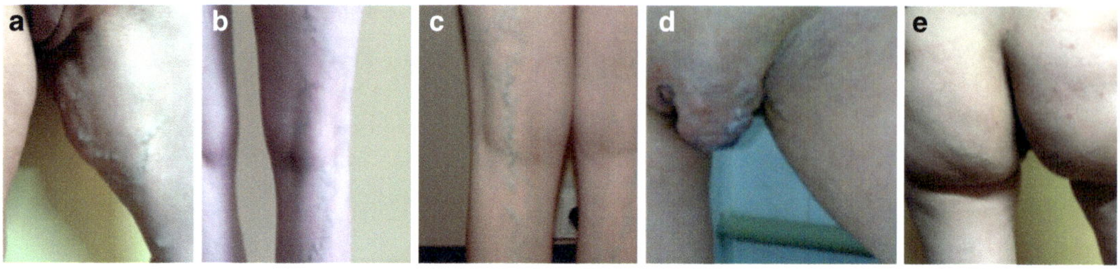

Fig. 13.1 Pelvic varices. (**a**) Perineal veins. (**b, c**) Posterior thigh veins with popliteal fossa communication. (**d**) Vulvar varicose veins with soft tissue enlargement. (**e**) Varicose veins of gluteal area bilaterally

drome, pelvic congestion syndrome, and May-Thurner syndrome, resulting in a more precise diagnosis that accounts for the underlying pathophysiology and anatomy (Fig. 13.1) [6].

PeVD is relatively new term which replaced old term "pelvic congestion syndrome." However, pelvic venous disorders (PeVD) and pelvic congestion syndrome (PCS) are closely related, but they are not synonymous. The difference is important conceptually and clinically. Pelvic venous disorders is the broad, pathophysiologic umbrella term. It refers to any abnormality of the pelvic venous system, including venous reflux, venous obstruction, or venous dilation. PeVD can exist with or without symptoms and may involve ovarian veins, internal iliac veins, renal vein compression, iliac vein compression, or pelvic and vulvar varices. Symptoms, when present, may be pelvic or extra-pelvic, such as vulvar varicosities or lower-extremity venous disease of pelvic origin. Pelvic congestion syndrome is a specific clinical syndrome within PeVD. PCS is diagnosed when pelvic venous abnormalities produce a characteristic symptom pattern, most notably chronic non-cyclical pelvic pain lasting more than 6 months, often accompanied by pelvic heaviness, dyspareunia, post-coital pain, or pain that worsens with standing or at the end of the day. In PCS, symptoms are central to the diagnosis.

3 Pathophysiology

The main mechanism in pathophysiology of PeVD is the development of venous hypertension in pelvic veins which is the result of retrograde flow and varicosities due to pelvic venous insufficiency from one side and flow obstruction in case of compression syndromes from another side. The ovarian plexus drains into the ovarian veins on both sides, whereas the hemorrhoidal, utero-ovarian, sacral, and vesicular venous plexuses drain into the internal iliac veins. The broad ligament has the internal iliac and ovarian veins running through it. In the majority of pelvic congestion syndrome cases, incompetency of the internal pudendal and broad ligament parametrial branches are involved. The pelvic venous reflux into the lower limb or vulvar varicosities is often associated with the incompetency of the branches of the circumflex femoral and obturator veins [7]. The primary vein insufficiency is due to either the absence of the venous valves or the incompetency of the valves. There are incompetent valves in 35% to 46% of women on the right and 41% to 43% on the left. The inclination of multiparous women to develop pelvic congestion syndrome can be due to the 50% increased pelvic vein capacity due to physiological changes during pregnancy. These changes can lead to retrograde blood flow and incompetency of the valves. Even 6 months after pregnancy, these vascular changes can persist [8]. Secondary pelvic vein incompetence is often due to external compression of the vein, leading to venous outflow obstruction. Different causes of external compression include the nutcracker phenomenon, also known as left renal vein entrapment syndrome. This phenomenon is due to the compression of the left renal vein between the superior mesenteric artery and the abdominal aorta. Similarly, the compression of the left common iliac vein by the right internal iliac artery in iliac vein entrapment syndrome can also lead to such results [9, 10]. Additionally, hormones play a role in the development of PeVD and improvement of symptoms after menopause indicates on it. Estrogen is a venous dilator and can thus produce the venous dilation implicated in the pathophysiology of pelvic congestion syndrome [11]. The exact etiology of pelvic congestion syndrome is unclear and is most likely dependent on multiple factors. The congestion of the pelvic veins can be due to hormones, venous insufficiency of the valves, venous obstruction, and secondary to concurrent medical conditions, such as peripheral artery disease. The release of pain-inducing substances due to increased dilatation of the veins along with stasis is a likely cause of the pain in pelvic congestion syndrome [12].

4 Clinical Work-Up

A detailed history, severity, and nature of symptoms, and a thorough physical examination are crucial for the management of any form of PeVD. The main patient population is women aged 20–45 (reproductive age), most of whom have had 2 or more pregnancies (multiparous). However, presence of PeVD in nulliparous women also well-recognized, which could be causing by congenital absence or incompetence of valves in ovarian veins and also due to presence of compression syndromes. In addition to the number of pregnancies and deliveries, the age at first pregnancy and the presence of spontaneous abortions in the anamnesis are of great importance. It is important to assess the patient's anthropological data—in patients of asthenic type with a low BMI, the likelihood of developing compression syndromes is much higher than in patients with a normal BMI. Nanavati et al., after investigated the data 100 patients with symptomatic forms of PeVD, concluded that "women with PCS are more likely to have a normal BMI with ovarian vein dilation compared with obese women, who are more frequently affected by leg varicosities." [13] The authors suggest that "dilated ovarian veins were more common in leaner patients. The abdominal compartment offers a greater volume than the compartments of the legs. This flexibility in space may allow intra-abdominal and pelvic fat to function as a cushion around veins, preventing their anatomic compression by surrounding structures. By occupying space, abdominal and pelvic fat may also prevent excessive dilation of pelvic veins and the subsequent pooling of blood." Except this, during physical examination it is important to pay attention to uterine tenderness, ovarian tenderness, and cervical motion tenderness on direct palpation during bimanual examination, which in a patient presenting with a complaint of chronic pelvic pain supports the diagnosis of pelvic congestion syndrome. In a study involving 57 females with pelvic pain, the combination of a history of post-coital pain with tenderness over the adnexa during physical examination demonstrated 77% specificity and nearly 94% sensitivity in differentiating pelvic congestion syndrome from other pathologies of pelvic origin [14]. Pelvic pain as a main symptom of PeVD is non-cyclical, chronic (more than 6 month) pain with gradual onset. By the quality of pain patients mostly described dull pain, heaviness in pelvic, dragging, or pressure-like feelings. Pain typically localized in lower abdomen or suprapubic area and can be irradiate to lower back, sacrum, groin, or thighs. However, not so rarely, it is poorly localized. The pain is worsening after standing, prolonged sitting and at the end of the day, which is resolving after lying down. Pain also could be worsening premenstrual period or during menstruation. Dyspareunia or post-coital pain is typical for patients with PeVD. The nature of dyspareunia in pelvic congestion syndrome (PCS) is quite specific and reflects the underlying venous congestion and reflux rather than inflammatory or structural gynecologic disease: Pain is felt deep in the pelvis (not at the vaginal introit), occurs with deep penetration. Pain builds gradually with continued or deep penetration, often worse in positions that increase pelvic venous pressure and could be lasting hours to days. Five or more points of pain intensity according to visual analogue scale (VAS) is significant for CPP of venous origin [15]. Except the pain, pelvic venous disorders could be manifesting by various symptoms which classically belong to other pathologies of pelvis: dysmenorrhea, dysfunction vaginal bleeding (gynecological), urinary urgency/frequency, bladder pressure, sensation of incomplete emptying (urological), nausea, bloating, rectal pressure or fullness, pain with defecation, IBS-like symptoms (gastrointestinal), fatigue, anxiety, sleep disturbance, reduced work productivity (psycho-emotional). An important step in physical examination is to evaluate varicose vein network, which may be present on perineal, vulvar, gluteal, or posterior thigh areas. Vulvar varicosities developed because of reflux in left and right ovarian and pudendal-obturator veins in case of pelvic floor insufficiency, whereas perineal, gluteal, and posterior thigh varicosities mostly generated by the reflux from internal iliac vein [16]. The pelvic escape points are peripheral tributaries of the IIVs and include the internal pudendal veins, obturator veins, round ligament (inguinal) veins, and inferior gluteal veins. These routes can lead to transmission of increased venous pressure in the pelvis to the superficial veins of the vulva and lower extremities, which may cause lower extremity symptoms with or without pelvic pain [17]. Vulvar varices occur in about 10% of pregnant women. They are rare during a first pregnancy and generally develop during fifth month of a second pregnancy. The risk is increases with the number of pregnancies. Vulvar varicosities tend to disappear spontaneously after delivery and rarely persists 1-month later [18]. Also, there is a strong association between hemorrhoids and internal iliac vein reflux. Untreated reflux may be a cause of subsequent symptomatic hemorrhoids [19].

5 Instrumental Examination

Standard instrumental work-up is starting with ultrasound examination. It is worth noting that the type of initial ultrasound examination (transabdominal or transvaginal) depends on which specialist the patient is being treated by: if the patient first consults a general practitioner or a vascular specialist, a transabdominal examination is performed first, whereas in gynecological institutions, a transvaginal ultrasound is predominantly performed as a screening examination. These types of examination have their advantages and limitations, and in high-level expert centers, both are usually performed to obtain maximum information. In addition, duplex sonographic examination of the veins of the lower extremities is necessary to create for a complete picture and make the right decision. As N. Labropoulos described, [20] the examination is performed after the patient has been fasting overnight. This decreases the likelihood of bowel gas obstructing the vascular structures and therefore increase the sensitivity of the examination. Additionally, partially filled bladder preferred for avoiding the compression of veins. The vessels examined are the inferior vena cava (IVC), left renal vein (LRV), iliac veins, ovarian veins, trans- and peri-uterine veins, and the tributaries of the internal iliac veins. The greatest benefit of this modality is the dynamic feature where patients are able to change positions from supine to standing as well as perform the Valsalva maneuver. The utilization of the standing position increases the hydrostatic pressure in the pelvic venous system, leading to the dilation of veins and revealing potential reflux. This enables real-time visualization of blood flow and possible reflux during these diagnostic maneuvers and may increase the diagnostic confidence. Criteria for sonographic diagnosis of PCS in the appropriate patients has been suggested by various authors. These included various ovarian vein diameter cut-offs starting above 4 mm, positive reflux, presence of pelvic varicosities, and reflux during Valsalva maneuver [21]. Till today is controversial the topic about correlation between vein diameter and venous reflux. During the transabdominal ultrasound examination necessary to check structural changes in uterus and ovaries: About half of patients with pelvic congestion syndrome had cystic changes in their ovaries, ranging from classic polycystic ovary syndrome to clusters of cysts in bilaterally enlarged ovaries [22]. Freitas et al. [23] presented newest version of protocol for transvaginal ultrasound (TVUS) for evaluation of PeVD, described that this "examination has undergone significant advances in accuracy and diagnostic precision. These advances have not only allowed a thorough examination of gynecologic pathologies, but have also facilitated the analysis of additional structures, including the pelvic veins." The patient should be placed supine, with the headboard elevated at 45°, knees flexed, and feet apart. This semi-upright posture is specifically recommended for the evaluation of PeVDs, because it increases venous distension and enhances the detection of reflux. The authors presented target parameters that should be assessed during the study: (1) *Venous Diameter*: Parauterine veins with a diameter of up to 5 mm are considered normal. However, diameter alone should not be the only factor used to assess these veins, because smaller veins may indicate reflux and larger veins may not indicate any signs of reflux; (2) *Definition of Reflux:* Reflux in pelvic varicose veins is defined differently than in peripheral veins. It can be characterized by the inversion of flow or increased flow during the Valsalva maneuver, considering that it is already reversed; (3) *Reflux Time*: There are few studies on reflux time in pelvic varicose veins…For both the internal and external iliac veins, we consider a reflux time of greater than 1 s, because these veins are part of the deep venous system; (4) *Leak Points*: Leak points are assessed when there is an insufficiency caused by the pelvic reflux connection that breaks the pelvic floor and drains into the perineal region or lower limbs. This assessment is not performed routinely, but rather when we detect this connection through venous mapping of the lower limbs. Authors described high diagnostic value of TVUS but also they draw attention that this method presents some limitations. It is an operator-dependent technique and does not provide an adequate assessment of more cranial venous structures, such as the gonadal veins in their abdominal course, iliac vein compressions, or in patients with anatomical variations. The examination is significantly more sensitive when appropriate provocative maneuvers are applied; their absence may lead to false-negative results, particularly in cases of intermittent reflux. Moreover, TVUS examination cannot be performed in patients for whom transvaginal access is contraindicated. Intensity of using of cross-sectional methods (CTV, MRV) is still controversial—they are generally used when there is suspicion of an obstructive type of PeVD, although in some centers these methods are used routinely. According to last protocol of contrast-enhanced CT, the scan is covered the area from the renal upper pole to the pelvic floor. Both plain CT scans and enhanced CT scans (including arterial, venous, and secretory phases) must be performed for all patients, because images during arterial phase are using to rule out possible reflux into ovarian veins, and images from venous phase is using for the assessment of pelvic and ovarian veins as well as identifying drainage locations of ovarian veins to renal vein or IVC. Also, the venous phase is using for assessment of abdominal and pelvic organs. The plain and secretory CT phases are using for assessment of the urinary system to exclude urological causes of the pain. The diagnosis of pelvic congestion syndrome is basing on presence of dilated ovarian veins (more than 5.5 mm) and para uterine venous plexus congestion (dilated veins more than 0.5 cm, tortuous, and difficult to see separately). Also, CT venography is useful in the assessment of outflow for the pelvic venous drainage through left renal and iliac veins [24]. MRI allows complete examination of the pelvic anatomy because of its multi-planar imaging capability. Dynamic subtraction MR angiograms can provide an overview of the vessels and demonstrate abdominal vascular anatomy and vessel occlusions. MRV allows assessment of the venous system in the pelvis and lower extremity with image quality comparable to that of conventional venography. However, due to its low specificity, MRV may underestimate venous pathology. This is because conventional cross-sectioned imaging studies are generally performed in the supine position and ovarian and pelvic varices may not be as prominent on such examinations. During MRV performed with the patient lying supine, gravity could not be used as an adjuvant to encourage reflux. Kim et al. described that TR-MRA is almost equal to conventional venography for detecting ovarian venous reflux, and TR-MRA is well suited as a screening method for the initial evaluation of patients with suspected pelvic venous congestion. In addition, TR-MRA may be more specific than conventional venography by virtue of its lack of disturbance of the normal physiological hemodynamics in the left renal vein and ovarian veins. They asserted that TR-MRA is a useful imaging technique for the detection of ovarian vein reflux, and it could become the gold standard for the evaluation of pelvic venous congestion and chronic pelvic pain [25]. Pelvic varicosities are identified as enlarged tortuous tubular structures in the trajectory of the ovarian veins, around the adnexa, and in the pelvic floor. Furthermore, the renal veins can be assessed for signs of compression (Nutcracker syndrome), as well as the common and/or external iliac vein [26]. The direct signs for renal vein compression on cross-sectional imaging are following: a) abrupt narrowing of the LRV between the aorta and SMA; b) Beak sign: sharp, triangular narrowing of the LRV at the compression point; c) Reduced aorto-mesenteric angle (typically <35°, often <25°), while in case of iliac vein compression following signs are noted: (a) Focal compression of the iliac vein (usually LCIV compressed between RCIA and spine); (b) Luminal narrowing ≥50%; (c) Flattened or slit-like vein appearance d) Intraluminal spurs (chronic MTS). Catheter-directed retrograde selective venography of ovarian and internal iliac veins is method of choice for the diagnosis of pelvic venous pathology. Confirmation of pelvic congestion syndrome via catheter-directed venography before embolization is essential. Access to pelvic veins could be done via cubital, jugular or femoral sites by using classic Seldinger method. Catheterization of bladder also recommend to avoid failure of visualization. For the catheterization of left renal vein various authors recommend different types of 4–6 F catheters (Simmons I, Simmons II, Cobra II, Multipurpose, etc.) over a hydrophilic guidewire. Manual ejection of iodinate contrast material must be done in semi-erect position of patient and/or during Valsalva maneuver. The right ovarian vein is catheterized directly via inferior vena cava and similarly assessed. Both internal iliac veins also must be evaluated very carefully [27]. Monedero et al. [11, 15] consider very important to measure reno-caval and ilio-caval pressure gradient to detecting left renal vein (Nutcracker) and left iliac vein (May-Thurner) compressive syndromes [28]. Diagnostic criteria for pelvic congestion syndrome are following: (1) an ovarian vein diameter more than 6 mm; (2) contrast retention more than 20 s; (3) congestion of the pelvic venous plexus and/or opacification of the ipsilateral (or contralateral) internal iliac vein, or (4) filling of vulvovaginal and thigh varicosities. Additionally, some invasive methods (intravascular ultrasound (IVUS), laparoscopy) could be using for confirmation of diagnosis.

6 Classification

Correct diagnosis is important step to make right decision. A revolutionary event on this path was the creation of a new classification. SVP classification is discriminative instrument which includes three domains: symptoms (S), varices (V), the primary sign of PeVD, and a composite anatomic-pathophysiologic domain (P) [29]. The composite P domain is composed of three subdomains, including the anatomy of the involved abdominal and pelvic veins (A), the associated hemodynamic abnormalities (H), and the underlying etiology (E), which are listed as subscripts after the P domain ($P_{A,H,E}$). An individual patient's pelvic classification is thus designated as $SVP_{A,H,E}$. Symptoms (S) and varices (V) associated with PeVD are considered to occur in 4 anatomic zones extending in a descending fashion from the renal veins to the lower extremities.

Three of these zones—(1) the left renal vein, (2) the gonadal and internal iliac veins and associated pelvic venous plexuses, and (3) the pelvic origin extra-pelvic transitional veins arising from reflux exiting the pelvis through recognized escape points—are included in the SVP classification. Although often communicating with zone 3, the fourth zone, the superficial and deep veins of the lower extremity and their tributaries, is optimally classified with CEAP and is not included in the SVP instrument. First domain "S" (symptoms) is divided by using subscripts: S_0—no symptoms of a PeVD (no renal, pelvic, or extra-pelvic symptoms); S_1—renal symptoms of venous origin; S_2—chronic pelvic pain of venous origin; S_3—extrapelvic symptoms of venous origin. The latter in turn includes three subgroups: a)—Localized symptoms (pain, discomfort, tenderness, itching, bleeding and superficial venous thrombosis) associated with veins of the external genitalia (vulva and scrotum); b)—Localized symptoms associated with pelvic origin non-saphenous veins of the leg. These include those related to pelvic origin varices of the posteromedial thigh (pain, discomfort, tenderness, itching, superficial venous thrombosis) as well as those related to sciatic/tibial nerve varices (pain, paresthesias). More generalized lower-extremity symptoms and signs, such as heaviness and swelling, are classified with CEAP not SVP. C)—Venous claudication. The venous system of the pelvis can be considered to consist of 3 reservoirs where varices may develop—(1) the renal hilum, (2) the venous plexuses of the pelvis, and (3) the pelvic origin extra-pelvic veins. The variceal reservoirs of the pelvis are designated V and are again denoted in a descending fashion: V_0—no abdominal, pelvic, or pelvic origin extra-pelvic varices on clinical or imaging examination; V_1—renal hilar varices; V_2—pelvic varices; V_3—pelvic origin extra-pelvic varices, which divided on 2 subgroups: (a) Genital varices (vulvar varices and varicocele) and (b) pelvic origin lower-extremity varicose veins arising from the pelvic escape points and extending into the thigh. Includes visible varicosities, typically over the posteromedial thigh, as well as sciatic varices and other refluxing veins transitioning the pelvic floor which are visualized only with ultrasound. The pathophysiology domain (P) is a composite of the anatomic (A), hemodynamic (H), and etiologic (E) subdomains. For the purposes of documenting reproducibility of the instrument and for recording data in clinical studies, all five domains and subdomains of S V P S, V, A, H, and E should be documented independently according to symptoms varices pathophysiology (SVP) classification scoring sheet.

7 Treatment

Treatment methods for PeVD include conservative (medical), surgical and endovascular options. Medical therapy of PeVD primarily involves pain management, with the strength of the medication used depending on the severity of the pain, but efforts should be made to avoid the use of opioids—usually, NSAID gives immediate good clinical effect. Faquhar and colleagues discovered that 30 mg of medroxyprogesterone acetate taken for 6 months effectively relieved pelvic symptoms, with 73% of women experiencing at least a 50% improvement, compared to 33% of women who received a placebo [30]. In another study, goserelin acetate (3.6 mg per month for 6 months) produced significantly better results than medroxyprogesterone [12]. Simsek et al. conducted a randomized controlled crossover trial of 20 patients, where randomization was performed in 2 groups of 10 patients. They either received MPFF 500 mg twice a day (treatment group) for 6 months or vitamin pills as placebo (control group) twice a day over the same period. Treatments were then crossed over for an additional 6 months. There was an improvement in pelvic pain scores starting at 2 months in the treatment group compared with the control group, which was significant ($P < 0.05$) at the time of the crossover [31]. However, the beneficial effects of all these treatments seemed to disappear once the treatment was discontinued. Various surgical methods have been reported for treatment of PeVD, such as ligation of the ovarian and/or IIVs, ligation of the ovarian and uterine arteries and veins, oophorectomy, and even total hysterectomy with bilateral salpingo-oophorectomy [32]. However, as these procedures are more invasive than endovascular embolization and they require a general anesthetic with a longer recovery period, they are rarely used at present. Furthermore, as surgical ligation can only interrupt the refluxing pathway at a limited number of locations, recurrences may be more common than after endovascular approaches. Hysterectomy with salpingo-oopherectomy has been performed in the past. However, its effect is not been proven convincingly and removal of the reproductive

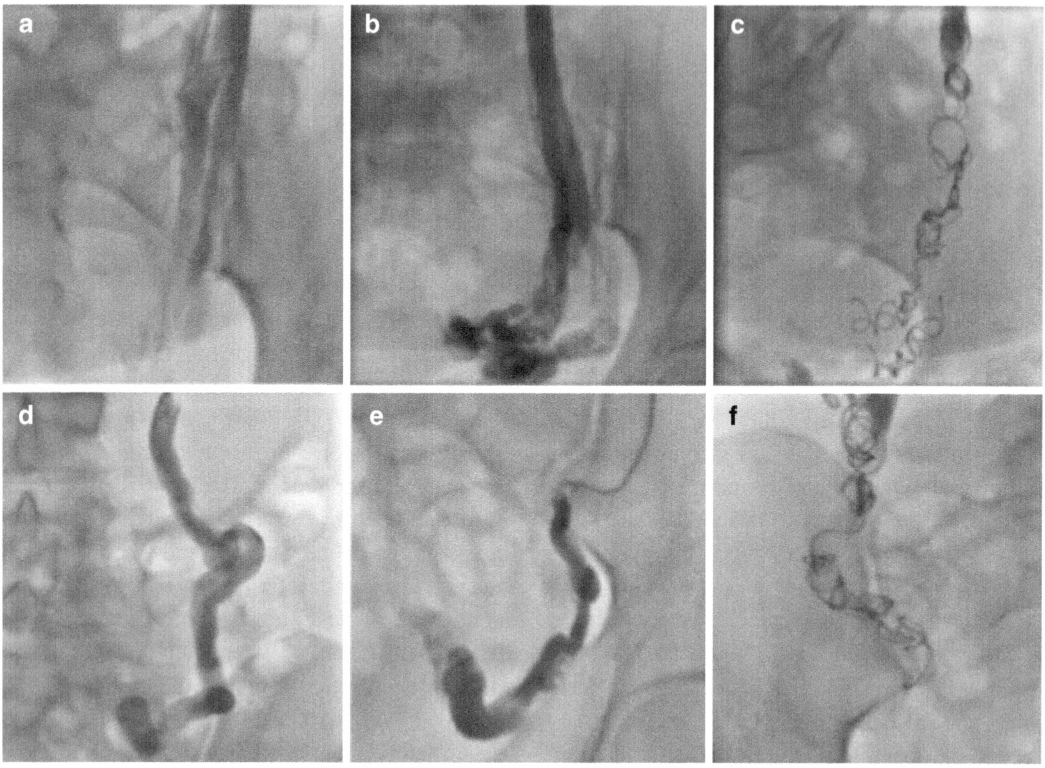

Fig. 13.2 Embolization of different types of pelvic reflux according to distribution of ovarian plexus: in "diffuse-type" dissemination (**a**, **b**, **c**), we prefer to use the "sandwich" technique (coil + sclerofoam) and in "stem-type" dissemination (**d**, **e**, **f**) coils can be used alone

organs is not advised. Ovarian vein embolization has a low rate of morbidity or complications and has largely replaced open surgical intervention for symptomatic ovarian vein incompetence. The first reported case of uterine-ovarian varices embolization was described by Edwards in 1993 [33]. Ovarian vein embolization is generally performed under local anesthesia or moderate sedation using fluoroscopic guidance on a radiological tilt table. A variety of access points have been utilized including the v. basilica, the right internal jugular vein and the femoral veins. As the course to the ovarian veins is shorter and straighter, many prefer the right internal jugular approach. The next step is to selectively cannulate the gonadal and internal iliac veins. The left gonadal vein is a tributary of the left renal vein and catheterization of this vein is usually performed first. The right gonadal vein is a tributary of the IVC just below the right renal vein and is often catheterized next. Contrast medium is injected in the vessel of interest and the patient (instructed before the procedure) is asked to perform a Valsalva maneuver, to evaluate for reflux. Tiling the table into a reverse Trendelenburg position can aid in this evaluation. Retrograde flow toward the pelvis is diagnostic of reflux. The internal iliac veins are subsequently studied using venography. In the internal iliac veins, the Valsalva maneuver will be very helpful to identify insufficiency and to define escape points to the lower limbs. However, even in the presence of internal iliac reflux, antegrade flow may preclude adequate visualization of caudal varices and escape points. A compliant occlusion balloon inflated in the internal iliac vein just proximal to the confluence with the external iliac vein can be very helpful in demonstrating the distal tributaries and pelvic escape points (Figs. 13.2 and 13.3).

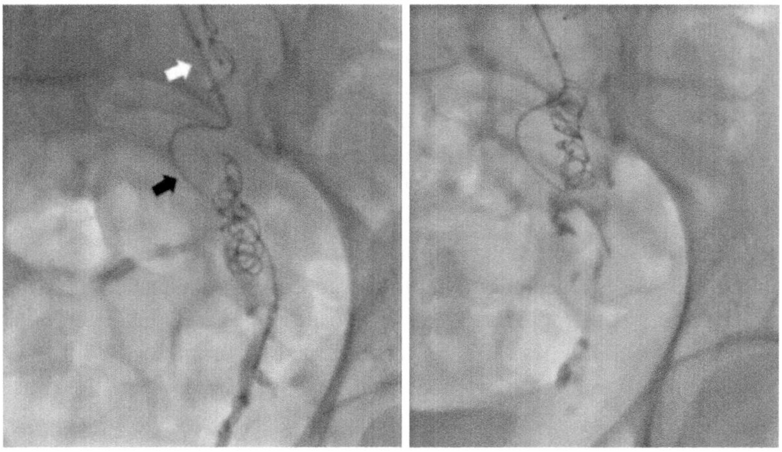

Fig. 13.3 Super-selective obliteration of internal iliac vein branch with sclerofoam using occlusion balloon (white arrow) and microcatheter (black arrow). Previously, left ovarian vein embolization was performed

8 Combined Embolization (Coils+Sclerofoam)

Embolization is typically performed using a "sandwich" mixed technique, which combines metallic devices with 3% aethoxysclerol foam (prepared according to Tessari's method during the procedure): [34] while allowing the sclerosant to dwell within the pelvic venous plexus, a cluster of appropriately sized coils are deployed at the caudal end of the dominant trunk just above the confluence of tributaries. The catheter is then withdrawn several centimeters within the ovarian veins and additional sclerosant instilled followed by a second cluster of coils. The procedure is then repeated at intervals with the last cluster of coils deployed just below the confluence of the ovarian vein with either the left renal vein or IVC. Although lacking robust supporting evidence, this technique offers the potential to treat the multiple small tributaries that are often associated with the ovarian veins and may function as a source of recurrence. *Reiner and colleagues* in 2009 presented the study of using "sandwich technique" for treatment of adolescent symptomatic varicocele: 3% sodium tetradecyl sulfate foam (STS) was placed distally in the ISV during compression so minimal foam entered the pampiniform plexus [35]. A second nest of coils was placed in the ISV at a position over the sacroiliac (SI) joint that occluded most of the parallel collateral vessels. Coils were not placed above the SI joint in most instances. Additional foam was injected in the ISV at the upper level of the SI joint. The upper ISV was left un-occluded. Our standard follow-up consisting of ultrasound and/or physical examination after varicocele occlusion was performed 2–12 months after the procedure. Authors described that all occlusions were technically successful, and 15 of 16 patients (94%) exhibited proven disappearance of the varicocele. All patients were asymptomatic except one who had pain despite disappearance of the varicocele. One patient with a bleeding disorder had 48 h of scrotal discomfort as a result of pampiniform phlebitis caused by the deliberate passage of foam into the pampiniform plexus. Monedero and colleagues presented treatment of pelvic venous reflux by using "sandwich" technique which combines metallic devices with 2% Aethoxisclerol foam (generally sodium tetradecyl sulfate mixed with contrast to result in a 1% to 1.5% concentration) [36]. Before sclerosis, the volume of the varicose pelvic venous plexus can be estimated by injecting contrast with the balloon inflated until normal veins start to be opacified. Generally, sclerosis is performed with a volume of sclerosant that is about 75% of the measured volume. After a few coils are placed in the lower part of the ovarian vein, the balloon is deflated and withdrawn a few centimeters, and the sclerosant injection is repeated utilizing a similar sandwich technique until about 5 cm from the termination of the gonadal vein. Following gonadal-vein closure, internal iliac veins should be investigated and, if necessary, treated. In the presence of leak points to the lower limbs or connections of internal iliac veins with lower periuterine varicose veins, selective cannulation and embolization with coils and/or sclerosants should be performed. The maximum dose of 3% STS recommended per procedure is 10 ml. STS is often injected in foam state mixed with room air, O2 or CO2. The higher concentration of nitrogen in room air poses a potential risk of air embolus and stroke when in Trendelenburg position (Tessari et al. 2001) [37]. Neimark and Shelkovnikova used "sandwich" technique for treatment of persistent dysuria and chronic pelvic pain in 16 women with pelvic varicose veins. They described that sclero-embolization was performed at the level of the lower third of the ovarian veins—this level was sufficient to stop the retrograde blood flow from the plexuses into the ovarian veins and eliminate blood flow in the underlying venous plexuses of the small pelvis, even with unilateral sclero-embolization due to the flow of the drug to the opposite side through the venous collectors. Positive therapeutic effect in the form of eliminating varicose pelvic veins, pain relief, disappearance of persistent dysuria, and the remission of chronic cystitis was achieved in 86% of women. This intervention provided the normal outflow of blood from the pelvic veins, contributed to the normalization of uroflowmetry data and restoration of normal microcirculation in the urinary bladder [38]. Hocquelet et al. presented retrospective study of 33 female patients undergoing pelvic venous embolization by using "sandwich" technique where pelvic veins and leakage points were embolized by lauromacrogol sclerosant in microfoam form (2% Aetoxysclerol) and coils, occasionally combined with the insertion of a plug [39]. They noted that no definitive technical failures occurred and only one patient required repeat treatment because of an inability to catheterize the left ovarian vein during the first embolization attempt. Each incompetent vein was embolized. Authors compared their own embolization technique with those reported in the literature and concluded: No studies have shown the use of coils alone to be superior to coils with a sclerosant or other liquid embolization agent, foam sclerosis has the advantage of spreading more readily into all of the venous collaterals and increasing the treatment surface area on the venous endothelium with a small amount of sclerosant, particularly, if concomitant venous dysplasia is present. Excellent results were presented by Venbrux AC et al. after combining (coils + sclerofoam) embolization in 56 female patient with chronic pelvic pain of venous origin: Percutaneous trans-catheter embolotherapy of ovarian and pelvic varices was technically successful in 56 of 56 patients (100%), the mean decrease in VAS was 5.1 (65% decrease) [40]. The clinical follow-up in this series ranged between 6 and 38 months; the mean was 22.1 months. Regarding the impact of embolization on menstruation, all patients responding to questionnaires indicated no change in menstrual cycle. Kim HC and colleagues also presented combine use of sclerosing foam with Gelfoam [41]. They described that the volume of sclerosant to be injected can be estimated based on a preliminary contrast agent injection into the cross-pelvic varices. To avoid non-target embolization, it may be appropriate to use a volume of embolic agent equal to or less than the volume of the contrast agent test injection. However, despite many authors demonstrated high efficacy and safety of "sandwich" technique, in 2022 Hongyu C and colleagues presented study of using proximal coil occlusion preceding distal sclerotherapy (PCODS) technique in comparison with "sandwich" technique [42]. Ninetyfour patients had undergone PCODS (study group), and 53 patients had been treated with the sandwich endovascular embolization technique (control group). During the procedure in patients from study group, proximal coil occlusion was applied at the ostium of the dilated and refluxing vein trunks. To prevent coil migration, coils with the diameter oversized by 30% were selected and deployed as a contained coil pack in a section shorter than the diameter of coils (i.e., dense coil packing) to allow the deployed coils to achieve stable anchoring. The pivotal step was cannulation through the coil packing with the catheter. A 0.035-in. hydrophilic-coated guidewire was introduced through the coils, followed by a catheter gently and angiography was done to identify the total area of venous varicosities and escape points. Finally, distal sclerotherapy with sclerosing foam was performed according to findings. With this technique, a compliant balloon was unnecessary to occlude the outflow of the diseased veins. Embolization was 100% successful in both groups. The clinical remission rates were stable without relapse evident within 12 months for both groups. The operative time and total fluoroscopy time were shorter for the PCODS group than for the control group (48.3 ± 5.2 min. and 37.7 ± 4.4 min. vs 53.9 ± 4.8 min. and 42.6 ± 4.1 min., respectively). The overall length of coils used per case was 19.8 ± 6.0 cm for the PCODS group and 31.7 ± 8.5 cm in the control group. Several reasons lie behind this effect, including sufficient venous mapping to ensure treatment effectiveness and stable anchoring, which was achieved by dense coil packing. Moreover, authors believed that the pressure cooker effect promoted diffusion of the foam to the distal tributaries, thoroughly embolizing the venous endothelium.

9 Sclerofoam Alone

Although the "sandwich" technique is considered superior for treatment of pelvic vein reflux, using of sclerosing agent alone (mainly in foam condition) also recommended as effective and safe method. In 2003, Pieri with authors reported successful treatment of pelvic congestion syndrome in 33 female patients using of percutaneous transcatheter embolization with 3% sodium tetradecyl sulfate [43]. According to the ultrasound examination, mean pre-procedural diameter of 4.5 mm for the right ovarian vein and of 6.3 mm for the left was reduced on 3.19 mm and 4.5 mm, respectively. At the 1-month follow-up, chronic pelvic pain was present in 13 patients (39%); the pain was continuous in three and intermittent in ten. At the follow-up after 6/12 months the symptoms were unchanged. It is important that symptoms persisted in women with pelvic varicosities measuring over 5 mm at ultrasound. Gandini et al. provided 2 series (total 64 patient) of sclero-embolization due to pelvic vein reflux. In first study, [44] they presented results 38 patients with left, right, or bilateral ovarian vein treated by trans-catheter foam sclerotherapy with 3% sodium tetradecyl sulfate foam (STSF). In the case of cross-pelvic varices, TCFS was only performed from the left ovarian vein using approximately 30 ml of STS foam. In the case of non-cross-pelvic varices, 30 ml of STS foam was selectively injected distally through the left ovarian vein into the varices. When ovarian varices were found also on this side, approximately 20 ml of STS foam was selectively injected distally through the right ovarian vein. Foam injection was continued until no refluxing into the varices was observed after manual injection of contrast agent through the catheter. STS foam was always injected while asking the patient to perform Valsalva's maneuver in order to avoid accidental dislocation of the sclerosing agent and to maximize its effects on the endothelial surface. After the procedure, the patient was invited to maintain a moderate Valsalva's maneuver for an additional 10 min. Two factors are noteworthy when considering this technique: (1) the volume of foam used in each case, especially for the treatment of bilateral ovarian vein lesions, significantly exceeded that reported in the literature; (2) the authors did not use a device to prevent retrograde foam spread (occlusion balloon) and this safety component of procedure is entirely entrusted to the patient (Valsalva maneuver). The authors suggested that compared to other endovascular procedures using sclerosing agents, the increased viscosity of STS foam allowed the use of smaller amounts of sclerosing agent and was associated with a lower risk of extravasation, systemic dispersion, and adverse reactions. They also noted that the use of STS in the form of foam is associated with several advantages. The foam spread on the endothelium with a larger surface contact, thus inducing more effective sclerosis. The foam's malleability allowed complete filling of the varices through the ovarian veins, without the need for selective catheterization and embolization of eventual collaterals draining into the internal iliac veins. In a second publication in 2014, [45] Gandini and colleagues presented a retrospective study of 26 patients with pelvic congestion syndrome (PCS) who had high-outflow venous collaterals treated by stop-flow foam sclerotherapy (SFFS). They presented following categories of high-flow pelvic varicocele: (a). Non-cross-pelvic (high-outflow through the ipsilateral hypogastric vein); (b). Cross-pelvic varicocele ((1). High-outflow through the contralateral hypogastric vein. (2). High-outflow through both hypogastric veins. (3). High-outflow through the contralateral ovarian vein. (4). High-outflow through all of the above veins). Presented technique had some changes compared to sclerotherapy of low-flow pelvic varicocele: After the retrograde venography, under the road mapping, the major venous vessels (hypogastric or ovarian veins) to which the high-outflow collaterals were tributary were selectively catheterized. A venographic control was then performed through the balloon catheter to confirm the retrograde opacification of the pelvic varices and to exclude the presence of other high-outflow venous collaterals requiring further balloon occlusion. After balloon occlusion and the complete filling of the pelvic varices with contrast medium, the patient was asked to perform the Valsalva maneuver while 20–40 ml of 3% STS foam were injected until the contrast medium present in the pelvic varices was completely washed out. The absence of contrast medium in the pelvic varices indicated their complete filling with 3% STS foam. In case of complete stagnation of contrast medium after multiple balloon occlusions, during injection of the foam one of the balloon catheters was deflated creating an obliged outflow route for the contrast medium. When the contrast medium was completely washed out, the balloon catheter was re-inflated. The balloon occlusion of the major veins to which the high-outflow collaterals were tributary was maintained for 30 min. After the follow-up period (12 month) authors described significant reduction of all important symptoms (pelvic pain, dyspareunia, menstrual pain, urinary urgency) without any severe complications. The main sclerosing agents, used for foam sclerotherapy of pelvic veins, are sodium tetradecyl sulfate (STS) and polidocanol (Aethoxysklerol) with various concentrations. In same time, last decade studies presented using of ethanolamine foam for occlusion of pelvic veins. Shahat et al. presented study with successful treatment of pelvic veins in 40 female patients by using ethanolamine foam for sclerotherapy of left ovarian vein [46]. The sclerotherapy procedure had a 100% technical success rate and a 97.5% primary clinical success rate as there was one case with recurrence during the 12 months follow up duration. Twenty-four of women (60%) had clinical improvement in the atypical lower limb varicosities (the veins became less apparent and disappeared in some cases). On the contrary, 16 (40%) women showed no improvement in the atypical lower limb varicosities. It is worth noting that one woman experienced post-procedural chest tightness and mild dyspnea that diagnosed as segmental and subsegmental pulmonary embolism and improved completely on anticoagulation. One of the most recent works, presented by Brazilian authors, was important in that two sclerosant foams were used for embolization purposes in 20 patients: monoethanolamine oleate 5% and/or polidocanol 3% (however, their use was not parity and, therefore, it was impossible to determine the superiority of any of them) [47]. The authors note a significant clinical effect and also a significant reduction in the diameter of the ovarian veins and reflux. Before the procedure, 80% ($n = 16$) of the patients had bilateral gonadal-vein reflux and 20% ($n = 4$) had reflux on the left only. After the procedure, bilateral reflux was found in 20% ($n = 4$) of cases, reflux on the left only was observed in 30% ($n = 6$) and reflux on the right only was observed in 15% ($n = 3$), while no reflux was observed in the Doppler study in the remaining 35% ($n = 7$) of patients. It is noteworthy that 95% of the patients ($n = 19$) reported pain before the procedure, whereas only 30% ($n = 6$) still complained of pain after the intervention.

10 Sclerofoam for Extra-Pelvic Veins

Foam sclerotherapy with or without miniphlebectomy is the method of choice for treatment of extra-pelvic varicose veins of pelvic origin. As we described above, pelvic veins are often interconnected with the superficial veins of the genitalia and the lower extremities, which can result in extra-pelvic symptoms. More than 90% of patients with VVs of pelvic origin do not have pelvic symptoms (such as chronic pelvic pain, dyspareunia, premenstrual pelvic pain) because the pelvic venous hypertension is transmitted through pelvic escape points directly to the veins of the vulva and/or lower extremity [48]. The most important factor in the management of extra-pelvic varicose veins is the correct decision making: when and how to do. Over the years, the question about necessity of pelvic vein embolization prior to treatment of extra-pelvic or recurrent varicose veins was disputable: Hartung et al. in 2015 presented the study with data of 119 female patient [49]. They described that Embolization led to improvement of PCS in 91% (60% without any pain) and of lower limb varicose veins in 51% by itself. If 82% need an additional treatment of lower limb varicose veins, embolization allowed a switch of strategy from surgery to sclerosis. In same time, Rabe and Pannier [50] presented review of literature and concluded that embolization is not essential in the treatment of leg varices of pelvic origin without pelvic congestive syndrome. Foam sclerotherapy or phlebectomy shows good results in patients with vulvar or pudendal varicose veins. For today, there are two approaches to how to treat these VVs. The first one, often referred to as the "top-down" strategy, involves addressing first the pathology of the pelvic veins. This can include pelvic vein embolization or treating the iliac or renal vein compression or post-thrombotic obstruction, particularly if they are identified as the underlying cause of PeVD. This method aims at correcting the hemodynamic abnormalities that contribute to the development of pelvic symptoms and extra-pelvic VVs of pelvic origin. The second approach, known as the "bottom-up" treatment, focuses on managing the peripheral, extra-pelvic manifestations of PeVD. The goal of this strategy is to alleviate extra-pelvic VVs through closing the incompetent pelvic escape points, and vulvar varicosities and also other lower limb VVs of pelvic origin, without direct management of the pathological pelvic veins [51]. This approach also recommended by the guidelines of the ESVS on managing chronic venous disease: "For patients with varicose veins of pelvic origin without pelvic symptoms requiring treatment, local procedures for varicose veins and related pelvic escape points should be considered, as initial therapeutic approach." [52] Authors noticed that as pelvic escape points played the same role as perforating veins, ultrasound guided foam sclerotherapy (UGFS) was an adequate method for treating upper thigh and vulvar VVs of pelvic origin, in patients without pelvic symptoms. Moreover, by accessing pelvic escape points, sclerosant foam may also reach the peri-uterine venous plexus. Brill and colleagues presented technical aspects UGFS for treatment of congenital (venous malformations) and acquired (extra-pelvic veins due to PeVD) varicose veins [53]. First of all, they pay attention that although most sclerotherapy procedures were performed under local anesthesia, sclerotherapy in the labial region was performed with sedation (analgosedation or general anesthesia) to avoid patient reaction and fear. The dysplastic vasculature was punctured (if not visible on the skin surface with the assistance of real-time ultrasound-guidance, linear probe, 20 MHz) using a 23G needle. Afterwards, blood aspiration and a venogram under fluoroscopy with iodinated contrast medium was performed to verify the correct intravascular position and dimension of the varicose veins, as well as to determine the volume of the sclerosant to be injected and to exclude a connection to the deep venous system. The sclerosing agent polidocanol was combined with a standardized microfoam using a 1:4 ratio (sclerosant to sterile air mixture) for treatment. Polidocanol 3% was chosen owing to its availability, low cost, low recurrence, and, most important, owing to its effectiveness (3% is more effective than 1% owing to less dilution) as a common sclerosant. The distribution of the sclerosant was controlled by fluoroscopy. Because the foam solution was not visible fluoroscopically, the lesion was filled with contrast agent first. Then, the foam was injected and replaced the contrast medium, providing visual control of the sclerosant's distribution. The volume of polidocanol used ranged from 1 to 15 mL (foam volume, mean 4.7 ± 14.1 mL) per patient. Jaworucka-Kaczorowska also noted that the use of the UGFS for PELVs also allowed foam to close incompetent peri-vaginal venous plexuses [51]. Marcellin and authors described that perineal varices of pelvic origin were often sclerotized after embolization if they persist [54]. Persistence was linked to superficial and deep anastomoses, which were identified by perineal varicography and treated by puncture of one or more varicose veins under ultrasound guidance. Sclerosis was performed with injection of 0.5% or 2% sclerosant foam. Kwon et al., after review the literature, concluded that there was currently no consensus regarding the optimal type, formulation, or concentration of sclerosant and, therefore, given the anatomical sensitivity of the vulvar region and the potential for cutaneous complications with high-concentration agents, foam or liquid formulations of sodium tetradecyl sulfate (STS) or polidocanol at concentrations of 0.5–1% were most commonly used [55]. However, foam sclerotherapy had some limitations for using due to sizes of targeting veins and surgical interventions like vein ligation and miniphlebectomy were recommended. This was particularly applicable for wide (>1 cm) and short extra-pelvic varicose veins.

11 Conclusions

Finally, we can conclude that foam sclerotherapy is an important, efficient, and safe tool for the treatment of various presentations and stages of PeVD related to refluxing pelvic veins, extra-pelvic varicose veins with atypical localization or lower extremities primary or recurrent varicose veins of pelvic origin. As reported already 10 years ago by Gianesini et al., in proper hands and with proper patient selection, adequate sclerotherapy can successfully manage a significantly percentage of pelvic venous disorders [56].

References

1. Sharp HT, Johnson JV, Lemieux LA, Currigan SM. Executive summary of the reVITALize initiative: standardizing gynecologic data definitions. Obstet Gynecol. 2017;129(4):603–7.
2. Dydyk AM, Singh C, Gupta N. Chronic pelvic pain. StatPearls Publishing; 2025.
3. Zondervan KT, Yudkin PL, Vessey MP, Jenkinson CP, Dawes MG, Barlow DH, Kennedy SH. The community prevalence of chronic pelvic pain in women and associated illness behaviour. Br J Gen Pract. 2001;51:541–7.
4. Rodrigues Barcelos P, Marques Conde D, de Deus JM, Martinez EZ. Quality of life of women with chronic pelvic pain: a cross-sectional analytical study. Rev Bras Ginecol Obstet. 2010;32(5):247–53.
5. Clark MR, Taylor AC. Pelvic venous disorders: an update in terminology, diagnosis, and treatment. Semin Intervent Radiol. 2023;40(4):362–71.
6. Kim HS, Malhotra AD, Rowe PC, Lee JM, Venbrux AC. Embolotherapy for pelvic congestion syndrome: long-term results. J Vasc Interv Radiol. 2006;17(2 Pt 1):289–97.
7. Lopez AJ. Female pelvic vein embolization: indications, techniques, and outcomes. Cardiovasc Intervent Radiol. 2015;38(4):806–20.
8. Ahlberg NE, Bartley O, Chidekel N. Right and left gonadal veins. An anatomical and statistical study. Acta Radiol Diagn (Stockh). 1966;4(6):593–601.
9. Birn J, Vedantham S. May-Thurner syndrome and other obstructive iliac vein lesions: meaning, myth, and mystery. Vasc Med. 2015;20(1):74–83.
10. Winer AG, Chakiryan NH, Mooney RP, Verges D, Ghanaat M, Allaei A, Robinson L, Zinn H, Lang EK. Secondary pelvic congestion syndrome: description and radiographic diagnosis. Can J Urol. 2014;21(4):7365–8.
11. Raffetto JD, Qiao X, Beauregard KG, Khalil RA. Estrogen receptor-mediated enhancement of venous relaxation in female rat: implications in sex-related differences in varicose veins. J Vasc Surg. 2010;51(4):972–81.
12. Soysal ME, Soysal S, Vicdan K, Ozer S. A randomized controlled trial of goserelin and medroxyprogesterone acetate in the treatment of pelvic congestion. Hum Reprod. 2001;16(5):931–9.
13. Nanavati R, Jasinski P, Adrahtas D, Gasparis A, Labropoulos N. Correlation between pelvic congestion syndrome and body mass index. J Vasc Surg. 2018;67(2):536–41.
14. O'Brien MT, Gillespie DL. Diagnosis and treatment of the pelvic congestion syndrome. J Vasc Surg Venous Lymphat Disord. 2015;3(1):96–106.
15. Lazarashvili Z, Antignani PL, Monedero JL. Pelvic congestion syndrome: prevalence and quality of life. Phlebolymphology. 2016;23:123–6.

16. Monedero J. Insuficienca venosa cronica dela pelvis y de los miembros inferiors. Madrid: Mosby/Doyma Libros SA; 1997.
17. Lemasle P, Greiner M. Duplex ultrasound investigation in pelvic congestion syndrome: technique and results. Phlebolymphology. 2017;24:79–87.
18. Beard RW, Reginald PW, Wadsworth J. Clinical features of women with chronic lower abdominal pain and pelvic congestion. Br J Obstet Gynaecol. 1988;95:153–61.
19. Holdstock JM, Dos Santos SJ, Harrison CC, Price BA, Whiteley MS. Hemorrhoids are associated with internal iliac vein reflux in up to one third of women presenting with varicose veins associated with pelvic vein reflux. Phlebology. 2015;30:133–9.
20. Labropoulos N, Jasinski PT, Adrahtas D, Gasparis AP, Meissner MH. A standardized ultrasound approach to pelvic congestion syndrome. Phlebology. 2017;32(9):608–19.
21. Park SJ, Lim JW, Ko YT, et al. Diagnosis of pelvic congestion syndrome using transabdominal and transvaginal sonography. AJR Am J Roentgenol. 2004;182:683–8.
22. Durham JD, Machan L. Pelvic congestion syndrome. Semin Intervent Radiol. 2013;30:372–80.
23. Freitas Fernandes F, Storino J, Souto Barros F, Barreto Silva M, Cardoso Oliveira N, Tavares IR. Transvaginal ultrasound approach for diagnosing pelvic venous disorders. J Vasc Surg Venous Lymphat Disord. 2025;13(6):102286.
24. Awad A, Taha M, Gad M, Mashhour S. Role of multi-detector CT venography in evaluation of pelvic congestion syndrome. Egypt J Radiol Nucl Med. 2020;51:159.
25. Kim CY, Miller MJ, Merkle EM. Time-resolved MR angiography as a useful sequence for assessment of ovarian vein reflux. AJR Am J Roentgenol. 2009;193:W458–63.
26. Robertson M, McCuaig R. Pelvic congestion syndrome. Australas J Ultrasound Med. 2013;16:26–9.
27. Antignani PL, Lazarashvili Z, Monedero JL et al. Diagnosis and treatment of pelvic congestion syndrome: UIP consensus document. Int Angiol. 2019;38(4):265–83.
28. Monedero JL, Ezpeleta SZ, Perrin M. Pelvic congestion syndrome can be treated operatively with good long-term results. Phlebology. 2012;27(Suppl 1):65–73.
29. Meissner MH, Khilnani NM, Labropoulos N, et al. The Symptoms-Varices-Pathophysiology classification of pelvic venous disorders: A report of the American Vein & Lymphatic Society International Working Group on Pelvic Venous Disorders. J Vasc Surg Venous Lymphat Disord. 2021 May;9(3):568–84.
30. Farquhar CM, Rogers V, Franks S, Pearce S, Wadsworth J, Beard RW. A randomized controlled trial of medroxyprogesterone acetate and psychotherapy for the treatment of pelvic congestion. Br J Obstet Gynaecol. 1989;96:1153–62.
31. Simsek M, Burak F, Taskin O. Effects of micronized purified flavonoid fraction (Daflon) on pelvic pain in women with laparoscopically diagnosed pelvic congestion syndrome: a randomized crossover trial. Clin Exp Obstet Gynecol. 2007;34:96–8.
32. Park YJ. Management of pelvic vein disorders. Ann Phlebology. 2024;22(1):1–5.
33. Edwards RD, Robertson IR, MacLean AB, Hemingway AP. Case report: pelvic pain syndrome—successful treatment of a case by ovarian vein embolization. Clin Radiol. 1993;47:429–31.
34. O'Brien MT, Gillespie DL. Diagnosis and treatment of the pelvic congestion syndrome. J Vasc Surg Venous Lymphat Disord. 2015;3:96–106.
35. Reiner E, Pollak J, Henderson K, Weiss R, Witte R. Initial experience with 3% sodium tetradecyl sulfate foam and fibered coils for management of adolescent varicocele. J Vasc Interv Radiol. 2008;19(2):207–10.
36. Monedero J, Ezpeleta S, Khilnani N. Treatment options for pelvic congestion syndrome. Phlebolymphology. 2016;23(3):144–51.
37. Tessari L, Cavezzi A, Frullini A. Preliminary experience with a new sclerosing foam in the treatment of varicose veins. Dermatologic Surg. 2001;27(1):58–60.
38. Nemark AI, Shelkovnikova NV. Endovascular treatment of persistent dysuria and chronic pelvic pain in women with pelvic varicose veins. [in Russian]. Urologiia. 2012;4(04):20–4.
39. Hocquelet A, Le Bras Y, Balian E, et al. Evaluation of the efficacy of endovascular treatment of pelvic congestion syndrome. Diagn Interv Imaging. 2014 Mar;95(3):301–6.
40. Venbrux AC, Chang AH, Kim HS, et al. Pelvic congestion syndrome (pelvic venous incompetence): impact of ovarian and internal iliac vein embolotherapyon menstrual cycle and chronic pelvic pain. J Vasc Interv Radiol. 2002;13:171–8.
41. Kim HS, Malhotra AD, Lee ML, Venbrux AC. Embolotherapy for pelvic congestion syndrome: long-term results. J Vasc Interv Radiol. 2006;17:289–97.
42. Chen H, Wu Z, Wu Z, et al. Proximal coil occlusion preceding distal sclerotherapy in patients with pelvic congestion syndrome: A multicenter, retrospective study. J Vasc Surg Venous Lymphat Disord. 2023 Jan;11(1):149–55.
43. Pieri S, Agresti P, Morucci M, de' Medici L. Percutaneous treatment of pelvic congestion syndrome. Radiol Med (Torino). 2003;105(1–2):76–82.
44. Gandini R, Chiocchi M, Konda D, et al. Transcatheter foam sclerotherapy of symptomatic female varicocele with sodiumtetradecyl-sulfate foam. Cardiovasc Intervent Radiol. 2008;31:778–84.
45. Gandini R, Konda D, Abrignani S, Chiocchi M, Da Ros V, Morosetti D. Treatment of symptomatic high-flow female varicoceles with stop-flow foam sclerotherapy. Cardiovasc Intervent Radiol. 2014;37(5):1259–67.
46. Shahat M, Hussein R, Ahmed A. Foam sclerotherapy in pelvic congestion syndrome. Vasc Endovasc Surg. 2023;57(5):451–7.

47. Gava NM, Silva AS, Maciel GSB, Assis MP, Santos CAD. Analysis of the efficacy of endovascular treatment with foam sclerotherapy for pelvic congestion syndrome with ultrasound assessment. J Vasc Bras. 2024;23:23.
48. Franceschi C, Bahnini A. Points de fuite pelviens viscéraux et varices des membres inférieurs. Phlebologie. 2004;57:37–42.
49. Hartung O. Embolization is essential in the treatment of leg varicosities due to pelvic venous insufficiency. Phlebology. 2015;30:81–5.
50. Rabe E, Pannier F. Embolization is not essential in the treatment of leg varices due to pelvic venous insufficiency. Phlebology. 2015;30(1 Suppl):86–8.
51. Jaworucka-Kaczorowska A. Pelvic escape points: bottom-up is the way to go. Turk J Vasc Surg. 2023;32(Suppl. S1):14–9.
52. De Maeseneer MG, Kakkos SK, Aherne T, Baekgaard N, Black S, Blomgren L, Giannoukas A, Gohel M, de Graaf R, Hamel-Desnos C, et al. Editor's choice—European Society for Vascular Surgery (ESVS) 2022 clinical practice guidelines on the management of chronic venous disease of the lower limbs. Eur J Vasc Endovasc Surg. 2022;63:184–267.
53. Brill R, Deistung A, Gussew A, et al. Safety and effectiveness of percutaneous sclerotherapy for venous disorders of the labia majora in patients with vascular malformations. J Vasc Surg Venous Lymphat Disord. 2020;8(6):1083–9.
54. Marcelin C, Le Bras Y, Molina Andreo I, Jambon E, Grenier N. Diagnosis and management of pelvic venous disorders in females. Diagnostics (Basel). 2022;12(10):2337.
55. Kwon S, Lee S, Kim H. Vulvar varicosities: a comprehensive review of pathogenesis, diagnosis, and treatment. Ann Phlebology. 2025;23(1):12–8.
56. Gianesini S, Antignani PL, Tessari L. Pelvic congestion syndrome: does one name fit all? Phlebolymphology. 2016;23(3):142–6.

Sclerotherapy for Vascular Malformations

14

Byung Boong Lee and Sergio Gianesini

1 Endovascular Therapy in General

Endovascular therapy with various embolization and sclerotherapy modalities is now fully accepted as the 'preferred' therapeutic option for the majority of 'extratruncular' congenital vascular malformation (CVM) lesions [1–4]. Indeed, CVM represents a group of unique vascular disorder of birth defect occurred during various stages of embryogenesis affecting throughout entire vascular systems: artery, vein, lymphatics, and capillary systems and 'extratruncular' lesions are one of them [5–8]. Hence, CVM lesions present an extreme variety with stigma of totally unpredictable behavior due to its unique embryological characteristics by 'extratruncular' lesions. Indeed, 'extratruncular' lesions are the outcome of defective development during the 'early stage' of embryogenesis before the vascular trunk is formed so that they maintain primitive reticular network structures in diffusely infiltrating condition in general, holding unique mesenchymal cell characteristics (cf. truncular lesion) [9–12]. Therefore, when the extratruncular form of CVM lesion is provoked/stimulated by various conditions (e.g., trauma, pregnancy, surgery, or hormone), it would continue to grow to make the condition worse; improper treatment strategy, therefore, only stimulates dormant extratruncular lesion to respond in an erratic way [13–16]. Therefore, through the last century, a cavalier approach based on then limited knowledge and experiences; mostly led by surgeons alone, often resulted in disastrous outcomes with high recurrence and high morbidity/complication. Hence, a contemporary concept was newly established for accurate diagnosis and advanced management based on various new technologies to compensate the earlier mistakes solely based on the open surgical treatment: ISSVA Classification and Hamburg Classification [17–20]. The endovascular approach with embolo-sclerotherapy was introduced as a new strategy for the CVM management through a long, evolving course with trials and errors for the last two decades; the endovascular therapy with various embolo-sclerotherapy now represents contemporary management of the CVMs across the board as the 'preferred' therapeutic option together with the conventional surgical for the majority of 'extratruncular' lesions [21–24]. Indeed, liquid agents with the ability to penetrate into the lesion/nidus are ideally suited for the treatment of amorphous structure of 'extratruncular' lesions as primitive lesions with potential to grow by its embryological characteristic. Such new approach opened the

B. B. Lee
Department of Surgery, George Washington University, Washington, DC, USA

S. Gianesini (✉)
Department of Translational Medicine, University of Ferrara, Ferrara, Italy

Department of Surgery, Uniformed Services University of Health Sciences, Bethesda, MD, USA
e-mail: gnssrg@unife.it

S. Gianesini, Y. W. Chi (eds.), *Sclerotherapy*, https://doi.org/10.1007/978-3-032-32794-9_14

door for 'endovascular therapy' as a new additional armamentarium to the traditional 'open surgical therapy' [25–28]. Endovascular/embolo-sclerotherapy is now fully accepted as the treatment of choice for surgically 'inaccessible' CVM lesions or the lesion with prohibitively high surgical risks such as CVM lesions that extend beyond the deep fascia and involve muscle, tendon, and bone as an independent therapy. Percutaneous injection of sclerosing agents without/with permanent outflow occlusion is the most common endovascular techniques to treating the venous malformations (VM) lesions [29–32]. Focal VM lesions are typically treated with sclerotherapy for usual indications for treatment including pain, swelling, disfigurement, bleeding, and consumption coagulopathy. Diffuse VMs often contain painful focal venous expansions that benefit from endovascular treatment. Hence, various liquid sclerosants are introduced to destroy the endothelial cell layer of the CVM lesions to become the major therapeutic tool for the treatment of low-flow vascular malformations (LFVMs) led by the VMs [33, 34].

The most commonly used sclerosants are absolute ethanol, sodium tetradecyl sulfate [STS], polidocanol, and bleomycin; the sclerosing agent selected is directly injected into the VM lesion in order to achieve endothelial cell death and subsequent fibrosis. In general, the efficacy of the therapy will depend upon the quality/extent of contact of the concentrated scleroagent solution with the endothelial lining of the VM [33, 34]. Careful selection of the sclerosing agent is, therefore, mandated especially for superficially located VM lesions (e.g., hand/palm, feet/sole, mucosae) because each liquid agent has its own unique property and side effects and further caution is indicated to the lesion located in anatomical regions with the risk to develop a compartmental syndrome secondary to the edema caused by the therapy [35, 36]. Now both modalities of the therapy are fully integrated through a multidisciplinary strategy to achieve an acceptable goal for the contemporary management of the CVMs [37–39]. However, this endovascular approach never became a panacea nor 'ultimate' solution to all the CVMs because an inherent risk of recurrence remains a major challenge to all the 'extratruncular' lesions due to their mesenchymal cell characteristics originated from the 'early' stage of embryogenesis [24, 40, 41]. Therefore, the endovascular treatment remains as one of the armamentaria within the boundary of a multidisciplinary approach to set up the treatment strategy together with traditional surgical treatment to challenge to the CVMs; both treatment modalities should be mutually complimentary and not to exclude/conflict to each other. New treatment strategy should be set accordingly with full integration of open surgery and endovascular surgery to improve the treatment outcome. But, the benefit of endovascular therapy can be maximized by *discriminating* use only to 'surgically inaccessible' lesions. Indeed, the endovascular therapy should remain as the treatment of choice only to 'surgically inaccessible' diffusely infiltrating lesion as an independent therapy within the boundary of a multidisciplinary team approach. Meanwhile, 'surgically accessible' lesions can be managed with open surgical/excisional therapy more effectively, providing a potential chance of 'cure' when the lesion is localized [17–19]. The role of endovascular therapy could be further expanded to the 'surgically accessible' lesions as a supplement to improve subsequent surgical/excisional therapy through preoperative as well as postoperative embolo-sclerotherapy. Such peri-operative, especially preoperative, therapy could reduce surgical morbidity as well as complications drastically so that such benefit can exceed the beyond the boundary for the traditional surgical approach. Nevertheless, the endovascular therapy based on various modalities of the embolo/sclerotherapy can provide only 'effective control' at best; it should not be abused overzealously aiming for a 'cure'. Therefore, the endovascular therapy is mandated for 'controlled' aggressiveness within the boundary of the 'palliative' concept only when the benefit should exceed the morbidity following the treatment and 'overkilling' by radical approach should be actively avoided. Preferred modality of embolo-sclerotherapy should be therefore, selected based on positive balance of benefit by the treatment over the morbidity accompanied by the treatment, unless the treatment is indicated for the life- if not limb-threatening condition (e.g., hemorrhage; high cardiac output failure). Critical role of careful assessment on benefit versus risk of morbidity before the commitment cannot be overemphasized, and the ultimate goal of the treatment has to be clearly defined with a realistic expectation [42, 43].

2 Indication for the Intervention

Not all CVM lesions are needed for the therapy; indeed, simple existence does not mean that the treatment is mandated and 'no treatment' should remain as one of the choices. The decision as well as the selection of the treatment modality should be made through multidisciplinary team assessment based on the indications. Indications for intervention, for example, may include the following conditions or complications of VMs and its associated conditions like lymphatic malformation (LM) [17]:

- Bleeding in various conditions/extents, from the skin or mucosa lesion to intra-muscular or retroperitoneal hematoma, hematuria, rectal bleeding, hematemesis, hemoptysis, or intracerebral or intraspinal bleeding.
- Signs and symptoms of CVI (painful varicosity, edema, skin changes, indolent ulcers, recurrent STP): Secondary complications of chronic venous hypertension.
- High output heart failure and/or secondary ischemic complications.
- Lesions located at a life-threatening region involving or close to vital structures (e.g., proximity to the airway), or located in an area threatening vital functions (e.g., sight, eating, hearing, or breathing).
- Disabling pain.
- Functional impairment (e.g., genital region).
- Cosmetically severe deformity.
- Lesions located at regions with potentially high risk of complications (e.g., hemarthrosis, thromboembolism).
- Lesions located at life-threatening region (e.g., proximity to the airway), or located at the region threatening vital functions (e.g., seeing, eating, hearing, or breathing).
- Lesions combined, producing the vascular bone syndrome (length discrepancy of the lower extremities, affecting the bone itself) or the destructive angiodysplastic arthritis (Hauert disease)
- Lesions obstructing the outflow and drainage of vital organ (e.g., liver, brain).
- Lesions generating a low perfusion and/or other relevant hemodynamic effects in the drained territory.
- Recurrent thrombosis of the affected area in extratruncular lesion.
- Pulmonary embolism (PE) from venous aneurysm or other venous dysplastic areas.
- Consumptive coagulopathy with clinically equivalent lesion.
- Persistent lymph leaks due to a combined LM lesions with/without infection.
- Recurrent sepsis, local and/or general, due to a combined LM lesion.

The UIP Consensus for the VM-2014 recommends further that the embryologic subtype of the VMs (extratruncular vs. truncular) should be identified before proceeding the treatment of any VMs through the proper appraisal of various symptoms and signs to indicate for the treatment. Careful assessment of the extent and severity of the VM lesion and identification of draining deep vein system is also mandatory. Besides, the presence of any other associated vascular malformations (e.g., AVM, LMs) if any should be also determined together [17].

3 Ethanol Sclerotherapy

Among various sclerosants, the most commonly used agent to treat the extratruncular CVM lesion is (absolute) ethanol since ethanol remains most effective with curative potential. Indeed, ethanol is powerful enough to cause the endothelial cell denuded from the vascular wall, its protoplasm precipitated, and the vascular wall fractured to the level of the internal elastic lamina resulting in permanent damage with no chance of recurrence [44–48]. Indeed, ethanol is a potent irritant sclerosant causing trans-mural destruction of the vessel wall. No other known agents were proven for equal potency to bring complete destruction of the 'extratruncular' lesions which possess the mesenchymal cell/angioblast characteristics to grow back when stimulated adequately (e.g., female hormone, puberty, pregnancy, trauma, and surgery). However, ethanol has been known for notoriously high risk of complications and morbidity in a wide range; from a simple skin breakdown and bullae/ulceration to extensive soft-tissue necrosis, peripheral nerve injury with severe neurologic complications, compartment syndrome, deep vein thrombosis, pulmonary embolism, and cardiopulmonary arrest/death [44–48]. But the majority of the complications can be preventable if not reducible to the acceptable range based on careful assessment of lesion location, lesion morphology, and the clinical circumstances. Lesion location is often the most important factor in determining which embolic/sclerosant agent to use. If a lesion is located near neurologic structures, then the use of ethanol may very well be contraindicated and the use of a different liquid embolic, such as N-butyl cyanoacrylate (NBCA) or Onyx may be preferable. Pulmonary hypertension as a potentially fatal complication of the ethanol to lead to subsequent cardiopulmonary arrest is also preventable; pulmonary arterial spasm induced by spilled over ethanol reaching to pulmonary vasculature can be managed safely with appropriate measures. Close cardiopulmonary monitoring with pulmonary artery catheter is therefore mandated during ethanol sclerotherapy; a total dose of ethanol per session should remain in less than 1 ml/kg and limiting ethanol injections to 0.14 ml ethanol/kg ideal body weight every 10 min is proven to be the best preventable measurement when anticipating large injections of ethanol in large lesions [44, 45]. Safe use of ethanol in AVM embolization requires accurate delivery into the nidus by precise placement solely in the AVM nidus vasculature. Proximal injection of ethanol into a feeding artery would cause severe tissue necrosis, and should be condemned. Therefore, the concerns regarding the liberal/casual use of ethanol for all CVMs are legitimate due to its significant risks of complications and morbidity. Treatment strategy based on ethanol should be set through multidisciplinary team approach to moderate its outcome/impact based on the anticipated risks. A discriminating use is therefore, mandated even to the AVM lesions which warrant aggressive control to risk the local or systemic complications in view of serious hemodynamic consequences caused by high-flow shunting/passing through dysplastic capillaries in the nidus as the remnant of non-involuting primitive vessels [47, 48]. Naturally, ethanol sclerotherapy has such high rate of complications and morbidity especially when the VM is located close to large nerves or skin, in the lip, tongue, gum/oral mucosa, the genital region, or in the hand at fingers, or in the foot at the toe, or palm, sole with or without transdermal extension. Indeed, the VM lesions with transdermal extension or in close proximity to the skin or mucosa are known to carry a high risk of skin or mucosa necrosis. 'Indiscriminate' use of the ethanol as the first line to treat the VM lesions therefore, has been called into question since the majority of VM lesions are seldom life or limb-threatening. Nevertheless, ethanol gel has been lately introduced in Europe for the treatment of LFVM lesions to get more effective local effects by ethyl cellulose allowing fewer systemic side effects in lower dose of ethanol [49]. Not all other CVMs are equally serious as AVM, and the VM or LM seldom becomes a limb or life-threatening condition. Therefore, the treatment of the VM and LM should aim to control the lesion with minimally possible complication and morbidity using less risky agents (e.g., sodium tetradecol sulfate/STS, polidocanol/POL, bleomycin and OK-432) first although the recurrence rate will be much higher than the ethanol [50–54]. Hence, the use of ethanol should be limited to the experienced specialists only for fully justified indication across the board, regardless. Indeed, the second-best policy is a lot better than ideal outcome of the 'cure' while paying prohibitively high price for this relatively safe CVM lesions [17]. Therefore, ethanol sclerotherapy requires special training and experience in order to minimize the risk of complication and subsequent morbidity. Although this agent still has a special role in the management of AVMs, it should be used only discriminately in the treatment of VM and LM [44–48]. Indeed, poor results of ethanol sclerotherapy with bad complications should be blamed on the inexperience by the ignorant user, and NOT on the innocent ethanol! Indiscriminating use of the ethanol with insufficient knowledge and experience has been a culprit of wrong prejudice against ethanol as the most controversial scleroagent for the CVM management. After all, the ethanol is a most effective sclerosagent so far across the board despite it has the highest rate of serious complications, such as peripheral nerve injury and cardiac arrest and remains de facto leading scleroagent till more advanced and safer agent to meet the mandate is available. Indeed, ethanol keeps best track records with the lowest recurrence rate by experienced specialists especially for the AVM.

4 Sclerotherapy in General with Other Agents

Proper selection of the embolo-scleroagent (e.g., bleomycin, STS, POL, absolute ethanol, Onyx, N-butyl cyanoacrylate (NBCA), coil and/or contour particles), therefore, should be made to fit best to each lesion with different location and severity. Most of presently available embolo-scleroagents are far from the perfect accompanying significantly high risk of complication and/or morbidity (e.g., absolute ethanol); a careful plan, from the diagnosis and treatment to the long-term follow-up assessment, is therefore mandated for each different agent with different limitation, risk, and morbidity (e.g., bleomycin). Bleomycin, originally an antitumor antibiotic, has been used extensively to various LMs for decades with excellent result for the macrocystic lesions in particular and still remains a major option when OK-432, also known as picibanil, which is made with attenuated streptococcal exotoxin, is not available for the LM [55–58]. Now, bleomycin is more popular as an effective agent for treating VMs as a single agent or combined with other compatible agent either in liquid or foam condition; its liquid form offers predictable systemic absorption and pharmacokinetics, but its foam modalities enhance local efficacy via improved stability and contact especially when combined with polidocanol and albumin [59, 60]. Bleomycin does not directly cause thrombosis but appears to recruit fibroblasts to cause mild sclerosing effect, consequently, causing the least amount of swelling after injection. Indeed, 'intralesional' bleomycin induces fibrosis by damaging endothelial cells and recruiting fibroblasts, leading to lesion regression with minimal pronounced post-sclerotherapy swelling seen with other agents like ethanol [61]. Therefore, bleomycin is the most appropriate agent for treating sites where swelling is poorly tolerated (e.g., the orbit, airway, and some muscle compartments). But the disadvantages of bleomycin are when used alone, it usually requires more procedures than other scleroagents, besides the concern for pulmonary fibrosis though fibrosis has not yet been reported as a complication of sclerotherapy. Nevertheless, bleomycin dose is generally limited to 0.5 mg/kg or 15 kg per procedure, with the lifetime limit of 300 mg. When used as the sole scleroagent, it works best when administered every 3 weeks. Bleomycin has been reported for similar efficacy in terms of symptom relief with less complications in comparison with ethanol, though required more procedures [62, 63]. Sclerotherapy is usually performed under the sedation or general anesthesia; all of these agents should be effective in obliterating a blood vessel or venous lake, but cure of a VM is usually not achieved, due to the nature of the malformation as an embryonic tissue remnant, after all.

Therefore, proper assessment on the response should be also included upon the decision on the subsequent session of the endovascular treatment for its agent to be used, the amount, and the delivery route, etc. Besides, endovascular treatment should be implemented only to the lesions which are indicated for the therapy. Indeed, not all the CVMs would need the therapy, and only those with fully assessed indications should be considered for the endovascular treatment. Potential risk of collateral damage to the surrounding tissues (nerve, vessel, cartilage, skin, and soft-tissue) by the embolo-scleroagent should be assessed ahead of the time. Endovascular treatment should be planned in multi-sessions with minimally possible amount for each session whenever possible in order to reduce potential risk of acute/chronic morbidity and complication. The embolo-sclerotherapy should be selected among the variety of options to fit best to the type of the CVM the lesion belongs. Because, not all the CVMs are same as one size fits to all. Different types of the CVM possess different embryological as well as hemodynamic characteristics so that their clinical significance, natural progress, response to the therapy, etc., are all different from each other. For example, VM and/or LM seldom become a life- or limb-threatening condition on the contrary to the AVM. Hence, implication of same indication for the AVM with same strategy to the VM and LM would bring more harm than good. Therefore, proper understanding on such complex nature of the CVMs: definition, classification, and diagnosis as well as the indication is the most critical precondition to provide right endovascular treatment. Indeed, the endovascular therapy to the AVM should be given based on different principles and guidelines from the rest of the CVMs because all the AVM lesions are potentially life-, if not, limb-threatening condition. Hence, early aggressive approach to all the AVM lesions is warranted in general, to reduce the impact as well as the consequence of the AVM lesion. But the aggressive approach must be tempered with realistic assessment of the long-term prospect of the treatment outcome. Precise control of the nidus of the lesion itself is essential to prevent recurrence and/or fast deterioration of all the CVM lesions, especially for the AVM lesion with much complicated hemodynamic consequences. For example, previous approach to the AVM only with the strategy to shut off the feeding artery, leaving the nidus of the lesion intact, is totally wrong; such mistake would provoke a more aggressive neovascular recruitment by this primitive lesion only to make the condition worse with no exception. Lastly, the majority of VM lesions seldom become a life or limb-threatening condition. Therefore, 'indiscriminating' use of the ethanol to a certain group of the VM lesions (e.g., transdermal extension and/or proximity to the skin/mucosa) is no longer tolerated due to extreme risk of skin/mucosa necrosis with severe morbidity by the ethanol. For example, the 'localized' VM lesions in the lip, tongue, gum/oral mucosa as well as those at finger, toe, palm, sole with/without transdermal extension should be tried with a low risk-accompanying scleroagent as the first option (e.g., foam sclerotherapy).

5 Embolotherapy

Embolotherapy in general is not ideal for the VM lesions with currently available embolization agents: coils, glue, and/or particles. Because micro particles and coils are usually not large enough to occlude these lesions generally with large diameter vascular channels effectively and often washed out in low-flow and high-volume status [17]. Besides, currently available agents for embolization are not able to deliver complete destruction of the vessel endothelium mandated to control these embryonic tissue remnants effectively. Indeed, incomplete endothelial cell destruction would rather stimulate primitive mesenchymal cell characteristics the extratruncular lesions possess as an embryonic tissue remnant following the developmental arrest in its early stage of embryogenesis, only provoking a significant risk of lesion recurrence [17]. Hence, these embolic agents can produce only mechanical compression of the lesion at most and the cessation of flow that results in thrombosis at best to allowing subsequent recanalization. The role of endovascular therapy is therefore relatively limited to deliver satisfactory long-term outcome. But, NBCA embolotherapy has a unique role, ideal as an adjunctive agent to fill up the VM lesion when done preoperatively to facilitate subsequent surgical excision, reducing the risk of bleeding and minimizing the sacrifice of collateral tissue to improve the safety and effectiveness of surgical excision [17].

6 Foam Sclerotherapy

Foam sclerotherapy is one form of sclerotherapies, well accepted for the treatment of LFVMs in general: VM and LM [30, 64–66]. Foam sclerotherapy is an effective treatment option for extratruncular as well as truncular VM lesions with the advantage of a better and longer-lasting contact of the sclerosing agent with the vessel wall which leads to a more effective treatment and to a reduction of concentrations needed in comparison to liquid sclerotherapy. Indeed, foam is significantly more effective than liquid as scleroagent and side effects with POL or STS foam are less in comparison with ethanol [67]. Foam sclerotherapy is therefore an effective treatment option for low-flow extratruncular and truncular venous malformations in general and either POL or STS foam sclerotherapy is now widely accepted as independent therapy for non to poor surgical candidate with surgically 'inaccessible' lesion, effectively reducing symptoms with an acceptable rate of complications [68, 69]. Besides, bleomycin-polidocanol foam (BPF) is also accepted as a safe and effective sclerosant for VMs, showing better efficacy and similar safety as commonly used mild sclerosants. With the addition of bleomycin, the half-lives of BPFs increased significantly and also achieved the smallest bubble diameter and wall thickness to increase BPF stability. Hence, BPF sclerotherapy as well is now considered an ideal alternative treatment to surgical resection together with the liquid-form sclerotherapy to deliver safe and effective control of diffuse infiltrating type of extratruncular form of VM in particular and recommended as a promising first-line treatment of VMs and also other LFVMs [60, 70, 71]. The foam therapy is therefore considered as the treatment of choice now to surgically inaccessible extensive lesions beyond deep fascia with involvement of muscle, tendon, and bone. Nevertheless, foam scleroagent can also cause tissue necrosis and swelling, but nerve injury is much less common, and cardiac arrest is extremely rare [72, 73]. Hence, it should be planned in multisessions with minimally possible amount for each session whenever possible in order to reduce potential risk of acute/chronic morbidity and complication.

7 Ultrasound-Guided Sclerotherapy (UGS) with Foam Sclerosants

Ultrasound-guided foam sclerotherapy (foam UGS) based on detergent-based sclerosants (e.g., STS, POL) has been reported to be well tolerated and improve the symptoms among LFVMs without the risks of more aggressive sclerosing agents (e.g., ethanol) [32]. Indeed, this new treatment approach for the treatment of VMs is now known to deliver satisfactory results with minimal morbidity especially to the 'diffuse infiltrating' VMs which would be otherwise treated with ethanol (31, 32, 69) and also the superiority of foam versus liquid sclerotherapy was reported through a prospective comparative randomized study by Yamaki et al. [31]. This treatment approach based on foam UGS is also reported to be useful especially for localized subcutaneous or intramuscular lesions as well as Klippel Trenaunay syndrome (KTS) patients for their LFVM lesions without associated risk of collateral damage seen with ethanol sclerotherapy (e.g., nerve injury, muscle) (Fig. 14.1) [74–76].

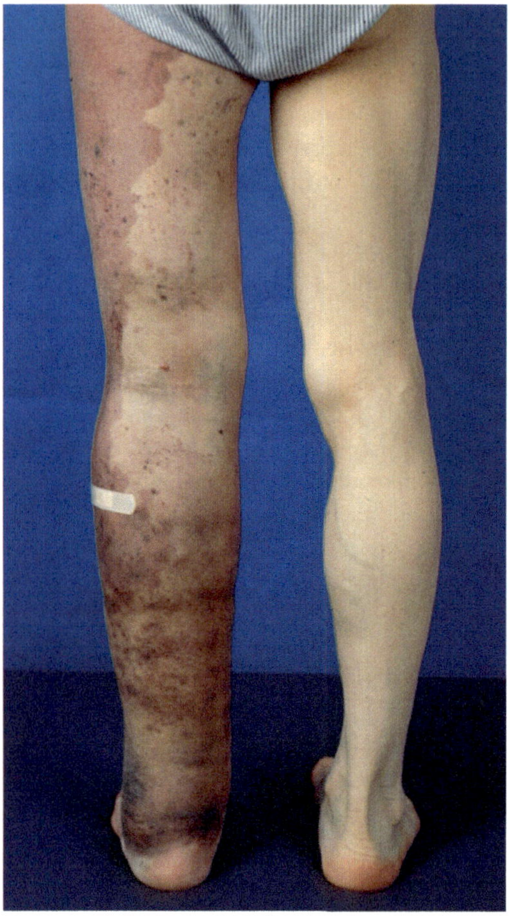

Fig. 14.1 *Klippel Trenaunay Syndrome*: Clinical photograph demonstrating typical features of Klippel–Trénaunay syndrome, characterized by a triad of capillary malformation (port-wine stain), venous malformations/atypical varicosities (often including a persistent lateral marginal vein), and limb overgrowth with soft-tissue and/or bony hypertrophy leading to asymmetry. This complex combined vascular malformation requires careful clinical and imaging evaluation to guide management and reduce risks such as pain, swelling, thrombophlebitis, bleeding, and thromboembolic events

Indeed, foam sclerotherapy can deliver good relief of symptoms and clinical improvement with minimal risk of complications, in this extended group of infiltrating VM lesions [32]. Besides, intradermal VMs and also Glomuvenous malformation lesions (GVMs) can be treated successfully with this new approach using foam or liquid agents under direct vision [77]. Foam sclerotherapy produces excellent short to mid-term control of small VM lesions. But higher recurrence remains the major disadvantage of foam sclerotherapy when treating large lesions, compared with ethanol sclerotherapy. Foam sclerotherapy of CVMs has been known to be associated rarely with stroke and transient ischemic attacks (TIA) [21, 78–80]. Indeed, a higher risk of neurological complications of foam can be associated with the patients with a known patent foramen ovale (PFO) or other right-to-left shunts. Precaution is warranted especially through large embryonic vascular spaces of LFVM lesions in view of unknown fluid mechanics and undefined rheology of foams with the possibility of drainage into the central venous system, and also the potential for systemic complications and cerebrovascular events [17]. Special care is also required in the injection of the marginal vein, due to the possible involvement of the deep venous and nervous systems (Fig. 14.2).

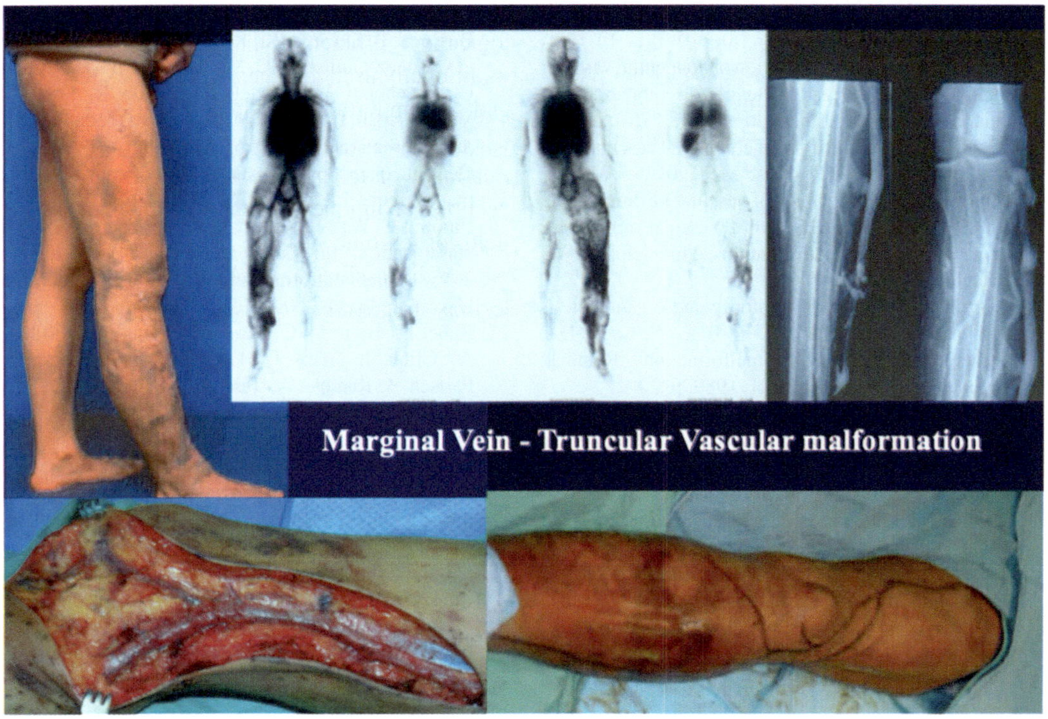

Fig. 14.2 Marginal vein: clinical photograph showing a marginal vein along the lateral aspect of the limb, consistent with a persistent embryonic superficial vein and part of a venous malformation rather than a simple varicose vein. This vessel is frequently associated with abnormal venous anatomy, including deep venous hypoplasia/obstruction and atypical perforator connections, and may represent an important (sometimes dominant) drainage pathway. Foam sclerotherapy must therefore be performed with particular caution, ideally after complete duplex and/or cross-sectional venous mapping, using low volumes and low concentration, slow injection under ultrasound guidance, and strict control of proximal outflow when indicated. Close monitoring is required to minimize complications such as skin necrosis, thromboembolism, nerve injury, and unintended deep venous thrombosis, and post-procedure compression and follow-up imaging are recommended

8 Fluoroscopic and Ultrasound-Guided Sclerotherapy (FUGS)

Combining approach with sonographic and fluoroscopic guidance sclerosants has a particular merit to the treatment of VM lesions to identify and localize the target vessels by ultrasound guidance and also visualization of the target lesion and the draining veins by contrast medium then injected on fluoroscopy [81, 82]. Hence, FUGS is particularly useful in treatment of intra-muscular VM lesions. Indeed, fluoroscopy allows a more comprehensive visualization of the target lesion and draining veins which is not possible with ultrasound imaging alone. On fluoroscopy, STS or POL foam introduced slowly into the lesion would appear radiolucent displacing most of the radiopaque contrast agent; the injection is then stopped when the draining veins to take up the foam sclerosant. Postoperatively, the compression should be applied for 7 days following the FUGS. Hence, FUGS is particularly useful in treatment of intra-muscular VM lesions [81, 82].

References

1. Yamaki T, Nozaki M, Fujiwara O, Yoshida E. Duplex guided foam sclerotherapy for the treatment of the symptomatic venous malformations of the face. Dermatologic Surg. 2002;28:619–22.
2. Cabrera J, Cabrera J Jr, Garcia-Olmedo MA, Redondo P. Treatment of venous malformations with sclerosant in microfoam form. Arch Dermatol. 2003;139:1409–16.

3. Belov S. Classification of congenital vascular defects. Int Angiol. 1990;9:141–6.
4. Lee BB, Laredo J. Classification of congenital vascular malformations: the last challenge for congenital vascular malformations. Phlebology. 2012;27(6):267–9.
5. Lee BB. New classification of congenital vascular malformations (CVMs). Rev Vasc Med. 2015a;3(3):1–5.
6. Mulliken JB. Classification of vascular birthmarks. In: Mulliken JB, Young AE, editors. Vascular birthmarks: hemangiomas and malformations. Philadelphia: WB Saunders; 1988. p. 24–37.
7. Bastide G, Lefebvre D. Anatomy and organogenesis and vascular malformations. In: Belov S, Loose DA, Weber J, editors. Vascular malformations. Reinbek: Einhorn-Presse Verlag GmbH; 1989. p. 20–2.
8. Lee BB. All congenital vascular malformations should belong to one of two types: "truncular" or "extratruncular", as different as apples and oranges! Editorial. Phlebological Rev. 2015b;23(1):1–3.
9. Belov S. Classification, terminology, and nosology of congenital vascular defects. In: Belov S, Loose DA, Weber J, editors. Vascular malformations. Reinbek: Einhorn-Presse; 1989. p. 25–30.
10. Belov S. Anatomopathological classification of congenital vascular defects. Semin Vasc Surg. 1993;6:219–24.
11. Sabin FR. Origin and development of the primitive vessels of the chick and of the pig. Cont Embriol Carnegie Inst. 1917;6–7:61–7.
12. Woolard HH. The development of the principal arterial stems in the forelimb of the pig. Contrib Embryol. 1922;14:139–54.
13. Lee BB, Laredo J, Lee TS, Huh S, Neville R. Terminology and classification of congenital vascular malformations. Phlebology. 2007a;22(6):249–52.
14. Lee BB. Critical issues on the management of congenital vascular malformation. Annals Vasc Surg. 2004;18(3):380–92.
15. Lee BB, Laredo J, Lee SJ, Huh SH, Joe JH, Neville R. Congenital vascular malformations: general diagnostic principles. Phlebology. 2007b;22(6):253–7.
16. Lee BB, Laredo J, Kim YW, Neville R. Congenital vascular malformations: general treatment principles. Phlebology. 2007c;22(6):258–63.
17. Lee BB, Baumgartner I, Berlien P, Bianchini G, Burrows P, Gloviczki P, Huang Y, Laredo J, Loose DA, Markovic J, Mattassi R, Parsi K, Rabe E, Rosenblatt M, Shortell C, Stillo F, Vaghi M, Villavicencio L, Zamboni P. Diagnosis and treatment of venous malformations consensus document of the International Union of Phlebology (IUP): updated 2013. Int Angiol. 2015a;34(2):97–149.
18. Lee BB, Antignani PL, Baraldini V, Baumgartner I, Berlien P, Blei F, Carrafiello GP, Grantzow R, Ianniello A, Laredo J, Loose D, Lopez Gutierrez JC, Markovic J, Mattassi R, Parsi K, Rabe E, Roztocil K, Shortell C, Vaghi M. ISVI-IUA consensus document – diagnostic guidelines on vascular anomalies: vascular malformations and hemangiomas. Int Angiol. 2015b;34(4):333–74.
19. Lee BB, Baumgartner I, Berlien HP, Bianchini G, Burrows P, Do YS IK, Kool LS, Laredo J, Loose DA, Lopez-Gutierrez JC, Mattassi R, Parsi K, Rimon U, Rosenblatt M, Shortell C, Simkin R, Stillo F, Villavicencio L, Yakes W. Consensus document of the International Union of Angiology (IUA)-2013. Current concept on the management of arterio-venous management. Int Angiol. 2013;32(1):9–36.
20. Enjolras O, Wassef M, Chapot R. Introduction: ISSVA classification. In: Color atlas of vascular tumors and vascular malformations. New York: Cambridge University Press; 2007. p. 1–11.
21. Rabe E, Breu F, Cavezzi A, Smith PC, Frullini A, Gillet J, Guex J, Hamel-Desnos C, Kern P, Partsch B, Ramelet A, Tessari L, Pannier F, For the Guideline Group. European guidelines for sclerotherapy in chronic venous disorders. Phlebology. 2013;29(6):338–54.
22. Lee BB. Congenital venous malformation: changing concept on the current diagnosis and management. Asian J Surg. 1999;22(2):152–4.
23. Dompmartin A, Vikkula M, Boon L. Venous malformations: update on etiopathogenesis, diagnosis & management. Phlebology. 2010;25(5):224–35.
24. Lee BB. Endovascular management of the congenital vascular malformation (CVM) is not a panacea: editorial. Damar Cer Derg. 2013;22(1):1–3.
25. Roh YN, Do YS, Park KB, Park HS, Kim YW, Lee BB, Pyon JK, Lim SY, Mun GH, Kim DI. The results of surgical treatment for patients with venous malformations. Ann Vasc Surg. 2012;26(5):665–73. >>>25
26. Lee BB. Commentary on "surgical treatment with or without embolotherapy for arteriovenous malformations". Ann Vasc Dis. 2013b;6(1):7–8.
27. Marji P, Laredo J, Lee BB. Surgical therapy combined with embolo/sclerotherapy-multidisciplinary approach. In: Lee BB, Gloviczki P, Blei F, Markovic J, editors. Vascular malformations: advances and controversies in contemporary management. Boca Raton: CRC Press, Taylor & Francis Group; 2020. p. 107–10.
28. Choi JCB, Laredo J, Lee BB. Excisional surgery: when and how much it can be incorporated? In: Lee BB, Gloviczki P, Blei F, Markovic J, editors. Vascular malformations: advances and controversies in contemporary management. Boca Raton: CRC Press, Taylor & Francis Group; 2020. p. 271–2.
29. Gelbert F, Enjolras O, Deffrenne D, Aymard A, Mounayer C, Merland JJ. Percutaneous sclerotherapy for venous malformation of the lips: retrospective study of 23 patients. Neuroradiology. 2000;42(9):692–6.
30. Rabe E, Pannier F. Sclerotherapy in venous malformation. Phlebology. 2013;28(Suppl 1):188–91.
31. Yamaki T, Nozaki M, Sakurai H, Takeuchi M, Soejima K, Kono T. Prospective randomized efficacy of ultrasound-guided foam sclerotherapy compared with ultrasound-guided liquid sclerotherapy in the treatment of symptomatic venous malformations. J Vasc Surg. 2008;47:578–84.

32. Blaise S, Charavin-Cocuzza M, Riom H, Brix M, Seinturier C, Diamand JM, Gachet G, Carpentier PH. Treatment of low-flow vascular malformations by ultrasound guided sclerotherapy with polidocanol foam: 24 cases and literature review. Eur J Endovasc Surg. 2011;41:412–7.
33. Burrows PE. Endovascular treatment of slow-flow vascular malformations. Tech Vasc Interv Radiol. 2013;16(1):12–21. https://doi.org/10.1053/j.tvir.2013.01.003. PMID: 23499128.
34. Burrows PE, Mason KP. Percutaneous treatment of low flow vascular malformations. J Vasc Interv Radiol. 2004;15(5):431–45. https://doi.org/10.1097/01.rvi.0000124949.24134.cf. PMID: 15126652.
35. Lee BB, Laredo J. Venous malformation: treatment needs a bird's eye view. Phlebology. 2013;28:62–3.
36. Lee BB. Changing concept on vascular malformation: no longer enigma. Ann Vasc Dis. 2008;1(1):11–9.
37. Lee BB, Bergan JJ. Advanced management of congenital vascular malformations: a multidisciplinary approach. J Cardiovasc Surg. 2002;10(6):523–33.
38. Lee BB. Critical role of multidisciplinary team approach in the new field of vascular surgery—endovascular surgery. J Kor Soc Vasc Surg. 2003a;19(2):121–3.
39. Lee BB, Do YS, Yakes W, Kim DI, Mattassi R, Hyun WS, Byun HS. Management of arterial-venous shunting malformations (AVM) by surgery and embolosclerotherapy. A multidisciplinary approach. J Vasc Surg. 2004;3:596–600.
40. Lee BB. Advanced management of congenital vascular malformation (CVM). Int Angiol. 2002;21(3):209–13.
41. Lee BB, Baumgartner I. Contemporary diagnosis of venous malformation. J Vasc Diagn. 2013;1:25–34.
42. Lee BB. Current concept of venous malformation (VM). Phlebolymphology. 2003b;43:197–203.
43. Lee BB. Not all venous malformations needed therapy because they are not arteriovenous malformations. Dermatol Surg. 2010;36(3):340–6.
44. Shin BS, Do YS, Lee BB, Kim DI, Chung IS, Cho HS, et al. Multistage ethanol sclerotherapy of soft-tissue aretriovenous malformations: effect on pulmonary arterial pressure. Radiology. 2005;235:1072–7.
45. Do YS, Yakes W, Shin SW, Lee BB. Ethanol embolization of arteriovenous malformations: interim results. Radiology. 2005;235:674–82.
46. Lee BB, Do YS, Byun HS, Choo IW, Kim DI, Huh SH. Advanced management of venous malformation (VM) with ethanol sclerotherapy: mid-term results. J Vasc Surg. 2003;37(3):533–8.
47. Jeon YH, Do YS, Shin SW, Liu WC, Cho JM, Lee MH, Kim DI, Lee BB, Choo SW, Choo IW. Ethanol embolization of arteriovenous malformations: results and complications of 33 cases. J Kor Radiol Soc. 2003;49:263–70.
48. Lee BB, Kim DI, Huh S, Kim HH, Choo IW, Byun HS, Do YS. New experiences with absolute ethanol sclerotherapy in the management of a complex form of congenital venous malformation. J Vasc Surg. 2001;33(4):764–72.
49. Dompmartin A, Blaizot X, Théron J, Hammer F, Chene Y, et al. Radio-opaque ethyl cellulose-ethanol is a safe and efficient sclerosing agent for venous malformations. Eur Radiol. 2011;21:2647–56.
50. Park JH, Kim DI, Huh S, Lee SJ, Do YS LBB. Absolute ethanol sclerotherapy on cystic lymphangioma in neck and shoulder region. J Korean Vasc Surg Soc. 1998;14(2):300–3.
51. Jeong HS, Baek CH, Son YI, Byun HS, Lee BB. Treatment for extracranial arteriovenous malformations of the head and neck. Acta Otolaryngol. 2006;126(3):295–300.
52. Kim KH, Kim HH, Lee SK, Seo JM, Chang WY, Lee BB. OK-432 intralesional therapy for lymphangioma in children. J Korean Assoc Pediatr Surg. 2001;7(2):142–6.
53. Park HS, Do YS, Park KB, et al. Clinical outcome and predictors of treatment response in foam sodium tetradecyl sulfate sclerotherapy of venous malformations. Eur Radiol. 2016;26:1301–10.
54. Lee BB, Laredo J, Neville R. Arterio-venous malformation: how much do we know? Phlebology. 2009;24:193–200.
55. Mathur NN, Rana I, Bothra R, Dhawan R, Kathuria G, Pradhan T. Bleomycin sclerotherapy in congenital lymphatic and vascular malformations of head and neck. Int J Pediatr Otorhinolaryngol. 2005;69:75–80.
56. Orford J, Barker A, Thonell S, King P, Murphy J. Bleomycin therapy for cystic hygroma. J Pediatr Surg. 1995;30:1282–7.
57. Ogita S, Tsuto T, Deguchi E, Tokiwa K, Nagahima M, Iwai N. OK-432 therapy for unresectable lymphangiomas in children. J Ped Surg. 1991;26:263–70.
58. Lee BB, Kim YW, Seo JM, Hwang JH, Do YS, Kim DI, et al. Current concepts in lymphatic malformation (LM). J Vasc Endovasc Surg. 2005;39:67–81.
59. Mack JM, Peterson EC, Crary SE, Moran JH, Neville K, Pierce CD, Richter GT. Pharmacokinetics of bleomycin sclerotherapy in 454 patients with vascular malformations. Pediatr Blood Cancer. 2022;69(8):e29733.
60. Sun Y, Gu H, Yang X, Cai R, Shang Y, Hu L, Wang Y, Chen H, Lin X. Bleomycin Polidocanol Foam (BPF) stability – in vitro evidence for the effectiveness of a novel sclerosant for venous malformations. Eur J Vasc Endovasc Surg. 2020;59(6):1011–8. https://doi.org/10.1016/j.ejvs.2020.01.023.
61. Abdelaty MH, Badran AI, Aborahma AM, Elheniedy MA, Kamhawy AH. Intralesional injection of bleomycin in the manage ment of low flow vascular malformations: results and factors affecting the outcome. J Vasc Surg Venous Lymphat Disord. 2024;12(2):101694.
62. Saitta P, Krishnamurthy K, Brown LH. Bleomycin in dermatology: a review of intralesional applications. Dermatologic Surg. 2008;34:1299–313.

63. Villavicencio JL, Scultetus A, Lee BB. Congenital vascular malformation: when and how to treat them. Semin Vasc Surg. 2002;15(1):65–71.
64. Mukul SK, Singh A, Kumar A, Pandey S, Singh S, Kumar A. Foam Polidocanol Sclerotherapy for Low-flow vascular malformations of tongue. Ann Maxillofac Surg. 2019;9(2):257–60. https://doi.org/10.4103/ams.ams_81_19. PMID: 31909004; PMCID: PMC6933997.
65. Lee BB, Bergan J. Transition from alcohol to foam sclerotherapy for localized venous malformation with high risk. In: Bergan J, Le Cheng V, editors. A textbook- foam sclerotherapy. London: The Royal Society of Medicine Press Ltd.; 2008. p. 129–39.
66. Blaise S. Le médecin vasculaire et l'échosclérothérapie à la mousse dans les malformations veineuses [Vascular medicine and foam sclerotherapy for venous malformations]. J Med Vasc. 2017;42(5):315–9. https://doi.org/10.1016/j.jdmv.2017.06.004. French. Epub 2017 Aug 2. PMID: 28964390.
67. Markovic JN, Nag U, Shortell CK. Safety and efficacy of foam sclerotherapy for treatment of low-flow vascular malformations in children. J Vasc Surg Venous Lymphat Disord. 2020;8(6):1074–82. https://doi.org/10.1016/j.jvsv.2019.11.023. Epub 2020 Apr 10. PMID: 32284312.
68. Arasakumar DRB, Pang C, Evans N, Papadopoulou A, Khalifa M, Tsui J, Hamilton G, Brookes J, Lim CS. Efficacy and safety of foam sclerotherapy with sodium tetradecyl sulfate as preferred sclerosant of venous malformations based on experience from a single specialist center. J Vasc Surg Venous Lymphat Disord. 2023;11(2):379–88. https://doi.org/10.1016/j.jvsv.2022.10.008. Epub 2022 Oct 31. PMID: 36328136.
69. Yang X, Chen H, Gu H, Jin Y, Hu L, Hua C, Wang Y, Sun Y, Yu W, Lin X. Interim results of bleomycin-polidocanol foam sclerotherapy as a highly efficient technique for venous malformations. J Vasc Surg Venous Lymphat Disord. 2020;8(6):1066–73. https://doi.org/10.1016/j.jvsv.2019.11.022. Epub 2020 Apr 10. PMID: 32284311.
70. He B, Yang B, Nie QQ, Zhang JB, Chen J, Liu P, Fan XQ, Ye ZD. Comparison of polidocanol foam versus bleomycin polidocanol foam for treatment of venous malformations. J Vasc Surg Venous Lymphat Disord. 2023;11(1):143–8. https://doi.org/10.1016/j.jvsv.2022.06.005. Epub 2022 Aug 5. PMID: 35940448.
71. Stuart S, Barnacle AM, Smith G, Pitt M, Roebuck DJ. Neuropathy after sodium tetradecyl sulfate sclerotherapy of venous malformations in children. Radiology. 2015;274(3):897–905.
72. Rautio R, Saarinen J, Laranne J, Salenius JP, Keski-Nisula L. Endovascular treatment of venous malformations in extremities: results of sclerotherapy and the quality of life after treatment. Acta Radiol. 2004;45(4):397–403.
73. McRae MY, Adams S, Pereira J, Parsi K, Wargon O. Venous malformations: clinical course and management of vascular birthmark clinic cases. Aust J Dermatol. 2012;54(3):188–94. https://doi.org/10.1111/j.1440-0960.2012.00959.x. [Epub ahead of print] PubMed PMID: 23082725.
74. Gloviczki P, Driscoll DJ. Klippel-Trenaunay Syndrome:current management. Phlebology. 2007;22(6):291–8. Venous Forum of the Royal Society of Medicine.
75. Lee BB, Vaghi M. Review on target treatment of Klippel-Trenaunay Syndrome. Ital J Vasc Endovasc Surg. 2021;28(1):42–9.
76. Lee BB, Laredo J. Hemo-lymphatic malformation: Klippel-Trenaunay syndrome. Rev Acta Phlebologica. 2016;17(1):15–22.
77. Parsi K, Kossard S. Multiple hereditary glomangiomas: successful treatment with Sclerotherapy. Aust J Dermatol. 2002;43:43–7.
78. Cavezzi A, Parsi K. Complications of foam sclerotherapy. Phlebology. 2012;27(Suppl 1):46–51.
79. Parsi K. Paradoxical embolism, stroke and Sclerotherapy. Phlebology. 2012;27:147–67.
80. Parsi K, Connor DE, Pilotelle A, Low J, Ma DD, Joseph JE. Low concentration detergent sclerosants induce platelet activation but inhibit aggregation due to suppression of GPIIb/IIIa Activation in vitro. Thromb Res. 2012;130(3):472–8.
81. Parsi K, Pereira J. Fluoroscopic ultrasound guided sclerotherapy. In: 16th international workshop on vascular anomalies, International Society for the Study of vascular anomalies. Milan; 2006. p. 66–7.
82. Van der Linden E, Overbosch J, Kroft LJ. Radiofrequency ablation for treatment of symptomatic low flow vascular malformations after previous unsuccessful therapy. J Vasc Interv Radiol. 2005;16:747–50.

15 Tips and Tricks in Sclerotherapy

Sergio Gianesini, Yasmina Chhih, Celine Eggen, and Rodrigo Rial

1 Strategic Indications and Case Selection

Among all venous interventions, sclerotherapy is probably the technique in which indication and case selection have the greatest impact on outcomes. In expert practice, technical execution is rarely the limiting factor; rather, success or failure is determined upstream, by how accurately the indication is defined and how realistically the treatment goal is framed. Unlike thermal or surgical techniques, sclerotherapy is inherently adaptable, operator-dependent, and iterative. These strengths can become weaknesses when indications are poorly chosen or insufficiently individualized. Modern guidelines provide a valuable reference framework, but they cannot fully account for the complexity of real-world venous disease. Experienced practitioners therefore use guidelines as a foundation, not a ceiling, integrating duplex-derived hemodynamics, vein morphology, patient phenotype, previous treatments, and patient priorities into a dynamic decision-making process. Most contemporary guidelines endorse sclerotherapy for telangiectasias, reticular veins, tributaries, perforators, and selected truncal veins, often with diameter-based thresholds. However, expert practice consistently demonstrates that diameter alone is a crude surrogate for treatment suitability. Vein compressibility, depth from skin, reflux pattern, drainage role, and positional behavior frequently provide more actionable information than static measurements. Expert refinement of indications also involves recognizing scenarios in which venous reflux is present but not clinically relevant. Segmental reflux without axial propagation, short reflux duration without symptoms or reflux confined to non-dominant drainage pathways should prompt caution. Treating such veins may improve ultrasound findings without meaningful symptomatic or cosmetic benefit, exposing patients to unnecessary risk. Conversely, strict adherence to guideline thresholds may result in under-treatment of symptomatic patients who would benefit from a minimally invasive approach. Experienced clinicians increasingly prioritize hemodynamic relevance and symptom correlation over rigid anatomic criteria, especially in patients with contraindications to thermal ablation or surgery. The decision to select sclerotherapy over endovenous thermal ablation or surgery

S. Gianesini (✉)
Department of Translational Medicine, University of Ferrara, Ferrara, Italy

Department of Surgery, Uniformed Services University of Health Sciences, Bethesda, MD, USA
e-mail: gnssrg@unife.it

Y. Chhih
Department of Internal Medicine, Ibn Sina University Hospital, Mohammed V University, Rabat, Morocco

C. Eggen
Centrum Oosterwal, Alkmaar, Netherlands

R. Rial
Vascular and Endovascular Department, University Hospital HM, Madrid, Spain

S. Gianesini, Y. W. Chi (eds.), *Sclerotherapy*, https://doi.org/10.1007/978-3-032-32794-9_15

should not be framed as a compromise, but as a strategic choice. Each modality has strengths and limitations and expert practice lies in matching the technique to the clinical scenario rather than defaulting to hierarchy-based algorithms. Sclerotherapy offers clear advantages in tortuous veins, superficial truncal segments, residual, or recurrent varicosities and in anatomies where catheter-based techniques are technically difficult or risky. It also plays a central role in patients with advanced age, frailty, anticoagulation, or intolerance to tumescent anesthesia. Comparative data suggest that while thermal ablation achieves higher immediate occlusion rates in large truncal veins, clinical improvement and patient-reported outcomes after sclerotherapy can be comparable when patients are appropriately selected [1, 2]. In recurrent varicose veins, where neovascularization, scar tissue and altered anatomy limit surgical and endovenous options, sclerotherapy allows precise targeting of pathological segments with minimal additional trauma. Importantly, expert use of sclerotherapy often occurs within hybrid treatment strategies, combining thermal ablation or surgery with sclerotherapy. Understanding when sclerotherapy should be primary, adjunctive, or staged is a key component of advanced venous practice. Sclerotherapy outcomes are profoundly influenced by patient-related factors, particularly expectations, compliance, and engagement with post-treatment care. Unlike single-session thermal procedures, sclerotherapy frequently requires multiple sessions and delayed result assessment, making expectation management essential. Compression therapy remains a cornerstone of outcome optimization, particularly after foam sclerotherapy. However, compliance varies widely and is strongly influenced by pre-procedural counseling. Clear explanation of the rationale, duration and expected benefits of compression improves adherence and reduces post-treatment complications such as hyperpigmentation and thrombophlebitis [3]. Expert clinicians also tailor treatment goals to patient priorities. For some patients, symptom relief is paramount, for others, cosmetic improvement dominates decision-making. Attempting to achieve cosmetic perfection in patients primarily seeking symptom relief may lead to unnecessary retreatments, while under-treating cosmetic concerns can result in dissatisfaction despite technically successful procedures. Over-indication remains one of the most common causes of suboptimal results in sclerotherapy. Treating veins with minimal hemodynamic significance, excessive pursuit of duplex "normalization" or aggressive retreatment of partially responsive veins increases complication risks without proportional benefit. Excess foam volumes and high concentrations used to compensate for poor indication selection are well-recognized risk factors for neurological symptoms, skin complications, and thrombotic events.

A frequent expert-level pitfall is the temptation to replace definitive axial treatment with repeated sclerotherapy sessions in veins that are unlikely to respond durably. While sclerotherapy is versatile, it is not universally appropriate and recognizing its limitations is as important as mastering its techniques. Under-indication is equally problematic. Rigid exclusion based on vein diameter, depth, or historical dogma may deprive patients of an effective, minimally invasive solution (Table 15.1). Ultimately, mastery in sclerotherapy lies in calibrated decision-making: knowing when to treat, when to defer, when to combine modalities, and when to stop. This balance, between confidence and restraint, defines expert practice, and distinguishes strategic sclerotherapy from purely technical execution.

Table 15.1 Practical suggestions for appropriate sclerotherapy indications

Practical suggestions	
Indication	1. Venous caliber is not the main feature
	2. Consider Hemodynamics
	3. Patients features matter
	4. Depth from skin
	5. Differentiate between methodologically sound evidence-based guidelines and consensus documents
	6. Patient compliance and reliability is pivotal

2 Pre-procedure Optimization

In advanced sclerotherapy practice, pre-procedure optimization represents a decisive therapeutic phase rather than a preliminary step. Many adverse events, technical failures, and disappointing outcomes attributed to sclerosant choice or injection technique are, in reality, the consequence of insufficient preparation. Pre-procedural planning is where risk is mitigated, efficacy is maximized, and treatment intent is clarified. A rigorously optimized pre-procedure phase transforms sclerotherapy from a technically simple act into a predictable, reproducible intervention with durable clinical benefit. Unlike thermal or surgical techniques, where energy delivery or anatomic correction dominates outcomes, sclerotherapy depends heavily on contextual variables: vein behavior under changing hemodynamic conditions, sclerosant–blood interaction and the surrounding tissue environment. Mastery lies in controlling these variables before the first injection is performed. Duplex ultrasound is the cornerstone of pre-procedure optimization, but its role extends far beyond confirming reflux. Ultrasound becomes a strategic mapping instrument, used to understand venous pathophysiology, hierarchy and interconnections rather than simply labeling veins as competent or incompetent. Advanced mapping begins with identifying the dominant reflux source and tracing its propagation pathways. This includes evaluating axial continuity, tributary inflow and outflow, perforator competence and potential deep venous interactions. Treating a vein without understanding its role within this network risks either incomplete treatment or disruption of compensatory drainage pathways. Dynamic maneuvers are essential. Reflux patterns often vary significantly between standing, sitting, and supine positions. Valsalva maneuvers, distal compression and release testing help distinguish true pathological reflux from transient or positional phenomena. Targeting precision is particularly critical in ultrasound-guided foam sclerotherapy. Mapping should identify not only refluxing segments but also optimal access points that allow controlled foam propagation. Antegrade filling, avoidance of perforator escape and containment within the target segment must be anticipated before injection. Pre-procedure skin marking of vein trajectories, junctions and access points improves procedural efficiency and reduces cognitive load during injection. A straightforward yet highly reliable ultrasound maneuver called Reflux Elimination Test can be used to confirm the saphenous reflux reversibility by simple digital compression of the incompetent tributaries. During the assessment, the Doppler probe must be positioned proximally to the evaluated tributaries. If the saphenous reflux induced by an active foot dorsiflexion disappears when the incompetent tributaries are compressed, the pathological pressure gradient can be restore by treating just the tributaries (Fig. 15.1) [4].

In recurrent disease, ultrasound mapping assumes even greater importance. Scar tissue, neovascularization and altered venous anatomy require meticulous identification of functional pathways. Failure to map these accurately is a leading cause of early recurrence and persistent symptoms after sclerotherapy. Moreover, rare but possible conditions of nerve proximity to the varices can favor a dedicated sclerotherapic approach [5]. Accurate vein characterization is fundamental to sclerosant selection, concentration adjustment and injection strategy. While vein diameter is commonly used as a decision-making parameter, expert practice recognizes that diameter is only one variable among many and often not the most predictive. Vein depth relative to the skin surface strongly influences both efficacy and complication risk. Superficial veins are more prone to skin necrosis, matting and hyperpigmentation, particularly when high sclerosant concentrations are used. In such cases, experts favor lower concentrations, staged treatments or liquid sclerosant rather than foam. Conversely, deeper veins may require higher sclerosant concentrations or foam formulations to ensure sufficient endothelial contact. However, depth alone does not determine response. Vein wall thickness, elasticity and surrounding tissue compliance all modulate sclerosant distribution and retention.

Flow dynamics are arguably the most under-appreciated component of vein characterization.

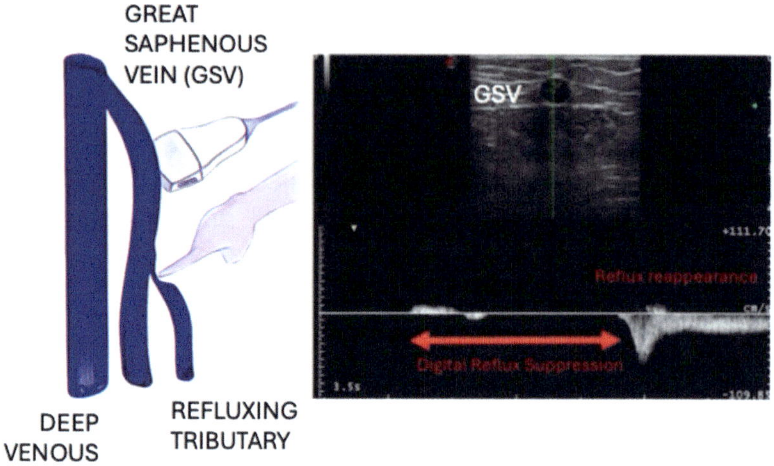

Fig. 15.1 Reflux elimination test: saphenous reflux suppression by digital compression, confirming the need to treat only the tributary, despite an eventually present reflux in the saphenous vein as it is fed by the refluxing tributary aspiration

Table 15.2 Ultrasound mapping practical suggestions

Practical suggestions	
Ultrasound mapping	1. Identify leaking and re-entry points of the reflux
	2. Perform the reflux elimination test
	3. Exclude pelvic sources
	4. Assess vessel caliber
	5. Assess hemoydnamic overload
	6. Assess flushing confluences

High-flow veins rapidly dilute sclerosant, reducing contact time, and increasing the likelihood of treatment failure. Experts anticipate this by implementing flow-reduction strategies such as limb elevation, proximal compression, or staged injections. In contrast, low-flow or static segments, common in recurrent disease, retain sclerosant longer but are at higher risk for inflammatory complications if overdosed. A careful evaluation also of the terminal and ilio-femoral valve must be included in case of sclerotherapy of this anatomical district because the incompetence of the same ilio-femoral tract is a recognized risk factor for recurrence [6]. Importantly, experts recognize that vein behavior is dynamic rather than static. Diameter and flow change with posture, temperature, hydration status, and even patient anxiety. Pre-procedure assessment should therefore be performed under conditions that approximate treatment circumstances as closely as possible (Table 15.2).

Patient positioning is a powerful but frequently underestimated determinant of sclerotherapy success. First of all, the patient must lie down comfortably, avoiding positions that could produce Valsalva maneuver and/or mobilization during the procedural time. The position must also favor the comfort of the healthcare professional and of the related injections site. The time used for proper positioning is always saved time and a further guarantee of treatment success. In case of ultrasound-guided procedures, it's also fundamental to properly line up the healthcare professional with the leg and the monitor, avoiding uncomfortable positions for the operator who should never assume unnatural postures to watch the screen. By manipulating gravity and venous filling, experts can significantly alter vein diameter, flow velocity and sclerosant distribution, often reducing the need for higher concentrations or volumes. Limb elevation prior to injection decreases venous pressure and diameter, enhancing sclerosant–endothelium contact and reducing dilution by residual blood. This strategy is particularly effective in truncal and large tributary veins. Standing or reverse Trendelenburg positioning remains valuable during diagnostic ultrasound, where gravitational loading unmasks reflux patterns not apparent in the supine position. However, experts often transition patients to a supine or mildly elevated position during injection to balance reflux visualization with treatment safety. Dynamic repositioning during

Table 15.3 Periprocedural practical suggestions

Practical suggestions	
Peri-procedural	1. Individual thrombotic risk assessment matters
	2. No candies/chewing gums during the treatment
	3. Naked arm for emergency vein access
	4. No compression stocking self-positioning (avoid Valsalva)

Table 15.4 Practical suggestion in patient and doctor positioning

Practical suggestions	
Position	1. Avoid Valsalva
	2. Comfortable for the patient and the doctor
	3. No rapid postural changes
	4. Line up the operator with the leg and the ultrasound monitor

treatment can be used to guide foam propagation along predefined pathways while minimizing escape into deep veins. Coordinating injection timing with respiratory cycles and avoiding immediate muscle activation further reduces unintended sclerosant migration, an especially important consideration in foam sclerotherapy. Post-injection positioning also matters. Almost immediate ambulation is encouraged to promote venous flow and reduce thrombotic risk, but excessive or premature muscle activation may displace sclerosant before adequate endothelial contact has occurred. Expert protocols balance these competing priorities through staged mobilization strategies. Before starting the procedure, it's a good practice to make sure the patient has no candies/chewing gum in the mouth and that, in case of emergency, an arm is ready for access. Indeed, the procedure is extremely safe and fast and office-based, yet underestimating the possible need to immediately take action could represent a major issue (Table 15.3).

Although sclerotherapy carries a low infection risk, meticulous skin preparation remains a cornerstone of expert practice, particularly in ultrasound-guided procedures involving multiple punctures or prolonged treatment times. Infection, when it occurs, is often the result of cumulative minor lapses rather than a single breach. Alcohol-based antiseptics provide effective skin disinfection when adequate contact time is respected. Overly aggressive antiseptic regimens offer little additional benefit and may increase skin irritation, particularly in patients with chronic venous skin changes Patients with eczema, lipodermatosclerosis, atrophie blanche or healed ulcers require special attention. Treating through inflamed or compromised skin significantly increases the risk of infection, necrosis, and poor cosmetic outcomes. Expert practice favors delaying sclerotherapy until skin integrity is restored, even if venous reflux is clearly present. Ultrasound probe hygiene is an often-overlooked aspect of infection prevention. The use of sterile gel or probe covers during ultrasound-guided injections reduces bacterial transmission, particularly in high-volume practices. Avoiding repeated needle passes through the same skin puncture further minimizes contamination risk (Table 15.4).

In expert sclerotherapy, pre-procedure optimization represents the convergence of diagnostic precision, hemodynamic control and procedural discipline. By mastering ultrasound mapping, vein characterization, patient positioning, and meticulous preparation, the clinician creates the conditions in which sclerosants can act predictably and safely. The more refined this preparatory phase becomes, the less aggressive and, paradoxically, the more effective the treatment itself needs to be.

3 Choice of Sclerosant: Practical Nuances

In sclerotherapy, the sclerosant is often mistakenly perceived as a fixed variable, a drug selected from a limited list and applied according to standardized concentration tables. In expert practice, however, the sclerosant functions as a highly adaptable therapeutic instrument, whose effect depends on formulation, concentration, volume, wetness, production and delivery method, and interaction with local hemodynamics. The same agent can behave as a gentle endothelial irritant or as a powerful obliterative toxin depending on how, where and in what context it is used. For the experienced clinician, the key question is rarely "which sclerosant is best", rather "which sclerosant configuration is optimal for this vein, in this patient, at this moment." Understanding the practical nuances of sclerosant selection is therefore central to achieving predictable efficacy while minimizing complications. Polidocanol and sodium tetradecyl sulfate are detergent sclerosants with broadly comparable efficacy, yet their clinical personalities differ in ways that meaningfully influence expert preference. These differences become particularly relevant in borderline indications, superficial veins, recurrent disease, and cosmetically sensitive areas. Polidocanol is widely favored for its excellent tolerability profile. Injection pain is minimal, inflammatory response is generally mild and the risk of severe tissue injury after extravasation is lower compared with sodium tetradecyl sulfate. These characteristics make polidocanol especially suitable for telangiectasias, reticular veins, superficial tributaries, and patients with low pain tolerance or heightened anxiety. Sodium tetradecyl sulfate, in contrast, is often described as more aggressive or potent, an attribute that can be advantageous in larger, fibrotic or previously treated veins. Its stronger detergent action may overcome resistance in veins with thickened walls or high-flow dynamics. However, this potency comes at the cost of increased risk of hyperpigmentation, post-treatment inflammation and skin necrosis in the event of extravasation or excessive concentration. It must be stated that this last observation is purely empirical and personal: no clear strong evidence in support of it is present in the literature to the authors' of this chapter knowledge.Expert practitioners rarely adopt an exclusive preference for one agent. Instead, many maintain parallel familiarity with both sclerosants, selecting polidocanol for superficial and cosmetic work and reserving sodium tetradecyl sulfate for deeper, larger, or refractory veins. Importantly, comparative studies suggest that when concentration, volume and technique are properly adapted, overall efficacy differences are modest, reinforcing the principle that operator judgment outweighs pharmacologic differences [1]. Concentration selection is one of the most consequential and most error-prone decisions in sclerotherapy. While guideline tables provide reference ranges, expert practice is guided by the principle of using the lowest concentration capable of achieving durable endothelial damage. Moreover, the provided tables do not take into consideration the production methods, the wetness and the possible hemodynamics variable: all factors that confound also the related scientific literature and that demand the high-level training before practicing sclerotherapy. In small-caliber veins such as telangiectasias and fine reticular veins, increasing concentration beyond minimal effective levels does not improve occlusion rates but markedly increases the risk of matting, hyperpigmentation and localized inflammation. As vein size increases, higher concentrations may be required, but diameter alone should not dictate dosing. Superficial large veins behave differently from deep large veins; low-flow recurrent segments behave differently from high-flow primary trunks. Experts therefore integrate depth, flow velocity, wall characteristics and venous pressure into concentration selection. A frequent expert adjustment involves reducing concentration when using foam rather than liquid sclerosant. Foam displaces blood and dramatically prolongs sclerosant–endothelium contact time, effectively increasing local potency. Failure to compensate for this effect is a common cause of overtreatment, particularly in superficial veins and perforators. Experienced practitioners also recognize that concentration selection is not static across sessions. As veins partially fibrose or decrease in caliber after initial treatment, subsequent sessions often require lower concentrations to avoid inflammatory sequelae. A fundamental principle is also to consider not the concentration and the sclerosing power inside the syringe, rather the final one injected into the vein, which depends on many material factors, such as the type and geometry of the syringe and of the needle and of the catheter. In this sense, even the choice of direct needle injection vs. butterfly with tube use can significantly change the final foam delivery. The introduction of foam sclerotherapy has profoundly altered the therapeutic landscape, expanding the range of veins amenable to sclerotherapy and reducing reliance on surgical or thermal techniques. Nevertheless, foam is not inherently superior to liquid sclerosant; rather, each formulation has distinct advantages and limitations. Liquid sclerosant remains the formulation of choice for very small veins, where intraluminal blood volume is minimal and precise dosing is essential. It offers excellent control, predictable spread, and a lower incidence of systemic side effects such as transient visual disturbances or migraine-like symptoms. Liquid is therefore preferred in cosmetic sclerotherapy and in patients with known or suspected right-to-left shunts. Foam sclerotherapy, by contrast, excels in larger veins. By displacing blood rather than mixing with it, foam allows prolonged, homogeneous contact with the endothelium, enabling effective treatment of truncal veins, perforators, and complex recurrent disease with relatively low drug doses. However, foam demands greater discipline. Volume control, bubble size, injection speed, appropriate material and patient positioning all influence systemic dispersion and safety. In expert practice, the choice between liquid and foam is rarely absolute. Many clinicians employ hybrid strategies, using foam for axial or deep segments and liquid sclerosant for superficial extensions or cosmetic finishing, thereby leveraging the strengths of both formulations. Beyond polidocanol and STS, several off-label sclerosants have been used historically or continue to be explored in niche applications. Among the currently most known ones, certainly there is Dextrose 75%, used in the CLACS strategy, for which the reader is invited to refer to Chap. 12. As tips and tricks herein we remind that it is a dense liquid for which the required injection pressure is higher. The same injection technique is different, particularly in CLACS where the vessel is already shrunk by the laser energy: rather than aiming at directly accessing the vein lumen, in this scenario the practitioner usually trespass the posterior wall, start injecting, and retract the needle until the access into the lumen is perceived. Current innovation in sclerotherapy focuses on providing a nitrogen-free multiple concentrations and gases combination foam, keeping the stability of nitrogen-based formulation, while guaranteeing the necessary safety (Table 15.5).

Table 15.5 Sclerosant agent practical suggestions

Practical suggestions	
Sclerosant	1. Sodium tetradecyl sulfate might be more aggressive than polidocanol
	2. Read concentrations and volume tables but take the final decision based on proper training as multiple factors are involved, higher concentation does not mean stronger occlusion
	3. A more stable foam does not always mean the best foam as it depends on the desired target anatomical and hemodynamic context
	Smaller more uniform bubbles produces more predictable and performing behavior
	4. Do not "remix" already coarsed foam
	5. Consider staging the procedure

Advances in foam preparation, gas composition, and injection devices aim to improve consistency, safety and endothelial contact while reducing systemic exposure. This reflects a broader maturation of the field, in which refinement and precision take precedence over pharmacologic novelty.

4 Foam Sclerotherapy: Technical Pearls

Foam stability is central to its therapeutic effect. Stable foam displaces blood effectively and maintains prolonged contact with the venous endothelium, while unstable foam collapses rapidly, behaving more like diluted liquid sclerosant. However, excessive stability is not inherently desirable: foam that persists too long increases the risk of systemic dispersion and post-procedural symptoms. Bubble size plays a critical role in both efficacy and safety. Smaller, more uniform bubbles provide a greater surface area-to-volume ratio, improving endothelial interaction and producing more predictable intraluminal behavior. Larger bubbles are prone to coalescence and fragmentation, increasing the likelihood of erratic propagation and unintended deep venous migration. Expert operators aim for a controlled intermediate stability: foam that persists long enough to achieve endothelial injury but dissolves promptly once its local action is complete. Achieving this balance requires careful attention to sclerosant concentration, sclerosant-to-gas ratio, gas solubility, and timing between preparation and injection.

Foam is inherently time-sensitive. Its physical properties degrade rapidly after preparation due to bubble coalescence and gas diffusion. Experts therefore inject foam immediately after preparation and discard unused foam rather than attempting to "recondition" it. Re-mixing partially degraded foam produces heterogeneous bubble populations with unpredictable in vivo behavior. Gas composition is one of the most debated aspects of foam sclerotherapy and a major determinant of systemic safety. Room air has historically been used because of its availability and ease of preparation. However, nitrogen-rich air produces foam with relatively long bubble persistence due to low solubility in blood, increasing the likelihood of foam reaching the pulmonary and systemic circulation. Carbon dioxide (CO_2) and CO_2/O_2 mixtures generate foam with much shorter bubble lifespan. These gases dissolve rapidly in blood, leading to faster foam collapse and reduced systemic persistence. The reduced stability of CO_2-based foam, however, introduces technical challenges. In high-flow veins or inadequately emptied segments, rapid foam degradation may compromise efficacy unless compensated by optimized positioning, flow reduction or adjusted sclerosant concentration. Expert operators recognize that gas choice and injection strategy are inseparable variables. In contemporary expert practice, CO_2 or CO_2/O_2 mixtures are increasingly favored for truncal veins, large volumes and high-risk patients (e.g., migraine sufferers or those with known or suspected right-to-left shunts). Foam standardization by fully automated devices able to produce nitrogen-free foam are therefore desired for safety, performance, and clinical governance validation. Foam volume management is the single most important determinant of safety in foam sclerotherapy. Unlike liquid sclerosant, foam acts as both a chemical irritant and a space-occupying embolic material. Excessive foam volume increases the risk of deep venous penetration, pulmonary passage and paradoxical embolization. Consensus recommendations often cite maximum foam volumes per session (commonly around 10 mL), but expert practice emphasizes individualized dosing rather than rigid numerical limits. This is particularly evident considering the discrepancies in the suggested volume reported by different documents: Australia doctors are suggested to inject less than 20 rather than 10 Ml [7]. The effective foam dose depends on vein capacity, degree of pre-injection emptying, flow dynamics and injection precision. Experts routinely demonstrate that large venous segments can be treated effectively with surprisingly small foam volumes when veins are adequately emptied through limb elevation, injection sites are strategically chosen and foam propagation is carefully monitored with ultrasound. Staged treatment is a hallmark of advanced foam sclerotherapy. Rather than attempting to treat extensive venous territories in a single session, experts deliberately divide treatment into multiple sessions, reducing cumulative foam exposure and improving control. This approach is particularly important for truncal veins, recurrent disease, and patients with elevated thromboembolic or neurological risk. Continuous ultrasound monitoring during injection allows real-time assessment of foam movement. Experts terminate injection immediately if foam approaches deep venous junctions or propagates beyond the intended segment. This disciplined restraint, knowing when *not* to inject, is one of the most distinguishing skills of expert foam sclerotherapy. In advanced practice, foam sclerotherapy is not defined by how easily foam can be produced, but by how precisely it is controlled, limited, and guided. Mastery lies in understanding foam as a transient, dynamic structure whose therapeutic value depends on preparation technique, physical properties, gas composition and, above all, volume discipline. When these elements are harmonized, foam sclerotherapy becomes not only more powerful than liquid sclerosant, but also safer, more predictable, and more elegant.

5 Injection Techniques and Access Tips

Among all steps in sclerotherapy, vascular access and injection technique represent the narrowest point of the therapeutic funnel. No amount of pre-procedure planning, sclerosant optimization, or foam refinement can compensate for imprecise access or poorly controlled injection dynamics. In expert hands, injection is not a mechanical delivery of a drug, but a real-time hemodynamic intervention, during which sclerosant behavior is actively shaped by needle choice, access strategy, pressure modulation, and continuous feedback from ultrasound and vein response. Injection-related errors account for a substantial proportion of complications (extravasation, skin necrosis, thrombophlebitis, pigmentation) and many apparent treatment failures. Conversely, refined injection technique allows experienced practitioners to achieve durable results with lower concentrations, smaller volumes and fewer sessions, underscoring the primacy of precision over aggressiveness. The choice of needle or catheter is often underestimated, yet it profoundly influences control, stability, and safety. Expert practice begins with the principle that the access device should be as small and as flexible as the vein will allow, without compromising control. For telangiectasias and very small reticular veins, ultra-fine needles (27–30 G) provide maximal precision and minimize tissue trauma. Larger needles in these veins increase the risk of extravasation and perivascular inflammation without improving sclerosant efficacy (Table 15.6).

In medium-sized reticular veins and superficial tributaries, 25–27 G needles often offer the best balance between stability and finesse. Foam injection through excessively fine needles can increase resistance, destabilize foam, and promote retrograde leakage at the puncture site. Experts therefore adapt needle size not only to vein diameter, but also to sclerosant formulation. Catheters provide stable intraluminal access, reduce the risk of displacement during patient movement or ultrasound probe manipulation, and allow controlled delivery of foam volumes. Yet, a consideration about the possible foam degradation through them must always be done. Crucially, expert practice avoids device escalation as a solution to resistance or difficulty. Increasing needle size or rigidity to "force" access often leads to endothelial injury, vein rupture, or extravasation. Instead, experts reposition, reassess vein filling, or change access site. Ultrasound-guided cannulation is indispensable in modern sclerotherapy, particularly for deep, non-visible, or recurrent veins. Yet, despite its apparent simplicity, it is associated with a distinct set of recurrent technical errors that can compromise both safety and efficacy. The most common error is loss of needle-tip visualization. Operators may believe the needle is intraluminal based on shaft visibility, while the tip lies outside the vein or has penetrated the posterior wall. Expert technique prioritizes continuous visualization of the needle tip, adjusting probe angle and insertion trajectory dynamically rather than advancing blindly. In this context, ultrasound longitudinal view allows to always visualize the tip of the needle, avoiding the risk of perforating the posterior wall of the vein. Ultrasound transverse view allows a 360-degree visualization of the perivenous area, yet it could generate the false image of a correctly positioned needle while, in reality, the image is related to the shaft rather than the tip (Fig. 15.2).

Table 15.6 Practical suggestions on materials

Practical suggestions	
Material	1. Rely on good quality ultrasound
	2. Consider sylicone component for detergent sclerosants degradation
	3. Consider the area of the plunger for final pressure
	4. Always assess the scientific validation of the eventually used foam production devices
	5. Consider nitrogen-free foam for safety
	6. Echogenic needles
	7. Consider foam degradation over 27 G
	8. Consider the foam degradation along butterly tubes/catheters

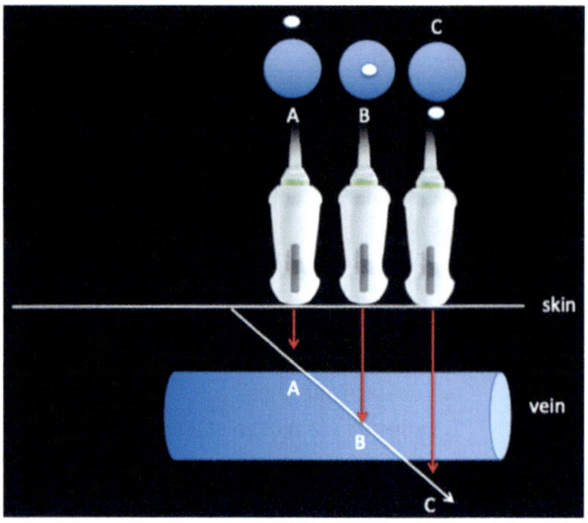

Fig. 15.2 Ultrasound transverse view producing the false image of a correctly positioned needle while it's actually visualizing the shaft (B) rather than the tip (A)

Not experts in ultrasound-guided procedures tend to move nervously fast with their hands while trying to access the vein. A good tip is the one of looking at our own hands to make sure they are poking lined up with the Doppler probe, rather than watching immediately the monitor. Once the first millimeters of poking are done, then it's appropriate to find the needle on the Doppler screen and move slowly while advancing, keeping the needle monitored. Tailing down the needle while piercing the vein can help in not trespassing the posterior wall.

Excessive probe pressure is another frequent pitfall. Compression may collapse the vein, falsely facilitating cannulation but predisposing to posterior wall puncture once pressure is released. Experts apply minimal probe pressure and allow the vein to maintain its physiologic shape during access. Aspiration of blood is an unreliable confirmation of intraluminal position, particularly in low-pressure venous systems or when using foam. Instead, experts rely on real-time ultrasound confirmation of sclerosant entry, observing immediate intraluminal filling and wall contact during the initial injection phase. Cannulation errors are especially consequential in foam sclerotherapy. Even minimal extravasation of foam can result in disproportionate tissue injury. For this reason, expert cannulation is deliberately slow, with low tolerance for uncertainty. When doubt exists, the needle is withdrawn and repositioned rather than advanced forcefully. Injection dynamics determine how sclerosant interacts with blood, vein wall and downstream venous pathways. Rapid injection increases intraluminal turbulence, raises venous pressure and promotes reflux into non-target veins or perforators. In foam sclerotherapy, excessive speed fragments foam, accelerating systemic dispersion and reducing local efficacy (Table 15.7).

Expert practice emphasizes slow, low-pressure injection, allowing sclerosant to replace blood gradually and uniformly. Injection pressure should barely exceed venous pressure: resistance

Table 15.7 Practical suggestions for injection

Practical suggestions	
Injection	1. Guarantee clean skin
	2. It's never about the concentration inside the syringe, rather the one getting into the vein after eventual degradation inside the delivery tool
	3. Teleangectasia total endothelial surface is wider than the varicose veins one, therefore do not underestimate aesthetic sclerotherapy complications
	4. Do not oversize the needle for teleangectasia, but consider possible foam degradation over 27 G
	5. Change access site rather than forcing the injection
	6. Watch your hands to confirm lining up with the probe
	7. Move slowly
	8. Do not over-pressure the skin with the probe
	9. The smaller the plunger the higher the generated pressure for the same applied force (Pressure = Force/Surface)
	10. Whenever in doubt, do not advance
	11. Treat feeding veins first
	12. Consider emptying the vein (limb elevation, manual compression and strategic positioning)
	13. Stop if the injection is painful or if there is immediate blanching or livedoid discoloration or swelling or delayed dusky erythema
	14. Favor short treatment segments/ multiple access points/small injection volumes

is interpreted as a warning signal rather than a challenge to be overcome. Increased resistance may reflect vein spasm, malposition, foam degradation or partial extravasation and should prompt immediate reassessment. Vein emptying prior to injection is one of the most powerful yet underutilized optimization strategies. Limb elevation, manual compression and strategic positioning reduce venous volume and flow, significantly enhancing sclerosant efficiency. Well-emptied veins require lower sclerosant concentrations and smaller volumes to achieve endothelial injury. Advanced sclerotherapy is frequently performed in anatomically challenging contexts (recurrent disease, elderly patients, obesity or chronic venous skin changes) where standard access strategies are insufficient. Expert practice is defined by adaptability rather than force. Tortuous veins complicate both access and sclerosant propagation. Experts favor short treatment segments, multiple access points and small injection volumes to maintain control. Attempting to treat long tortuous segments from a single access site often results in incomplete treatment or unintended sclerosant migration. Deep veins require meticulous ultrasound guidance and heightened discipline. Increased depth amplifies the consequences of malposition and extravasation may go unnoticed until symptoms develop. Experts often accept partial treatment rather than aggressive pursuit of complete occlusion when access is unstable. Lower sclerosant concentrations are frequently sufficient due to improved foam efficiency and controlled flow reduction. Fragile veins, common in elderly patients or those with long-standing venous disease, are prone to rupture, spasm, and inflammation. Gentle cannulation, minimal needle manipulation and very low-pressure injection are essential. Experts resist the temptation to "salvage" fragile veins with higher concentration or forceful injection, recognizing that restraint prevents complications without compromising overall outcome (Fig. 15.3).

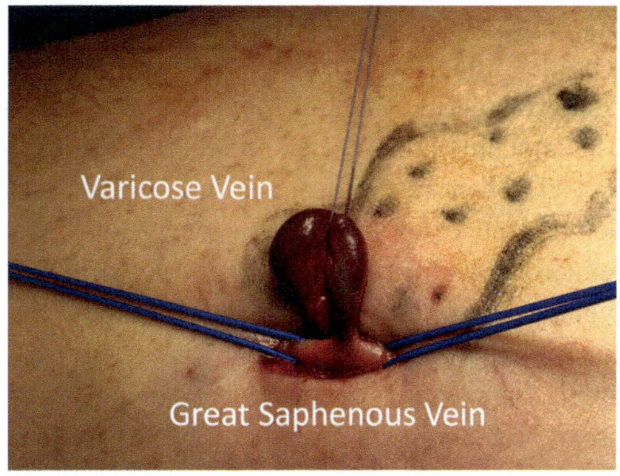

Fig. 15.3 Macroscopic evident difference between the consistency of the saphenous vein wall and the nearby varicose tributary, characterized by a far more fragile wall

Across all difficult anatomies, expert practice emphasizes goal adjustment. Partial closure, symptom reduction or staged treatment may represent success, whereas aggressive pursuit of anatomical perfection often leads to complications. In expert sclerotherapy, injection technique is not about delivering sclerosant efficiently, but about controlling the interaction between sclerosant, vein wall and venous flow. Mastery lies in precise access, disciplined injection dynamics and continuous responsiveness to real-time feedback. When injection technique is refined, sclerotherapy becomes safer, more predictable and paradoxically more effective and achieving more with less. In sclerotherapy, compression is frequently described as an adjunctive or supportive measure, yet in expert practice it should be regarded as a continuation of the therapeutic act itself. Compression directly influences post-injection hemodynamics, vein wall apposition, thrombus organization, inflammatory response and ultimately the durability and cosmetic quality of the result. An otherwise impeccably executed sclerotherapy session can be undermined by inadequate compression, while a well-conceived compression strategy can compensate for the need to use lower sclerosant concentrations and volumes, reducing complications without sacrificing efficacy. For vascular specialists, moving "beyond the basics" means abandoning rigid, protocol-driven compression prescriptions in favor of adaptive, goal-oriented strategies that reflect vein characteristics, treatment intent and patient-specific constraints. The choice of compression modality (elastic stockings, multilayer bandaging or adjustable compression devices) has a direct impact on pressure distribution, reproducibility and patient adherence. Elastic compression stockings are the most commonly used modality due to ease of application and predictable pressure profiles. Multiple studies have demonstrated improved vein occlusion rates, reduced inflammation, and lower rates of hyperpigmentation when compression is applied after sclerotherapy, particularly following foam treatment. Bandaging systems may provide higher initial pressures and are sometimes favored immediately after truncal or extensive foam sclerotherapy. However, they are more operator-dependent and often less well tolerated, particularly outside specialized centers. Adjustable compression systems offer flexibility but require patient education and engagement to be effective. Compression level must be calibrated carefully. Excessively high pressures increase discomfort, reduce compliance and may exacerbate skin irritation or ischemic symptoms in susceptible patients. At the same time, it should be remembered that the interface pressure at the tight is inversely related to the radius of the limb (Laplace law), therefore dropping significantly. Duration of compression remains controversial. Historically, prolonged compression was advocated across all indications, but strong evidence-based data on the topic are missing. In contrast, larger tributaries and truncal veins, especially after foam sclerotherapy, benefit from longer compression to stabilize thrombus formation and promote fibrosis. Expert practice therefore favors graduated compression duration, with both pressure and length of use scaled to vein size, depth and treatment complexity rather than dictated by uniform protocols. Compression strategies should always be designed around a clearly articulated treatment goal. Cosmetic improvement, symptom relief, reflux abolition, and prevention of recurrence each impose different mechanical and biological requirements. For telangiectasias and very small reticular veins, the primary objective is cosmetic optimization with minimal inflammatory response. Light to moderate compression applied for a limited duration reduces bruising and pigmentation while maintaining patient comfort. Over-compression in this context provides little additional benefit and may increase intolerance In medium-sized reticular veins and superficial tributaries, compression serves to maintain vein wall apposition after sclerosant-induced endothelial injury and to reduce residual intraluminal blood, thereby limiting post-treatment thrombophlebitis and pigmentation. Moderate compression for several days is usually sufficient to achieve these goals. In truncal veins and perforators treated with foam sclerotherapy, compression assumes a more decisive role. Sustained external pressure reduces vein diameter, limits early recanalization and promotes organized fibrosis. Expert protocols often combine immediate post-procedural bandaging with subsequent stocking use, tailoring duration to vein caliber, treated length, and patient tolerance. Importantly, experienced clinicians recognize that compression is not a corrective tool for poor indication or technique. Attempting to compensate for excessive foam volume or inappropriate vein selection with prolonged or high-pressure compression often increases patient burden without improving outcomes.

Similarly to compression, validated venous active drugs, particularly the ones demonstrating anti-inflammatory and potentially anti-hyperpigmentation effects, must be taken into serious consideration.

6 Managing and Preventing Complications

In expert sclerotherapy practice, complications are not viewed as unpredictable mishaps but as biologically plausible, largely preventable events that arise from the interaction between sclerosant properties, venous anatomy, hemodynamics, and post-procedural care. While sclerotherapy has an excellent overall safety profile, its complications, particularly cosmetic and thrombotic, carry a disproportionate impact on patient satisfaction and medico-legal exposure. For vascular experts, complication management begins long before the needle enters the vein. Appropriate indication, vein selection, sclerosant choice, foam discipline, injection control and compression strategy collectively define the complication risk profile. When adverse effects occur despite best practice, early recognition, accurate pathophysiological interpretation and proportionate intervention are essential to prevent progression and long-term sequelae. Post-sclerotherapy hyperpigmentation is the most frequent complication encountered in clinical practice and a leading cause of patient dissatisfaction, particularly in cosmetic indications. It results primarily from hemosiderin deposition following erythrocyte extravasation or intraluminal thrombus degradation, rather than direct melanocyte stimulation or sclerosant toxicity. The incidence of hyperpigmentation varies widely, reported in up to 10–30% of treated veins depending on vein size, depth, sclerosant concentration, formulation, and compression strategy. Superficial veins, reticular veins and foam-treated segments are particularly susceptible when residual blood trapping occurs. Prevention begins with minimizing intraluminal thrombus formation. Experts favor adequate vein emptying before injection, conservative sclerosant concentration, controlled foam volumes and early, well-fitted compression. Excessive sclerosant concentration and prolonged blood–sclerosant mixtures promote inflammatory thrombosis, increasing the likelihood of pigment deposition. Early evacuation of trapped thrombus, either through spontaneous drainage or targeted needle aspiration within 2–4 weeks, can significantly reduce both severity and duration of pigmentation. Once established, hyperpigmentation should be managed conservatively. Most cases fade gradually over 6 to 18 months and premature intervention often worsens outcomes. Persistent pigmentation may respond to topical depigmenting agents, chemical peeling, or laser therapy, but evidence remains limited and outcomes variable. Expert counseling is critical. Patients should be informed pre-procedurally that hyperpigmentation is usually transient, benign, and self-limiting and that aggressive retreatment of pigmented veins is contraindicated. Different is the case of the telangiectatic matting, the development of fine, reddish, lace-like networks of new vessels adjacent to treated veins, typically appearing several weeks after sclerotherapy. Although medically benign, matting is aesthetically distressing and often interpreted by patients as treatment failure. The pathophysiology of matting is multifactorial and incompletely understood. It is thought to involve angiogenic stimulation, local inflammatory mediators, estrogenic influence and unresolved venous hypertension (https://pubmed.ncbi.nlm.nih.gov/10928579/). Matting is more common in women, obese patients and individuals with hormonal therapy or underlying reflux. A critical expert insight is that matting often reflects incomplete treatment of feeding veins rather than a primary skin-level reaction. High sclerosant concentrations in superficial veins, aggressive cosmetic treatment without addressing underlying reticular or truncal reflux and inadequate compression are to be avoided. Prevention focuses on treating hemodynamic sources before cosmetic veins, avoiding excessive sclerosant concentrations, using staged treatment and ensuring appropriate compression. Persistent matting warrants reassessment with duplex ultrasound to identify untreated feeders or residual reflux. Low-concentration sclerotherapy, transcutaneous laser therapy, or combined approaches may be used once inflammation has resolved. Aggressive early retreatment often exacerbates matting and should be avoided. Skin necrosis is a rare but potentially devastating complication of sclerotherapy. It most commonly results from extravasation of sclerosant, intra-arterial injection, or use of excessively high concentrations in superficial veins. Early recognition is paramount. Warning signs include severe pain disproportionate to injection, immediate blanching, livedoid discoloration, swelling, or delayed dusky erythema. Injection should be stopped immediately at the first sign of abnormal pain or resistance. Expert immediate management includes aspiration of residual sclerosant if possible, dilution with saline infiltration, topical nitroglycerin in suspected arterial spasm and close observation. Prevention remains the most effective strategy. This includes meticulous ultrasound-guided cannulation in high-risk areas, low-pressure injection, avoidance of force when resistance is encountered and conservative sclerosant concentration in superficial veins. Established necrosis requires prolonged wound care and may result in scarring. Early referral to wound specialists improves outcomes. Transparency, documentation, and patient support are essential components of expert management. Transient neurological and visual symptoms are among the most distinctive complications of foam sclerotherapy. These include scintillating scotomas, blurred vision, migraine-like aura, dizziness, and transient sensory disturbances. Symptoms typically resolve within minutes to hours but can be alarming. The prevailing mechanism involves microembolic passage of foam bubbles into the cerebral circulation, often facilitated by right-to-left shunts such as patent foramen ovale. Risk increases with larger foam volumes, air-based foam, rapid injection, and inadequate flow control Prevention strategies in expert practice include strict limitation of foam volume, preference for nitrogen-free gas, slow ultrasound-guided injection, avoidance of Valsalva maneuvers, and almost immediate ambulation during injection. In high-risk patients, those with migraine with aura or known shunts, liquid sclerosant, or alternative treatment modalities should be considered. Management is supportive. Patients should be placed supine, reassured and monitored until symptom resolution. Persistent or focal neurological deficits warrant formal neurological evaluation. Pre-procedure counseling significantly reduces patient anxiety and improves tolerance of transient symptoms. Deep vein thrombosis after foam sclerotherapy are rare but clinically significant complications. Incidence remains low in experienced hands but increases with extensive truncal treatment, excessive foam volume, proximity to deep venous junctions, and patient-specific thrombophilic risk factors. Prevention relies on meticulous technique and patient selection. Experts limit foam volume, avoid forceful injection near junctions, use ultrasound to monitor foam propagation in real time, encourage early ambulation and appropriate compression. Routine post-procedure duplex ultrasound is recommended after truncal foam sclerotherapy or in high-risk patients. Early detection of non-occlusive thrombus extension allows conservative management with surveillance or anticoagulation when indicated. Crucially, experts distinguish clinically significant DVT from benign, localized thrombosis within treated veins. Overdiagnosis leads to unnecessary anticoagulation and patient anxiety, whereas under-recognition may delay critical intervention. It's fundamental to always obtain a proper individual thrombotic risk assessment, highlighting each and every single patient characteristics. In expert sclerotherapy practice, complications are neither inevitable nor entirely avoidable. They are signals of imbalance between sclerosant effect, vein biology and post-treatment conditions. Mastery lies in anticipating these imbalances, minimizing their occurrence, recognizing them early, and responding with informed, proportionate strategies. When managed skillfully, even complications can reinforce patient trust, demonstrate clinical expertise and ultimately improve long-term outcomes.

7 Special Clinical Scenarios

In advanced venous practice, sclerotherapy reveals its greatest value not in straightforward primary disease, but in complex, heterogeneous, and non-standard clinical scenarios. These situations challenge rigid algorithms and reward adaptability, precision, and clinical judgment. Recurrent disease, obesity, perforator incompetence and cosmetic microvascular pathology each present unique anatomical, hemodynamic and patient-related constraints that fundamentally alter treatment strategy. For vascular experts, these scenarios highlight sclerotherapy's defining strength: its capacity to be tailored. When applied with insight and restraint, sclerotherapy becomes not a fallback option, but the most logical and effective intervention where other modalities lose precision or increase morbidity. Recurrent varicose veins constitute one of the most technically demanding and conceptually complex indications in venous disease management. Unlike primary varicosities, recurrence is rarely driven by a single dominant reflux source. Instead, it reflects a combination of altered venous anatomy, adaptive hemodynamics and prior intervention–related changes. After surgical stripping, recurrence is frequently associated with neovascularization at former junctional sites. These neovessels are characteristically tortuous, thin-walled and low-flow, making them poorly suited to repeat surgery or thermal ablation. Duplex ultrasound typically demonstrates irregular, serpiginous channels with limited axial continuity. Ultrasound-guided foam sclerotherapy (UGFS), when performed with low volumes and careful flow control, allows selective targeting of these vessels with minimal trauma. Following endovenous thermal ablation, recurrence more often results from untreated tributaries, perforator incompetence or segmental recanalization rather than true neovascularization. In this context, sclerotherapy enables focused treatment of residual reflux without re-entering fibrotic or ablated segments, reducing procedural complexity and patient discomfort. Expert management of recurrence begins with exhaustive duplex mapping. Treating all reflux indiscriminately risks disrupting compensatory drainage and exacerbating symptoms. Instead, experts prioritize hemodynamically relevant targets correlated with symptoms, often accepting residual reflux in non-dominant pathways. Staged, low-volume foam injections are favored to maintain control and minimize complications. Obesity introduces a constellation of challenges that significantly influence sclerotherapy strategy. Increased subcutaneous adiposity alters vein depth, reduces ultrasound resolution and increases venous pressure, all of which affect sclerosant distribution and durability of closure. Additionally, calf muscle pump inefficiency and reduced mobility contribute to persistent venous hypertension. From a technical perspective, ultrasound guidance is essential. Visual cues are unreliable and veins that appear superficial may in fact be deeply embedded. Longer needles are often required, increasing the importance of precise needle-tip visualization and low-pressure injection to avoid extravasation. Foam sclerotherapy is frequently preferred due to its superior efficacy in larger, deeper veins, but strict volume discipline is mandatory. Compression therapy is often less effective or poorly tolerated in obese patients due to fit issues, discomfort and difficulty donning garments. Expert practitioners compensate by optimizing vein emptying, adjusting sclerosant concentration conservatively and favoring staged treatments rather than attempting extensive correction in a single session Equally important is expectation management. While symptomatic improvement is commonly achievable, cosmetic outcomes may be limited by vein depth and overlying tissue. Experts align treatment goals with physiological realities, emphasizing function over appearance when appropriate, which improves patient satisfaction despite inherent limitations. Incompetent perforator veins occupy a nuanced position in venous disease management. While many incompetent perforators are clinically insignificant, selected perforators contribute meaningfully to localized venous hypertension, recurrent varicosities, and chronic venous skin changes. Sclerotherapy, particularly ultrasound-guided foam sclerotherapy, offers a minimally invasive option for perforator treatment, especially in patients unsuitable for surgical ligation or thermal ablation. Foam allows effective endothelial contact within short, often tortuous multi-branched perforator segments embedded in fibrotic tissue. Expert technique emphasizes precise localization, minimal foam volume and continuous ultrasound monitoring. Limb elevation and manual compression reduce flow and enhance sclerosant efficacy. Injection is halted immediately if foam approaches the deep venous system, reinforcing the principle that perforator treatment demands restraint. Outcome assessment should be clinical rather than purely anatomical. Symptom improvement, reduction in localized edema, and stabilization of skin changes are more meaningful endpoints than complete perforator obliteration. Experts accept partial closure or functional improvement as success, particularly in advanced chronic venous disease.

8 Telangiectasias vs. Reticular Veins: Different Tactics

Although frequently addressed together, telangiectasias and reticular veins represent distinct therapeutic targets requiring different strategies. Failure to differentiate between them is a common cause of suboptimal cosmetic outcomes and patient dissatisfaction. Telangiectasias are superficial, low-volume vessels treated almost exclusively for cosmetic reasons. Liquid sclerotherapy with very low sclerosant concentrations remains the gold standard. Foam is generally unnecessary and may increase the risk of matting and pigmentation. Precision, minimal volume, and gentle injection technique are paramount. Reticular veins are larger, deeper, and often serve as feeder vessels for telangiectatic networks. Treating telangiectasias without addressing underlying reticular veins frequently leads to recurrence or matting. Expert practice therefore prioritizes reticular vein treatment first, often using slightly higher concentrations or foam, followed by delayed cosmetic treatment of residual telangiectasias. Staged treatment and patience are essential, as aggressive pursuit of immediate cosmetic perfection often worsens outcomes. In expert sclerotherapy practice, special clinical scenarios are not deviations from standard care but tests of clinical maturity and judgment. Recurrent disease, obesity, perforator incompetence, and cosmetic microvascular pathology each demand tailored strategies that balance efficacy, safety, and patient expectations. Sclerotherapy's unique strength lies in its adaptability; when applied with insight and discipline, it becomes the modality of choice precisely where rigid techniques reach their limits.

9 Post-procedure Follow-Up and Retreatment

In expert sclerotherapy practice, the post-procedural phase is not an epilogue but a decisive continuation of treatment. Unlike thermal ablation or surgery, where success is often judged immediately, sclerotherapy is intrinsically biological, progressive, and iterative. Vein closure, fibrosis, recanalization, and hemodynamic redistribution unfold over weeks to months, and the final clinical outcome is shaped as much by post-treatment decisions as by the injection itself (Table 15.8).

Table 15.8 Post-procedural practical suggestions

Practical suggestions	
Post-procedural	1. Certified compression matters
	2. Validated venous active drugs matters
	3. Life-style matter
	4. Follow-up in 2–3 weeks with eventual trapped blood drainage
	5. Do not act aggressively immediately after hyperpigmentation
	6. Do act rapidly after matting to find the eventually left behind feeding veins
	7. Customized follow up based on the specific case, yet it's appropriate to have at leat one in the first few weeks

For vascular specialists, follow-up is therefore an active interpretive process, integrating duplex findings, symptom evolution, cosmetic change and patient expectations. Poor follow-up strategy is a common source of overtreatment, unnecessary complications, and dissatisfaction. Conversely, thoughtful observation and selective retreatment allow sclerotherapy to reach its full therapeutic potential with minimal intervention. Duplex ultrasound is indispensable after sclerotherapy but its value depends entirely on when it is performed and how its findings are interpreted. Inexperienced use of ultrasound risks transforming a powerful tool into a driver of overtreatment. Early post-treatment ultrasound, typically within 7–14 days, is most useful for safety assessment rather than efficacy judgment. At this stage, ultrasound allows exclusion of deep vein thrombosis or junctional thrombus extension, identification of excessive retained thrombus within treated veins, confirmation of correct target engagement after ultrasound-guided foam sclerotherapy, particularly in truncal veins, perforators or high-risk patients. However, expert clinicians recognize that early ultrasound findings are provisional.

Residual flow, partial compressibility or echogenic intraluminal material at this stage often reflects normal post-sclerotherapy evolution rather than failure. Inflammatory thrombosis, early organization and partial recanalization may still progress to durable fibrosis over subsequent weeks. Delayed ultrasound assessment, commonly at 6–12 weeks, provides a more reliable evaluation of treatment durability and hemodynamic impact. At this time point, experts assess persistence or abolition of reflux, degree of vein shrinkage, collateral formation or flow redistribution and relationship between duplex findings and clinical improvement. Crucially, duplex findings must never be interpreted in isolation. Asymptomatic residual reflux or partial recanalization often warrants observation, not intervention. Multiple studies demonstrate poor correlation between complete duplex occlusion and patient-reported outcomes, particularly in cosmetic and tributary treatments. Expert follow-up protocols therefore individualize ultrasound timing based on vein type and size, foam volume and proximity to deep veins, patient thrombotic risk and clinical response. One of the clearest markers of expertise in sclerotherapy is the ability to resist unnecessary retreatment. The temptation to pursue anatomical perfection, particularly when duplex abnormalities persist, is a common driver of complications, including hyperpigmentation, matting and thrombophlebitis. Expert clinicians prioritize clinical endpoints: symptom relief, functional improvement, stabilization or improvement of skin changes and patient-perceived cosmetic benefit. If these goals have been achieved, observation is often the correct choice, even when residual veins or reflux remain detectable on ultrasound. Evidence consistently shows that complete anatomical closure is neither necessary nor sufficient for patient satisfaction. Retreatment becomes appropriate when residual or recurrent veins are clearly symptomatic, hemodynamically dominant on duplex, cosmetically unacceptable to the patient or associated with progression of chronic venous disease. Timing is critical. Retreatment performed too early, before inflammation subsides and vein remodeling stabilizes, significantly increases complication risk. Experts generally wait at least 6–8 weeks before retreating the same venous segment, unless intervention is required to manage complications such as painful thrombosis or retained clot. Before retreatment, experts reassess the original strategy rather than simply escalating dose or volume. Persistent disease often reflects untreated feeder veins, underestimated flow dynamics, suboptimal access points or insufficient post-procedural compression. Retreatment without addressing these factors merely repeats the same limitations. Partial or suboptimal responses are not failures, but expected outcomes in a biologically variable treatment. Vein wall characteristics, flow velocity, patient activity level, hormonal factors and compliance with compression all influence response magnitude and speed. Expert management begins with classification of the response partial occlusion with symptom resolution, partial occlusion with persistent symptoms, early recanalization after initial closure, cosmetic persistence without functional relevance. Each category requires a different approach. Observation alone is often sufficient in cases where symptoms have resolved, as continued fibrosis may occur over time. In contrast, persistent symptoms with partial occlusion may justify targeted retreatment. When retreatment is indicated, experts do not simply repeat the original protocol. Instead, they analyze why the response was incomplete and adapt accordingly. This may involve modifying sclerosant concentration, switching between liquid and foam, altering gas composition or foam volume, improving vein emptying and positioning, selecting alternative access points or staging treatment more conservatively. Patient communication is central to managing partial responses. Clear explanation that sclerotherapy is often a process rather than a single event improves satisfaction and reduces pressure for premature retreatment. Unrealistic expectations of immediate or total anatomical resolution are among the most common causes of dissatisfaction and unnecessary intervention In expert sclerotherapy practice, post-procedure follow-up is where technical intervention is translated into durable clinical success. Duplex ultrasound must be used judiciously, retreatment decisions must be guided by symptoms and hemodynamics rather than imaging alone and partial responses must be analyzed rather than reflexively corrected. Mastery lies in recognizing that effective sclerotherapy is defined not by immediate closure but by sustained symptom relief, acceptable cosmetic outcome and the disciplined avoidance of unnecessary treatment.

10 Expert Tricks and Personal Practice Insights

Expert practice is not defined by technical bravado, but by economy of action, consistency of reasoning and disciplined restraint. One of the most powerful expert adjustments is temporal discipline. Experts slow down at every critical step: ultrasound mapping, access, injection, and follow-up decisions. This deliberate pacing allows subtle cues (vein recoil, foam behavior, patient discomfort) to guide micro-adjustments in real time. Rushing is one of the most consistent predictors of avoidable complications. Another high-impact adjustment is doing less per session. Treating shorter vein segments, using smaller sclerosant volumes and staging interventions reduces inflammatory burden and improves long-term outcomes. Experienced practitioners often achieve better closure rates with multiple conservative sessions than with a single aggressive treatment. Vein emptying is frequently underestimated. Minor changes in limb elevation angle, manual compression technique, or patient posture immediately before injection can dramatically alter sclerosant efficiency. Experts reassess vein filling immediately before injection rather than relying on ultrasound findings obtained minutes earlier. Access strategy refinement also yields disproportionate benefits. Selecting puncture sites that favor controlled, antegrade propagation, even if technically more demanding, reduces unintended spread and improves uniform endothelial contact. Experts are willing to reposition, re-puncture or abandon suboptimal access rather than compromise control. A further subtle adjustment is session closure discipline. Experts resist the urge to "use up" prepared foam or sclerosant. The decision to stop injecting is treated as a technical skill in itself. When foam behavior becomes unpredictable, resistance increases or patient feedback changes, experts end the session, even if theoretical capacity remains. Experience reduces novice errors but introduces more subtle risks. One of the most common is ultrasound absolutism: the tendency to treat every visible reflux signal. Experts periodically recalibrate by prioritizing symptoms, hemodynamic relevance and patient goals over duplex perfection. Treating ultrasound findings in isolation is a leading cause of overtreatment. Another frequent pitfall is dose escalation reflex. When outcomes are suboptimal, even experienced operators may instinctively increase sclerosant concentration or foam volume. In reality, incomplete response more often reflects flow dynamics, access limitations, vein depth or compression issues rather than insufficient chemical potency. Dose escalation frequently increases complications without improving efficacy. Inconsistency is another expert-level hazard. Minor variations in foam preparation, injection speed, or compression advice may seem trivial but accumulate across sessions and patients. Experts strive for high internal consistency, so that when outcomes differ, the cause is easier to identify. Premature retreatment remains a persistent error. Even seasoned practitioners may feel pressure, internal or patient-driven, to act before biological remodeling has stabilized. Retreatment in an inflamed or partially thrombosed vein increases the risk of pigmentation, matting and thrombophlebitis. Finally, experts may underestimate the need for repetitive patient education. Familiarity with the procedure can lead clinicians to abbreviate explanations. However, sclerotherapy's iterative nature makes repeated reinforcement of expectations, timelines, and limitations essential, even for returning patients. While sclerotherapy expertise cannot be rushed, the learning curve can be made safer and more efficient. One of the most effective accelerators is structured self-review. Experts regularly analyze cases with suboptimal outcomes or complications, focusing not on blame but on identifying modifiable variables. This reflective practice is far more valuable than reviewing successes alone. Developing a personal system early is another shortcut. Standardizing foam preparation ratios, preferred access devices, injection pacing, and compression/venous active drugs prescriptions reduces cognitive load and highlights deviations that correlate with outcomes. Flexibility is preserved, but within a stable baseline. Mentorship remains irreplaceable. Observing experienced practitioners reveals non-verbalized skills (probe pressure modulation, needle angulation, injection rhythm) that are rarely captured in textbooks. Conversely, teaching sclerotherapy to trainees forces experts to articulate implicit knowledge and often exposes their own habits to scrutiny. Simulation and deliberate practice, particularly for ultrasound-guided access in difficult anatomy, significantly reduce early complication rates. Experts also advise starting conservatively: lower concentrations, smaller volumes, shorter segments. Confidence should grow from pattern recognition, not from early technical ambition. A critical psychological milestone in the learning curve is accepting that not every vein should be treated. Developing the confidence to defer treatment, recommend observation or redirect patients to alternative modalities is a hallmark of maturation. Mastery includes knowing when intervention adds no value. In advanced sclerotherapy practice, expertise is defined less by expanding technical repertoire and more by refining judgment. Small, experience-driven adjustments, applied consistently, have a greater impact than dramatic technical changes. Awareness of subtle pitfalls prevents complacency, while reflective practice accelerates growth. Ultimately, the most valuable expert insight is learning to do *just enough*: never considering teleangectasia as a starting easy point for beginners, treating veins with precision, patients with clarity and complications with foresight, while resisting the impulse to intervene simply because one can.

11 Clinical Example

11.1 Foam Sclerotherapy of the Great Saphenous Vein Using a Standard Central Venous Catheter (Practical and Personal Tips and Tricks to Improve Clinical Outcomes)

11.1.1 Clinical Case and Iconography Provided by Rodrigo Rial

A 53-year-old patient presents with great saphenous vein (GSV) insufficiency, 6 mm in diameter, from sapheno-femoral junction (SFJ) to the upper third of the leg. The patient wishes to avoid any sick leave. Cyanoacrylate glue closure was offered as an option but was declined due to financial reasons. We proceeded with foam sclerotherapy using a central venous catheter.

The required materials are easy to obtain. A single- or double-lumen central venous catheter is used, typically measuring 20 cm in length. To utilize this technique, a minimum length of the insufficient saphenous vein segment is required to allow the catheter tip to be positioned approximately 8–10 cm from the SFJ (Fig. 15.4).

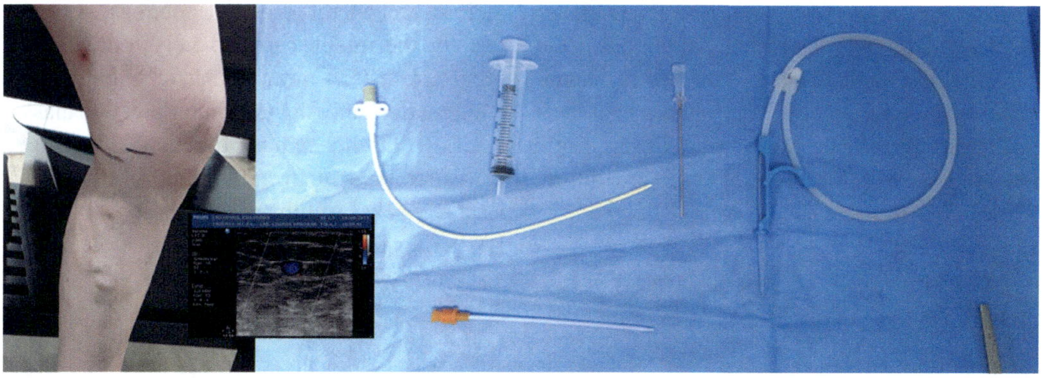

Fig. 15.4 Tributaries with marked saphenous puncture site. Single-lumen central venous catheter

The puncture is performed using a standard Seldinger venin canalization (local anesthesia), advancing the guidewire and the catheter until they are positioned within the safety margin (8–10 cm).

Trick: An *elastic tourniquet* (those used for vein puncture for blood test) is utilized to reduce flow through the saphenous vein; this way, the foam remains more stationary by decreasing the yield stress (Fig. 15.5).

Trick: Since foam degrades upon contact with blood, the lumen intended for injection is *flushed with saline solution* prior to the procedure. If possible, chilled, to induce moderate vasospasm. The use of heparinized saline is optional (Fig. 15.2).

Tip: The standard Tessari technique (air/gas ratio 1:4 and 20 passes between the 10 ml syringes) is performed using 3% polidocanol and a *small amount of glycerin* (easily obtained as a compounded formula from pharmacies) to achieve a solution with 1.6% glycerin. The recommendation is to add 0.2 ml of the 20% glycerin compounded formula to 2 ml of 3% polidocanol. This yields a 1.6% glycerin solution while the sclerosant concentration does not effectively decrease, remaining at practically 3%.

Tip: In the last passes the foam can be passed through a *0.5-micron filter* to improve homogeneity and reduce bubble size and increase stability.

First injection with 3 ml of foam (catheter takes almost 1 ml). Ultrasound monitoring the correct progression of foam to the SFJ is mandatory. Once a clear acoustic shadow has been produced at the SFJ, apply transverse gentle compression with the probe 2 cm below during 1 min.

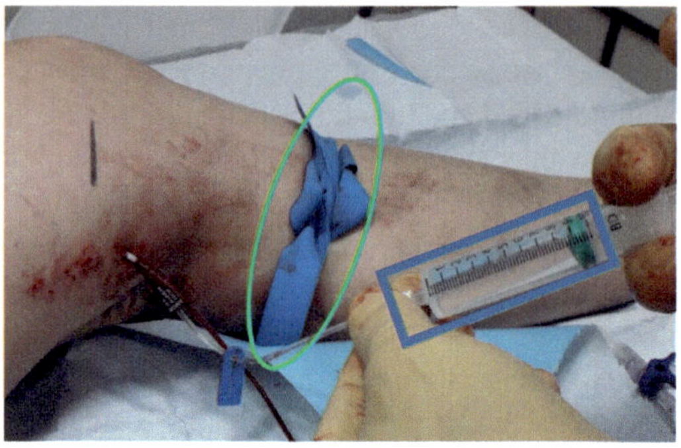

Fig. 15.5 Tourniquet and flushing the vein with normal saline

Tip: After the first injection, withdraw the catheter 5–10 cm, wait *one or two minutes before proceeding with the second one*. This will induce significant vasospasm of the saphenous vein, which will help prevent the foam from entering the deep venous system during subsequent injections of 2 ml each (Fig. 15.3).

Trick: Before proceeding with subsequent injections (1–2 min interval), the Tessari technique should be repeated. This ensures that freshly prepared foam is used at each injection site (Fig 15.6).

Excessive Trendelenburg positioning during injection is controversial because it may favor distal migration of the foam, thereby reducing effective contact with the proximal part of GSV.

Tip: My recommendation is a *maximum of 10° Trendelenburg* or a horizontal position.

Post-procedural recommendations: Relative rest for the minutes immediately following the procedure (5 min). Elastic thigh-length compression stocking (AG), compression class II (CCL-2). Do not remove during the first night; thereafter, wear it from morning to night for at least 2 weeks. Antithrombotic prophylaxis with LMWH or DOACs depends on risk scale.

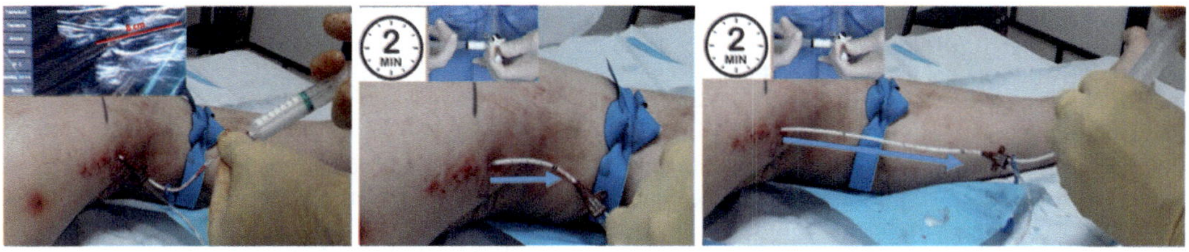

Fig. 15.6 Withdraw the catheter between 5 and 10 cm after each injection, with a wait time of 1–2 min, repeating the Tessari technique each time

12 Discussion

There is limited material specifically designed for catheter-directed foam sclerotherapy, and it is not always available. The off-label use of central venous catheters for this purpose does not pose any risk. Introducer sheaths can also be used. Intravenous catheters may be utilized for insufficient saphenous veins with a shorter course. This procedure is very similar to previously published ones, but without the use of tumescence and with some added contributions. While tumescence undoubtedly must have a positive effect, it is difficult to determine its actual impact on the final outcome. What is certain is that it lengthens the procedure and increases patient discomfort. We have been modifying the technique, evolving from a simultaneous catheter withdrawal and continuous foam injection to the current technique, which we consider to be more refined and precise. Aids for increasing foam stability, whether physical (such as the filter) or chemical (such as glycerin or surfactants in general), are simple to use and reproducible. Procedure safety is essential, and controlling foam volumes is very important. A precise calculation of the foam volume (square radius $\times \pi \times$ length) is not necessary, as it also depends on positioning; however, in cases of significantly larger or smaller diameters, it may be necessary to make adjustments to the described volumes. The use of antithrombotic prophylaxis with anticoagulant drugs at prophylactic doses will depend on the Caprini risk score and the recommendations made by sclerotherapy consensus guidelines. Related readings are suggested [8–13].

References

1. Gianesini S, Chi YW, Agüero C, et al. Fake-news-free evidence-based communication for proper vein-lymphatic disease management. Int Angiol. 2023;42(2):89–189.
2. Gianesini S, Danese M, AlQedrah D, et al. Multi-specialty recommendations for the appropriate and affordable lower limb vein-lymphatic disorders management. Int Ang. 2026;45(1):1–64.
3. Tan MKH, Salim S, Onida S, et al. Postsclerotherapy compression: a systematic review. J Vasc Surg Venous Lymphat Disord. 2021 Jan;9(1):264–74.
4. Gianesini S, Occhionorelli S, Menegatti E, et al. CHIVA strategy in chronic venous disease treatment: instructions for users. Phlebology. 2015;30(3):157–71.
5. Gianesini S, Menegatti E, Tacconi G, et al. Echo-guided foam sclerotherapy treatment of venous malformation involving the sciatic nerve. Phlebology. 2009 Feb;24(1):46–7.
6. Gianesini S, Occhiorelli S, Menegatti E, et al. Femoral vein valve incompetence as a risk factor for junctional recurrence. Phlebology. 2018;33(3):206–12.
7. Gianesini S, Obi A, Onida S, et al. Global guidelines trends and controversies in lower limb venous and lymphatic disease: narrative literature revision and experts' opinions following the vWINter international meeting in phlebology, lymphology & aesthetics, 23–25 January 2019. Phlebology. 2019;34(1 Suppl):4–66.
8. Rabe E, Breu FX, Cavezzi A, et al. Guideline Group. European guidelines for sclerotherapy in chronic venous disorders. Phlebology. 2014;29(6):338–54. https://doi.org/10.1177/0268355513483280. Epub 2013 May 3. PMID: 23559590.
9. Wong M, Parsi K, Myers K, et al. Sclerotherapy of lower limb veins: indications, contraindications and treatment strategies to prevent complications – a consensus document of the International Union of Phlebology-2023. Phlebology. 2023;38(4):205–58. https://doi.org/10.1177/02683555231151350. Epub 2023 Mar 14. PMID: 36916540.
10. Cavezzi A, Mosti G, Campana F, et al. Catheter foam sclerotherapy of the great saphenous vein, with perisaphenous tumescence infiltration and saphenous irriga-

tion. Eur J Vasc Endovasc Surg. 2017;54(5):629–35. https://doi.org/10.1016/j.ejvs.2017.08.004. Epub 2017 Sep 18. Erratum in: Eur J Vasc Endovasc Surg. 2018;55(5):745. doi:10.1016/j.ejvs.2018.03.001. PMID: 28927554.
11. Shirazi AR, Goldman M. The use of a 5-microm filter hub increases foam stability when using the double syringe technique. Dermatologic Surg. 2008;34:91–2.
12. Peterson JD, Goldman MP. An investigation on the influence of glycerin on sclerosant foam stability. Phlebology. 2011;26(6):232–4. https://doi.org/10.1258/phleb.2010.010028. Epub 2011 Mar 17. PMID: 21415429.
13. Rial R, Hervas LS, Monux G, Galindo A, Martin A, Hernando M, Martinez I, Hernando A, Serrano FJ. Polidocanol foam stability in terms of its association with glycerin. Phlebology. 2014;29(5):304–9. https://doi.org/10.1177/0268355513477858. Epub 2013 May 3. PMID: 23470491.

16 Considerations on Medical Technological Advancement and Their Regulation

Javier Palma, Yung Wei Chi, and Sergio Gianesini

1 Introduction

The development of new medical technology often begins with the identification of an unmet clinical need. In the field of venous disease, this need became evident in the early 1990s: conventional sclerotherapy achieved satisfactory results in small vessels but proved inadequate for larger veins. From this limitation emerged an innovative process combining clinical observation, pharmaceutical insight, and technical development.Over the past fourteen years, our work has focused on creating a system capable of generating safe, homogeneous, pharmaceutical-grade, and reproducible sclerosant microfoam. The M-FOAMER was conceived to expand the therapeutic potential of sclerotherapy through controlled and standardized preparation.

The origin of this development traces back to the work of Drs. Juan Cabrera Garrido and Juan Cabrera García-Olmedo, who together described and patented in 1993 the technique of sclerosant microfoam (U.S. Patent 5,676,962) [1]. Their joint contribution marked both a technical milestone and a conceptual transformation: venous insufficiency could now be treated with precisely prepared microfoam under reproducible safety parameters.

Since then, sclerotherapy has evolved from a manual, operator-dependent procedure into a controlled process defined by measurable variables such as pressure, flow rate, and gas composition. The replacement of atmospheric air with physiological gas mixtures free of nitrogen concentrations potentially harmful to patients was a decisive step in improving safety and tolerance. The current objective is to produce microfoam with a consistent pharmaceutical profile, minimizing procedural variability.

Such progress has been made possible through collaboration between clinicians, formulation experts, and engineers, a synergy that has reshaped the conception of therapeutic technologies. Several international research groups, including those led by Cavezzi, Morrison, Coleridge-Smith, Guex, and Gillet, demonstrated that gas optimization, microfoam stability, and reproducibility are key determinants of both safety and efficacy [2–5].

The evolution of sclerotherapy illustrates how technological innovation acquires its fullest meaning when it enhances clinical practice, while keeping the patient at the center of progress (Fig. 16.1).

J. Palma
Independent Lawyer, Granada, Spain

Y. W. Chi
Department of Cardiovascular Medicine, University of California, Davis Vascular Center, Sacramento, CA, USA
e-mail: ywchi@ucdavis.edu

S. Gianesini (✉)
Department of Translational Medicine, University of Ferrara, Ferrara, Italy

Department of Surgery, Uniformed Services University of Health Sciences, Bethesda, MD, USA
e-mail: gnssrg@unife.it

S. Gianesini, Y. W. Chi (eds.), *Sclerotherapy*, https://doi.org/10.1007/978-3-032-32794-9_16

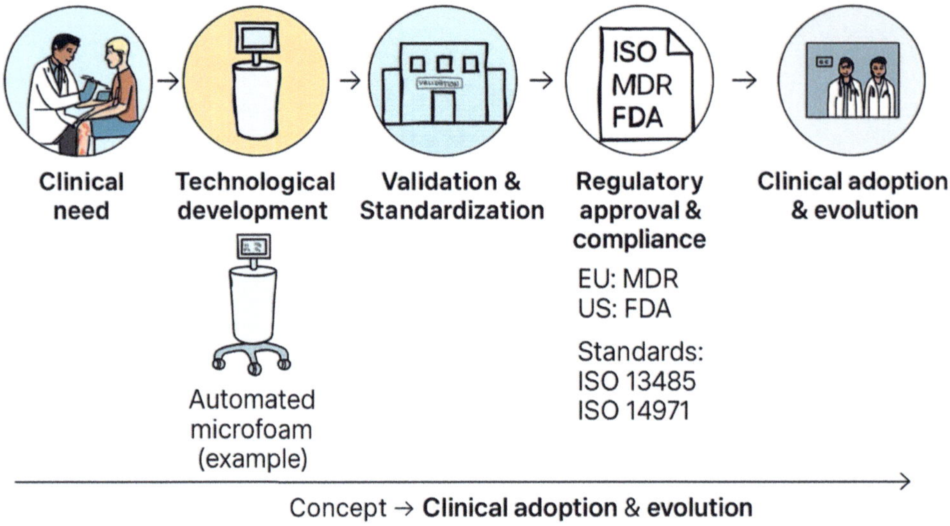

Fig. 16.1 Technological integration pathway in sclerotherapy

This figure summarizes the evolution of sclerotherapy technology—from clinical observation and identification of therapeutic limitations to the development of automated systems for controlled microfoam preparation. It highlights how medical need, engineering design, validation, and regulatory coordination converge toward reproducible and standardized treatment.

The diagram illustrates the conceptual pathway that leads from initial clinical observation toward the regulated and automated generation of microfoam in sclerotherapy.

2 Technological and Conceptual Evolution of Sclerotherapy

Following the first clinical experiences of the 1990s, led by the Cabrera group, various manual methods for preparing sclerosant foam became widespread. The most popular was the Tessari method (2000), which used two syringes connected by a three-way stopcock and controlled agitation to obtain a stable microfoam [6]. Its simplicity encouraged rapid adoption, although variability persisted in bubble size and foam density. In most cases, atmospheric air was employed as the gas phase—rich in nitrogen, a poorly soluble gas that prolongs bubble persistence within the venous system. This persistence increased the risk of gas microemboli or paradoxical passage into the arterial circulation in patients with right–left shunts. Replacing air with physiological gases—mixtures of carbon dioxide and oxygen—greatly improved solubility and clinical safety. In the early 2000s, research groups from Harvard Medical School, the University of Oxford, the University of Ferrara, and Imperial College London performed in-depth studies on the physics and hemodynamics of sclerosant foams [7, 8]. Their findings established a clear relationship between bubble size, temporal stability, and clinical efficacy, confirming that the physicochemical quality of the foam determines therapeutic outcomes.

The need for reproducibility led to the development of closed systems capable of precisely controlling gas-to-liquid ratio, pressure, and mixing temperature. A decisive turning point came in 2013, when the U.S. FDA approved Varithena® (BTG plc), the first endovenous microfoam authorized for therapeutic use [9]. Varithena was developed in direct collaboration with the Cabrera group, translating clinical expertise into an industrially reproducible pharmaceutical for-

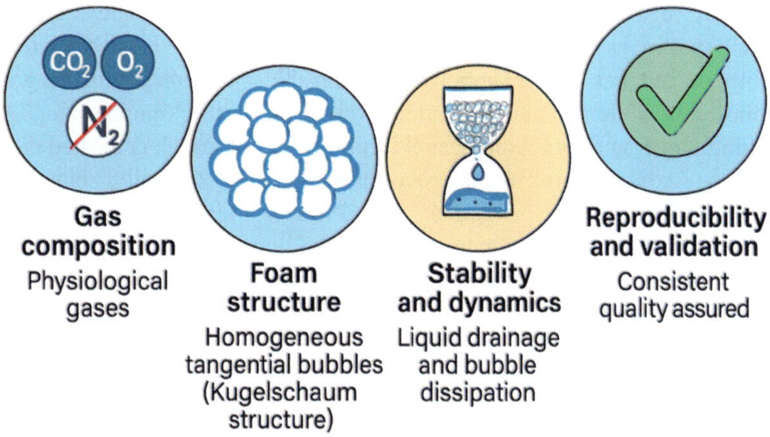

Fig. 16.2 Controlled microfoam generation: Key parameters

mulation. This achievement demonstrated that sterile, stable, and consistent microfoam could be produced under pharmaceutical-grade conditions. The use of physiological gases (CO_2/O_2) further improved safety and marked the transition from manual practice to controlled, validated production.

Over the past decade, digital technologies and computational modeling have provided tools to characterize microfoam generation and performance with greater precision.

Multidisciplinary teams across Europe, North America, and Asia have applied controlled-pressure systems, data logging, and algorithmic analysis to quantify stability, reproducibility, and other quality parameters under laboratory conditions. Although no system currently performs real-time telemetry or clinical traceability during microfoam preparation, these studies form the scientific basis for future automated systems ensuring consistent therapeutic results (Fig. 16.2).

This figure identifies the parameters that determine the quality of sclerosant microfoam: bubble size and distribution, half-life, drainage velocity, gas-to-liquid ratio, gas composition (CO_2/O_2, excluding N_2), and injection conditions. Together, these define foam stability, safety, and reproducibility.

Alt text: Infographic showing the key physical and chemical parameters that govern sclerosant foam generation.

3 Regulatory Framework and Certification of Medical Technologies in Sclerotherapy

The regulation of medical technologies seeks to ensure patient safety and consistent performance. In sclerotherapy, where pharmaceutical science, engineering, and clinical application converge, regulation must integrate all these dimensions. Over the last decade, the international regulatory environment has evolved toward harmonized systems that assess innovation proportionally to risk—encouraging progress without compromising safety. In the European context, Regulation (EU) 2017/745 (MDR) provides the main legislative framework for medical devices. Technologies related to sclerotherapy fall under several categories, depending on their intended use:

- *Laboratory equipment*, designed for microfoam preparation or testing without patient contact, certified under CE marking (IEC 61010-1, Directives 2014/35/EU and 2014/30/EU).
- *Medical accessories*, assisting during the procedure and classified according to intended use (MDR, Article 2.2).
- *Active medical devices*, directly involved in treatment and subject to MDR conformity assessment pathways according to their risk class.

This regulatory differentiation ensures that each system is evaluated according to its true purpose and risk level, supporting responsible innovation while maintaining patient protection. Within this framework, polidocanol formulations such as Aethoxysklerol® are approved as medicinal products whose Summary of Product Characteristics explicitly permits their use in foam form for venous disease [10]. This provides a well-defined pharmaceutical basis for clinical foam preparation and represents a distinctive feature of the European regulatory landscape. In the United States, the FDA follows a parallel philosophy of risk-based evaluation. Two regulatory pathways apply to technologies related to sclerotherapy:

- *Drug–device combination products*, such as Varithena® (BTG plc, NDA 205098), evaluated through a pharmaceutical regulatory process that includes the device component.
- *Independent preparation devices*, such as automated microfoam generators using previously approved drugs. These fall under 21 CFR 880.5440 (Intravascular Administration Set, product code NEP), classified as Class II devices exempt from premarket notification [11].

Both pathways coexist, reflecting complementary strategies for technological advancement—one integrating drug and device components, the other emphasizing reproducibility and safety through dedicated engineering.

Globally, convergence among regulatory systems is progressing through standards such as ISO 13485, ISO 14971, ISO 10993-1, IEC 62304, IEC 62366-1, and IEC 61010-1, which establish shared principles for quality, safety, and usability. Initiatives such as the International Medical Device Regulators Forum (IMDRF) promote mutual recognition of audits and documentation, reducing redundancy and streamlining regulatory approvals. Validation of microfoam-generation systems focuses on reproducibility, compatibility, and process control in accordance with these standards. The assessment of parameters such as bubble characteristics, gas-to-liquid ratio, gas composition, and injection conditions provides measurable evidence of safety and stability. These parameters bridge engineering precision with clinical reliability and lay the foundation for the next phase: scientific validation (Fig. 16.3).

This infographic compares the European regulatory framework under MDR 2017/745—characterized by device classification, conformity assessment, and CE marking—with the U.S. FDA

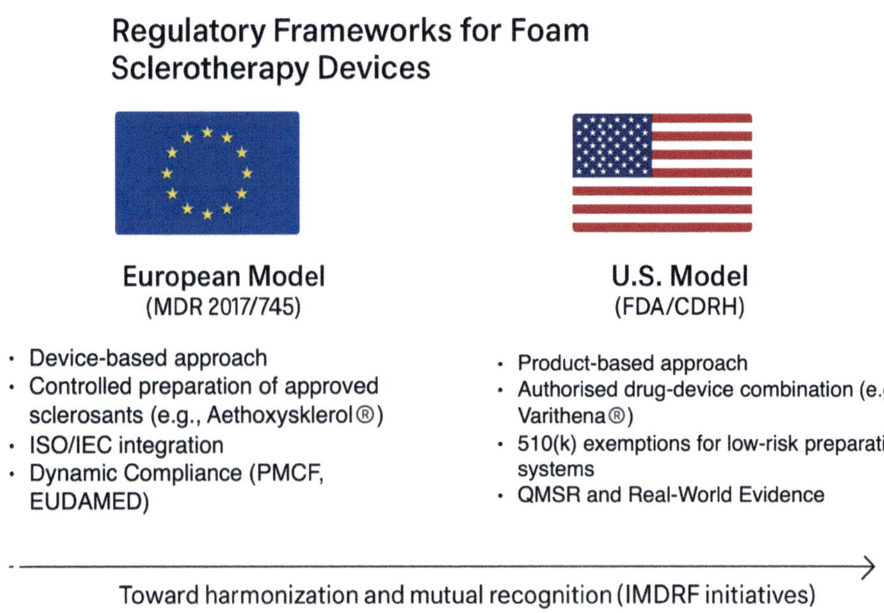

Fig. 16.3 Comparative regulatory models: EU and U.S. approaches

pathways that differentiate drug–device combinations from independent preparation systems. The figure also highlights areas of convergence through ISO/IEC harmonization and IMDRF initiatives.

Alt text: Diagram comparing European and U.S. regulatory models for microfoam-related devices, illustrating differences in regulatory pathways and points of convergence through international standards.

4 Validation, Standardization, and Reproducibility

After establishing the regulatory frameworks that govern microfoam technologies, the next step is validation—verifying through rigorous experimentation that engineering design translates into predictable and safe clinical performance. Validation in medicine is not a simple procedural step; it is the process of ensuring that performance is stable, measurable, and consistent under controlled conditions. In sclerotherapy, where therapeutic efficacy depends on finely tuned physical and chemical parameters, validation forms the bridge between technical design and clinical reliability. A system developed for controlled microfoam preparation must ensure uniform product quality, generating homogeneous, reproducible, and clinically safe microfoam. Validation transforms technical design into verifiable evidence, connecting engineering precision with patient safety and clinical trust. Technological validation of microfoam systems focuses on the control and measurement of key parameters internationally recognized as indicators of quality and stability. The most relevant include:

- *Mean Bubble Diameter (MBD)* (determines uniformity and gas retention)
- *Bubble Size Distribution (BSD)* (describes variability of bubble population)
- *Half-life ($t^{1/2}$)* (duration of structural integrity before drainage or coalescence)
- *Drainage Velocity* (rate of liquid–gas phase separation)
- *Gas-to-liquid Ratio* (defines density and compressibility)
- *Gas Composition* (solubility of CO_2/O_2 mixtures vs. nitrogen-rich air)
- *Injection Conditions* (pressure, rate, temperature influencing bubble formation and dispersion)

Each parameter must be assessed under repeatable laboratory conditions to ensure that microfoam characteristics remain consistent across production cycles and environments. Modern validation relies on advanced analytical tools. Dynamic foam analyzers, laser diffraction systems, and high-speed microscopy provide objective data on bubble structure and decay. These measurements correlate physical behavior with therapeutic effect, establishing a quantitative foundation for safety and performance evaluation. Compliance with international quality standards—including IEC 61010-1 (laboratory safety), IEC 60601-1 (electromedical safety), ISO 13485 (quality systems), and ISO 14971 (risk management)—ensures that design and documentation remain auditable and reproducible within the manufacturer's quality management system. Validation transcends mechanical verification; it generates scientific knowledge. By studying how physical and design parameters influence clinical outcomes, validation transforms empirical practice into structured understanding. Experimental data become reproducible evidence, and applied engineering evolves into a discipline grounded in measurable certainty. When laboratory results are reproducible and correlate with clinical observations, technology reaches scientific maturity. Validation thus unites technical rigor, therapeutic safety, and physician confidence. Validation, standardization, and reproducibility constitute the essential triangle of scientific credibility in microfoam technologies. They ensure that results arise not from chance but from controlled, documented, and repeatable processes. Regulatory oversight becomes the mechanism that transforms innovation into clinical confidence, consolidating the link between technology, evidence, and patient safety. These principles create the framework on which current pharmacological developments build, linking physical control with optimization of the biological response (Fig. 16.4).

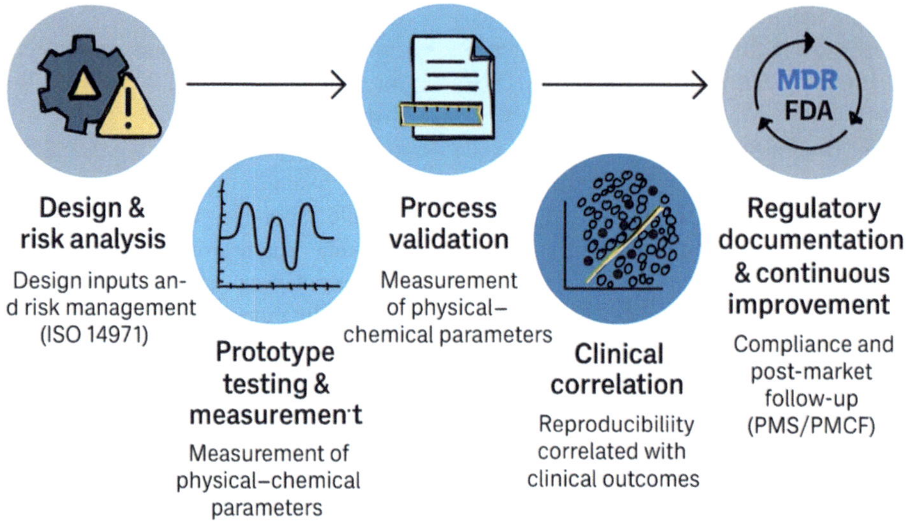

Fig. 16.4 Validation and standardization workflow

This diagram outlines the workflow for validation of microfoam systems—from design control and reproducibility testing to compliance with ISO/IEC standards and final conformity assessment.

Alt text: Flowchart showing stages of device validation, standardization, and regulatory conformity in medical microfoam technology.

5 Recent and Future of Pharmacological Research Applied to Microfoam

Over the past two decades, pharmacological research applied to microfoam has advanced considerably, providing a clearer understanding of how different sclerosant agents behave within the venous segments being treated. Foundational work from leading European and North American groups—including Cavezzi, Labropoulos, Morrison, Rabe, Guex, and Coleridge-Smith—has described the relationship between sclerosant concentration, contact time, and controlled endothelial injury [2–5, 7, 8]. These investigations, conducted through in vitro and ex vivo models, reproduce the interaction between the preparation and the venous wall under controlled conditions and have generated increasingly robust data on endothelial response.

In parallel, the physical behavior of microfoam has emerged as a key determinant of therapeutic consistency. Bubble size and uniformity, temporal stability, and the proportion between gas and liquid phases influence sclerosant distribution and the intensity of its pharmacological effect [2–4, 7]. Systematic observation of these variables has defined a technical process based on verifiable measurements, reducing variability and supporting a more predictable and standardized approach in clinical practice.

Current lines of research aim to refine the behavior of microfoam across different anatomical settings. Investigations include the use of physiological gas mixtures, modifications in density or viscosity, and agents capable of influencing the early inflammatory response [2–5]. These developments seek to adapt the preparation to the morphology and flow characteristics of each venous territory, enabling more precise and homogeneous applications in real-world practice.Complementing these advances, digital tools are providing an additional layer of knowledge. The aggregation of large multicenter datas-

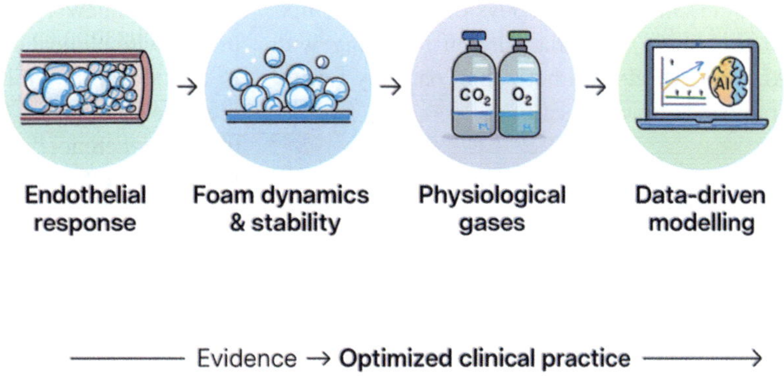

Fig. 16.5 Pharmacological research and future directions in microfoam

ets and their analysis using algorithmic methods enables the identification of patterns that previously escaped clinical observation. Artificial intelligence assists in linking anatomical characteristics, disease patterns, sclerosant concentrations, and preparation conditions with outcomes observed in daily practice [12, 13]. This approach broadens the clinician's ability to adjust treatment decisions to specific patient profiles and contributes to a more personalized application of microfoam techniques.

Feedback between laboratory work and clinical experience remains a central driver of progress. The systematic comparison of large series, the evaluation of treatment outcomes, and collaboration among centers generate insights that inform adjustments in preparation and administration [6]. As these data are incorporated into more structured working models, the technique becomes more stable and its variability decreases, translating into greater consistency and safety. Technological development in this area requires a structured and sustained process encompassing research, validation, manufacturing, certification, and clinical use. Each stage depends on resources, continuity, and the ability to maintain quality over time. Economic viability plays a decisive role in this progression by influencing the capacity to meet regulatory requirements, scale production, and sustain ongoing investigation [14, 15]. Designing a technological project with sustainability criteria from its earliest stages allows scientific advances to mature into practical, accessible solutions for clinicians, ensuring continuity within healthcare systems.

Regulatory frameworks evolve alongside these developments by requiring evidence that supports safety, stability, and reproducibility. Pharmacological research applied to microfoam is generating the parameters that may define future performance standards used by regulatory agencies [7, 9, 11, 16–18]. The combination of experimental data, process engineering, and multicenter analysis provides a solid foundation for establishing measurable criteria of efficacy and safety.

The convergence of pharmacology, engineering, and sustainability defines a strong framework for the future evolution of this technology. Integrating these perspectives into rigorous validation systems will support the development of more stable, reproducible, and clinically aligned methods [14, 15]. This evolution strengthens the foundations of technologies that persist and become naturally integrated into modern healthcare practice (Fig. 16.5).

This figure illustrates the main domains that underpin current and emerging pharmacological research in microfoam sclerotherapy. It integrates four key areas: the interaction between sclerosant foam and the venous endothelium, the physical behavior and stability of microfoam formulations, the use of physiological gas mixtures (CO_2/O_2), and data-driven modeling supported by large clinical datasets.

Together, these elements define the scientific basis for improving reproducibility, safety, and personalized application in therapeutic practice.

Alt text: Diagram showing four circular icons representing endothelial interaction, microfoam dynamics and stability, physiological gas mixtures (CO_2/O_2), and data-driven modeling with AI, arranged along a horizontal pathway toward optimized clinical practice.

6 Conclusions

Technological innovation in medicine arises from coordinated knowledge across disciplines—clinicians, engineers, pharmacists, jurists, and regulatory experts. This convergence forms a responsible ecosystem in which the creation of new therapeutic tools carries an ethical commitment to both patients and society [14]. Transformative projects reflect this plural vision through structured operation. In sclerotherapy, progress emerges from the combined contributions of those who design, generate, validate, and implement microfoam technologies. When clinical expertise, process engineering and regulation work in parallel, ideas evolve into safe, reproducible therapies. Cross-disciplinary collaboration strengthens each component—scientific, technical, legal, and entrepreneurial—and transforms innovation into shared, meaningful knowledge. The future of medical technology increasingly depends on effective coordination among stakeholders. Developers, clinicians, investors, manufacturers, regulatory bodies, and healthcare systems each shape different stages of the life cycle of a device. When these perspectives align—scientific evidence, clinical need, regulatory clarity, manufacturing capacity, and sustainable financing—innovation advances with purpose and stability. Public–private partnerships contribute decisively to this alignment, combining agility, resources, and creativity with equity, traceability, and efficient technology transfer [15].

Digital infrastructures and data-driven systems reinforce this collaborative model. Large clinical datasets, algorithmic analysis, and real-world performance feedback support continuous refinement of design and preparation conditions. This transparency strengthens trust among developers, regulators, and clinicians, and creates an iterative framework in which technology evolves in step with clinical experience.

Sustainability in biomedical innovation has multiple dimensions. Technical consistency, regulatory coherence, and economic viability reinforce each other. A project that anticipates its production demands, quality requirements, market constraints, and regulatory obligations is more likely to reach clinical adoption and remain accessible over time. Incorporating sustainability into the earliest stages of development ensures that scientific ambition is matched with practical conditions for long-term continuity and patient benefit.

Technological progress rarely follows a linear path. Many promising concepts stall in the "Valley of Death," the stage where scientific efficacy is demonstrated but clinical translation remains incomplete [8]. Our own experience—built over more than fifteen years of continuous work—shows that excellence endures when supported by operational discipline, structural robustness, and a long-term vision. Financing remains a critical factor: biomedical innovation requires sustained investment that often exceeds the stability of conventional funding cycles. Commitment frequently demands personal sacrifice, sometimes extending to family. Yet innovation thrives when those who pursue it find not only vocation, but also a legitimate and sustainable way to continue their work.

The most valuable resource in innovation is time. Each year dedicated to research, validation, or refinement represents a deliberate investment—a conscious renunciation of other paths. That effort, often unseen by those who witness only the final result, gives true value to applied science. The future belongs to those who understand that scientific excellence and social responsibility are complementary dimensions of the same purpose: rigor ensures results, and purpose gives them meaning.

Knowledge built upon time leaves a mark that transcends those who create it, transforming individual effort into service to others (Fig. 16.6).

This diagram illustrates the conceptual framework that supports responsible technological

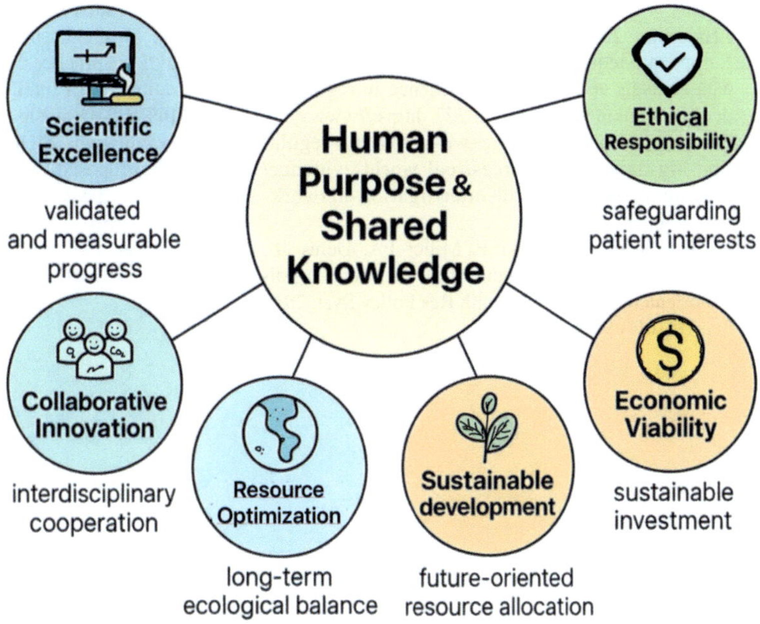

Fig. 16.6 Pillars of innovation in sclerotherapy

progress in sclerotherapy. The outer pillars represent the scientific, regulatory, ethical, collaborative and sustainability dimensions that enable a technology to mature in a consistent and clinically meaningful way. All elements converge toward a central principle—shared purpose and shared knowledge—which ultimately guides the translation of innovation into durable patient benefit.

Alt text: Circular diagram showing six pillars of innovation connected to a central concept of shared purpose and knowledge

References

1. Cabrera J, Cabrera J Jr, Garcia-Olmedo MA, Redondo P. Treatment of venous malformations with sclerosant in microfoam form. Arch Dermatol. 2003 Nov;139(11):1409–16.
2. Bottaro E, Paterson J, Zhang X, et al. Physical Vein Models to Quantify the Flow Performance of Sclerosing Foams. Front Bioeng Biotechnol. 2019 May 21;7:109.
3. Albanese G, Kondo KL. Pharmacology of sclerotherapy. Semin Intervent Radiol. 2010 Dec;27(4):391–9.
4. Alder G, Lees T. Foam sclerotherapy. Phlebology. 2015 Nov;30(2 Suppl):18–23.
5. Guex JJ. Foam sclerotherapy: an overview of use for primary venous insufficiency. Semin Vasc Surg. 2005 Mar;18(1):25–9.
6. Cavezzi A, Tessari L. Foam sclerotherapy techniques: different gases and methods of preparation, catheter versus direct injection. Phlebology. 2009 Dec;24(6):247–51.
7. Eberhardt RT, Raffetto JD. Chronic venous insufficiency. Circulation. 2014 Jul 22;130(4):333–46.
8. Joyce DP, De Freitas S, Woo EY, Tang TY, Tubassam M, Walsh SR. Ultrasound-guided foam sclerotherapy as a therapeutic modality in venous ulceration. Surgeon. 2022 Oct;20(5):e206–13.
9. FDA. Varithena® (polidocanol injectable foam) prescribing information. NDA 205098. Silver Spring; 2013. https://www.accessdata.fda.gov/drugsatfda_docs/nda/2013/205098Orig1s000Lbl.pdf.
10. Kreussler Pharma. Aethoxysklerol® (polidocanol) – summary of product characteristics. EMA; 2023. https://aethoxysklerol.co.uk/wp-content/uploads/2020/09/Aethoxysklerol-Key-Characteristics-14062019.pdf.
11. FDA. Pharmacy compounding systems—class II special controls guidance for industry and FDA staff. Silver Spring; 2001. https://www.fda.gov/medical-devices/guidance-documents-medical-devices-and-radiation-emitting-products/pharmacy-compounding-systems-final-class-ii-special-controls-guidance-document-industry-and-fda.
12. Chiasakul T, Lam BD, McNichol M, et al. Artificial intelligence in the prediction of venous thromboem-

bolism: A systematic review and pooled analysis. Eur J Haematol. 2023 Dec;111(6):951–62.
13. European Medicines Agency. Big data task force: data analysis and real-world evidence in regulatory decision-making. EMA; 2022. https://www.ema.europa.eu/en/about-us/how-we-work/data-regulation-big-data-other-sources/real-world-evidence/data-analysis-real-world-interrogation-network-darwin-eu.
14. Pacifico Silva H, Lehoux P, Miller FA, Denis JL. Introducing responsible innovation in health: a policy-oriented framework. Health Res Policy Syst. 2018 Sep 10;16(1):90.
15. Esmaeilzadeh P. Challenges and strategies for wide-scale artificial intelligence (AI) deployment in healthcare practices: A perspective for healthcare organizations. Artif Intell Med. 2024 May;151:102861.
16. IMDRF. Software as a Medical Device (SaMD): clinical evaluation. IMDRF/SaMD WG/N41FINAL:2017.
17. FDA. Proposed regulatory framework for modifications to AI/ML-based software as a medical device (SaMD). Silver Spring; 2019.
18. European Medicines Agency. Adaptive pathways: key principles. EMA/CHMP/ 233604/2016.

17 Similarities and Controversies in International Sclerotherapy Guidelines

Sergio Gianesini and Armando Mansilha

1 Introduction

Among all interventions in contemporary venous practice, sclerotherapy is perhaps the one that most clearly reveals how international guidelines can differ from country to country and even from document to document. A 2019 large publication of our group highlighted similarities and discrepancies in different vein-lymphatic recommendations documents around the world [1]. Such differences are not based on a globally shared methodologically-sound analysis of the available evidence followed by the related nationalization of the recommendation based on appropriateness and affordability principles [2]. The origin of such heterogeneity in the different documents providing recommendation on sclerotherapy is more to be found in the creation of independent groups from different regions, specialties and expertise, mixing consensus documents with methodological literature analysis (Table 17.1).

A typical example can be found in the evident discrepancies of the maximum foam volume recommended in Australia (20 ml) [7] compared to the European indication (10 ml) [6]. As this textbook previous chapters demonstrated, many are the variables involved in the production of a properly performing sclerotherapy act. Recommendations on sclerotherapy should always be based on studies guaranteeing the investigation only of appropriate sclerotherapy specifics use (appropriate concentrations, volume, foam production methods, wetness, materials, injection techniques). Unfortunately, the vast majority of the available scientific literature does not even specify these aspects, therefore diminishing the reliability of the data. The goal of this chapter is not to adjudicate which guideline is "correct", rather to explore why convergence occurs in some domains and persistent divergence in others and what this tells us about both sclerotherapy and the nature of guideline development itself.

S. Gianesini (✉)
Department of Translational Medicine, University of Ferrara, Ferrara, Italy

Department of Surgery, Uniformed Services University of Health Sciences, Bethesda, MD, USA
e-mail: gnssrg@unife.it

A. Mansilha
Department of Angiology and Vascular Surgery, Faculty of Medicine of University of Porto, São João University Hospital, Porto, Portugal

S. Gianesini, Y. W. Chi (eds.), *Sclerotherapy*, https://doi.org/10.1007/978-3-032-32794-9_17

Table 17.1 Comparison among recommendations provided by the American Venous Forum (AVF)/American Vein Lymphatic Society (AVLS) in 2022–23, [3, 4] by the European Vascular Surgery Society (ESVS) in the same year [5], and by the 2013 Consensus of 23 European Societies of Phlebology [6]

USA				Europe						
AVF/AVLS (2022)				ESVS (2022)				23 European Phlebology Societies (2013)		
Anatomical district	Recommendation	Clinical significance		Anatomical district	Recommendation	Clinical significance	Notes	Anatomical district	Recommendation	Notes
Great saphenous vein	For patients with symptomatic varicose veins and axial reflux in the great saphenous vein who place a high priority on the long-term outcomes of treatment (quality of life and recurrence), we suggest treatment with endovenous laser ablation, radiofrequency ablation, or high ligation and stripping over physician-compounded ultrasound-guided foam sclerotherapy	Symptomatic GSV reflux with long term outcomes desire, physician compounded foam to be discarded in favor of laser/ radiofrequency/ surgery		**Great saphenous vein**	For patients with great saphenous vein incompetence requiring treatment, endovenous thermal ablation is recommended as first choice treatment, in preference to high ligation/stripping and ultrasound-guided foam sclerotherapy	Highest evidence in thermal tumescent vs scleortherapy	The similar scenario in the American document is rated 2C vs. IA	**Saphenous trunks**	Sclerotherapy is indicated for saphenous trunks without caliber limitations	Opposite indication compared to the 2022 European document
	2B				**IA**				**IA**	

Small saphenous vein	For patients with symptomatic varicose veins and axial reflux in the small saphenous vein who place a high priority on the long-term outcomes of treatment (quality of life and recurrence), we suggest treatment with laser ablation, radiofrequency ablation, or ligation and stripping from the knee to the upper or mid-calf over physician-compounded ultrasound-guided foam sclerotherapy	Symptomatic SSV reflux with long term outcomes desire, physician compounded foam to be discarded in favor of laser/ radiofrequency/ surgery		**Small saphenous vein**	For patients with small saphenous vein incompetence requiring treatment, endovenous thermal ablation is recommended in preference to surgery or foam sclerotherapy	Endovenous thermal ablation is indicated over sclerotherapy for the small saphenous vein with a grade IA, while in the American document it's 2C				
	2C				**IA**					

(continued)

Table 17.1 (continued)

USA				Europe						
AVF/AVLS (2022)				ESVS (2022)				23 European Phlebology Societies (2013)		
Anatomical district	Recommendation	Clinical significance		Anatomical district	Recommendation	Clinical significance	Notes	Anatomical district	Recommendation	Notes
Anterior or posterior accessory saphenous vein	For patients with symptomatic varicose veins and axial reflux in the anterior accessory or posterior accessory great saphenous vein who place a high priority on the long-term outcomes of treatment (quality of life and recurrence), we suggest treatment of the refluxing superficial trunk with endovenous laser ablation, radiofrequency ablation, or high ligation and stripping, with additional phlebectomy, if needed, over physician-compounded ultrasound-guided foam sclerotherapy	In axial reflux + varicosities, phlebectomy to be preferred to physician compounded foam		**Sapheonus trunk**	For patients with saphenous trunk incompetence undergoing treatment, ultrasound-guided foam sclerotherapy may be considered for treating saphenous trunks with a diameter less than 6 mm	Sclerotherapy MAY BE considered only for saphenous trunk <6 mm	The American document does not mention vein diameter cut off			
	2C				**IIbB**					

Axial reflux + varicose tributaries	For patients with symptomatic reflux in the great or small saphenous vein and associated varicosities, we recommend ablation of the refluxing venous trunk and concomitant phlebectomy or ultrasound-guided foam sclerotherapy of the varicosities with physician-compounded foam or commercial polidocanol endovenous microfoam	No difference among phlebectomy, ultrasound-guided foam sclerotherapy of the varicosities with physician compounded foam or polidocanol endovenous microfoam		**Great saphenous vein**	For patients with great saphenous vein incompetence requiring treatment, catheter directed foam sclerotherapy with or without the use of peri-venous tumescent solution may be considered	Catheter-directed foam sclerotherapy MAY BE considered, with no difference if with or without tumescence			
	1C				**IIbB**				
Varicose tributaries	For treatment of symptomatic varicose tributaries, we recommend mini-phlebectomy or ultrasound-guided sclerotherapy using physician compounded foam (PCF) or polidocanol endovenous microfoam (PEM)			**Varicose tributaries**	For patients with chronic venous disease requiring treatment of varicose tributaries, ambulatory phlebectomy, *ultrasound-guided* foam sclerotherapy or a combination of both are recommended	No discrimination between phlebectomy and ultrasound-guided foam *sclerotherapy* or a combination of both. No mention about the staging in regard to the axial reflux			

(continued)

Table 17.1 (continued)

USA				Europe						
AVF/AVLS (2022)				ESVS (2022)				23 European Phlebology Societies (2013)		
Anatomical district	Recommendation	Clinical significance		Anatomical district	Recommendation	Clinical significance	Notes	Anatomical district	Recommendation	Notes
	1B				**IB**					
Great, anterior or posterior accessory saphenous vein	For patients with symptomatic reflux in the anterior accessory or posterior accessory great saphenous vein, we suggest ablation of the refluxing venous trunk and concomitant phlebectomy or ultrasound-guided foam sclerotherapy of the varicosities with physician-compounded foam or commercial polidocanol endovenous microfoam	Staged procedures only for specific anatomic and medical reasons (no difference between phlebectomy and physician compounded foam or polidocanol endovenous microfoam)		**Anterior saphenous vein**	For patients with incompetence of the anterior accessory saphenous vein requiring treatment, ultrasound-guided foam sclerotherapy may be considered	The American document supports the use endovenous laser or radiofrequency or surgery for the anterior saphenous vein				
	2C				**IIbC**					
Reticular veins	For patients with symptomatic telangiectasias and reticular veins we recommend sclerotherapy with liquid or foam	Liquid or foam sclerotherapy is recommended for both teleangectasia and reticular vein	No discrimenation between reticular veins and telangectasia, differently from the same year European document.	**Reticular veins**	For patients with reticular veins, where treatment is planned, sclerotherapy is recommended, as the first choice treatment	Sclerotherapy, independently by liquid or foam, is the first choice treatment		**Reticular veins**	Sclerotherapy is indicated for reticular veins	
	1B				**IA**				**1A**	

				Teleangectasia	For patients with telangiectasias, where treatment is planned, sclerotherapy should be considered	For reticular veins, sclerotherapy is recommended as first choice, while for teleangectasia it can just be considered. No mention of this in the American document		**Teleangectasia**	Sclerotherapy is indicated for teleangectasia with a grade 1A	The 2022 European document indicates only that sclerotherapy should be considered and with a IIaA indication
					IIaA				**1A**	
				Foot and nkle veins	For patients presenting with foot and ankle varicose veins, phlebectomy, sclerotherapy, and foot perforating vein ligation may be considered during or after ablation of proximal reflux	Phlebectomy, perforating vein ligation or sclerotherapy may be equally considered for foot and ankle varicose veins				
					IIbC					

(continued)

Table 17.1 (continued)

USA				Europe						
AVF/AVLS (2022)				ESVS (2022)				23 European Phlebology Societies (2013)		
Anatomical district	Recommendation	Clinical significance		Anatomical district	Recommendation	Clinical significance	Notes	Anatomical district	Recommendation	Notes
Recurrent varicosities	For patients with symptomatic recurrent varicosities due to persistent or recurrent reflux at the groin, either EVLA or RFA can be used if there is a straight GSV stump, long enough for thermal ablation. Sclerotherapy or phlebectomy should be performed for recurrence due to neovascularization			**Recurrent varicosities from saphenous trunks**	For patients with symptomatic recurrent varicose veins due to saphenous trunk incompetence, endovenous thermal ablation or ultrasound-guided foam sclerotherapy with or without phlebectomy should be considered	Same indication for surgery, thermal tumescent, foam sclerotherapy in recurrent varicosities				
	Consensus statement				**IIaB**					
Recurrent small saphenous vein	For patients with symptomatic recurrent varicosities due to persistent or recurrent reflux of the SSV, ultrasound-guided foam sclerotherapy should be performed			**Recurrent varicosities NOT from saphenous trunks**	For patients with symptomatic recurrent varicose veins without truncal incompetence, ultrasound-guided foam sclerotherapy and/or ambulatory phlebectomy should be considered	Scleortherapy and phlebectomy equally considered in non saphenous recurrent varicosities		**Recurrent varicosities with/out saphenous trunks involvement**	Indication to sclerotherapy with a 1B grade	In the 2022 European document the indication is IIaB
	Consensus statement				**IIaC**				**1B**	

				Ulcer	For patients with active venous leg ulceration, ablation of thesub-ulcer venous plexus using ultrasound-guided foam sclerotherapy should be considered as part of the treatment strategy			**Ulcer**	Sclerotherapy is indicated with grade 1B	In the 2022 European document sclerotherapy for ulcer plexuses received a IIaC indication
					IIaC				**1B**	
Bleeding	For patients presenting with acute bleeding from varicose veins, leg elevation, direct compression and sclerotherapy should be attempted before suture ligation to control bleeding			**Bleeding**	For patients with chronic venous disease who have suffered from an episode of acute bleeding of superficial veins or telangiectasias, local foam sclerotherapy should be considered to prevent recurrent bleeding					
	Consensus statement				**IIaC**					

(continued)

Table 17.1 (continued)

USA				Europe						
AVF/AVLS (2022)				ESVS (2022)				23 European Phlebology Societies (2013)		
Anatomical district	Recommendation	Clinical significance		Anatomical district	Recommendation	Clinical significance	Notes	Anatomical district	Recommendation	Notes
Great, anterior or posterior accessory saphenous vein	For patients with symptomatic reflux in the great or small saphenous vein, we suggest ablation of the refluxing venous trunk and staged phlebectomy or ultrasound-guided foamsclerotherapy of the varicosities only if anatomic ormedical reasons present. We suggest shared decision-making with the patient									
	2C									

Major superficial venous trunks	For patients with symptomatic reflux in the major superficial venous trunks and associated varicosities undergoing initial ablation alone, we recommend that patients be followed up for >3 months to assess the need for staged phlebectomy or ultrasound-guided sclerotherapy for persistent or recurrent symptoms. Longer follow-up is recommended for patients with recurrent symptoms and for patients who participate in clinical trials.	3 months follow up for staging (no difference if phlebectomy or sclerotherapy)								
	Good clinical practice									
Symptomatic GSV/SSV reflux	For patients with symptomatic reflux in the great or small saphenous vein, we suggest ablation of the refluxing venous trunk and staged phlebectomy or ultrasound-guided foamsclerotherapy of the varicosities only if anatomic or medical reasons present. We suggest shared decision-making with the patient	Staged procedures only for specific anatomic and medical reasons (no difference between phlebectomy and physician compounded foam or polidocanol endovenous microfoam)								
	2C									

2 Historical Context

The historical roots of sclerotherapy exert a subtle but powerful influence on guideline language. In continental Europe, sclerotherapy developed as a central pillar of phlebologic practice long before the advent of endovenous thermal techniques. European phlebology therefore tends to view sclerotherapy not as an "alternative" but as a foundational modality, adaptable across disease stages and anatomical contexts. This historical continuity is reflected in the detailed, technique-oriented nature of European sclerotherapy guidelines, which specify sclerosant concentrations, volumes and indications with a granularity rarely seen in North American documents [6]. In contrast, in North America, sclerotherapy evolved alongside a strong surgical tradition and later within an office-based procedural model that emphasized safety, standardization and medico-legal defensibility. As endovenous thermal ablation became dominant for truncal reflux, sclerotherapy was increasingly repositioned as an adjunctive or secondary therapy, particularly for tributaries and cosmetic disease. This historical pathway helps explain why North American guidelines often frame sclerotherapy in algorithmic terms, where it fits relative to other interventions, rather than as a standalone discipline with its own internal logic [3]. An exception to this concept is represented by the American introduction of Polidocanol Endovenous Microfoam (PEM, Varithena™). It's introduction into the market in 2013 revoluzionized the positioning of foam sclerotherapy, placing it as a possible alternative even to thermal tumescent options for saphenous ablation. The evidence produced led the United States to recognize a reimbursability code dedicated to its use. The process was feasible for this unique foam generator because it involved a fully automated system with less than 0.8% nitrogen, allowing therefore an extremely standardized, reproducible, safe, yet effective, foam administration. Yet, the limitation of Varithena™ remains in the only available concentration (polidocanol 1%) and gas mixture (O_2 65%; CO_2 35%). The indication provided by FDA ranges from great and anterior saphenous vein to visible varicosities (5 ml per injection and 15 ml per session maximum, repeatable after 5 days). Nevertheless, a wider versatility and a more precise indication is needed to cover all the possible everyday clinical scenarios in vein treatment. Moreover, the Varithena™ role in small saphenous vein treatment was not enough investigated to obtain approval [8]. Ongoing investigations are exploring the possibility of reproducing the same safety and efficacy in a wider range of concentraitons and biocompatible gasses percentages.

3 Similarities and Discrepancies

One of the clearest areas of international agreement is the recognition that sclerotherapy is not a single intervention, but a spectrum of related techniques. Guidelines consistently distinguish between liquid sclerotherapy for telangiectasias and reticular veins, foam sclerotherapy for larger varices and ultrasound-guided foam sclerotherapy for non-visible or deeper venous segments. This conceptual framework is explicit in European sclerotherapy guidance and implicitly adopted in broader chronic venous disease guidelines worldwide [5, 6]. This shared framing matters because it allows guideline panels with very different clinical cultures to speak a common language. Even when recommendations diverge, they do so within a mutually understood taxonomy of disease severity and treatment modality. Another strong point of convergence is the role of duplex ultrasound. Across international guidelines, ultrasound guidance is treated as essential when sclerotherapy is applied to anything beyond the superficial dermal plexus. Moreover, even for the more superficial aesthetic sclerotherapy treatment, a previous ultrasound scanning and mapping of the eventually feeder veins is recommended by the V.A.L.I.D. (Venous And Lymphatic International Document) clinical governance publication [2]. The rationale is both technical and ethical: ultrasound improves accuracy, enables hemodynamic assessment and reduces the risk of inadvertent arterial injection or deep venous extension. While early sclerotherapy literature often relied on visual targeting alone, modern guidelines uniformly regard ultrasound-guided foam sclerotherapy as the appropriate approach for treating larger veins and perforators [9, 10]. International guidelines also converge on the idea that no single outcome metric adequately captures the success of sclerotherapy. Instead, they endorse a multidimensional assessment incorporating patient-reported symptoms, quality of life, visual improvement and duplex-defined anatomic outcomes. This reflects a mature understanding of venous disease as a condition in which hemodynamic correction, symptom relief and cosmetic satisfaction are related but not interchangeable goals [3–5]. Extreme care must be put in the identification of what outcome measures were chosen by the authors of the guidelines to provide the related recommendation. This is important both clinically to steer the right everyday practice, but also in the meta-analysis data extraction, otherwise falling into the flaw of heterogeneous forms of recurrence/treatment failure discussion. Perhaps the most visible area of apparent agreement, but underlying controversy, is the positioning of sclerotherapy relative to endovenous thermal ablation for truncal reflux. Many guidelines, particularly those from the UK and North America, prioritize endothermal ablation as first-line therapy when anatomy is suitable, relegating foam sclerotherapy to a secondary role [3, 4, 11]. However, this alignment is more superficial than it appears. In NICE guidance, the hierarchy is heavily influenced by health-economic modeling and cost-effectiveness analysis within a publicly funded system. In contrast, North American documents are shaped by comparative effectiveness frameworks that weigh randomized trial data against regulatory constraints. European documents, particularly those from the ESVS, adopt a more pluralistic stance. While acknowledging the durability of thermal ablation, they emphasize individualized decision-making based on anatomy, comorbidity and patient preference, and they explicitly recognize foam sclerotherapy as an acceptable alternative in selected contexts, more than often using statements such as "should/may be considered", which are not really providing a real guidance/recommendation, neither in the clinical practice nor in the weighted evidence certainty. Worthy of notice is how UK NICE indicates thermal tumescent as first option for saphenous trunks, followed by sclerotherapy and then by surgery, while the American document includes surgery with endovenous thermal option [3, 4, 12]. Where international consensus is strongest is in the treatment of tributary veins and recurrent varicosities. Across guideline systems, sclerotherapy, liquid or foam, is consistently endorsed as a primary or adjunctive therapy in these settings. This convergence reflects both evidence and experience: tributary networks are anatomically variable, recurrence is often multifactorial and sclerotherapy offers unmatched flexibility and repeatability [1]. Notably, in these scenarios, guideline language becomes less hierarchical and more permissive. Rather than prescribing a single preferred modality, documents emphasize clinician judgment and patient-centered decision-making, implicitly acknowledging the limits of comparative trials in such heterogeneous disease states. Moreover, sclerotherapy is mentioned together with phlebectomies as two equally alternative options, generating confusion on what the best choice among the two might be. Future indications should highlight the eventually different performance of the two, providing clear recommendation on when to prefer one rather than the other. Although guidelines clearly differentiate liquid and foam sclerotherapy, they diverge on how strongly to favor one over the other in specific contexts. For telangiectasias and reticular veins, most agree that liquid sclerotherapy remains the standard, with foam reserved for selected patterns or operator preference. In truncal disease, however, the debate becomes more complex. Evidence suggests that foam sclerotherapy may have lower long-term occlusion rates than surgery or thermal ablation in some settings, yet it offers advantages in invasiveness, cost and applicability to tortuous anatomy. Guidelines differ in how they weigh these trade-offs, leading to divergent recommendations that reflect differing tolerances for reintervention and differing definitions of "success" [1]. Few areas illustrate the limits of evidence-based standardization more clearly than foam preparation. International consensus documents acknowledge that foam characteristics (bubble size, stability, gas composition) matter, yet they stop short of mandating a single preparation method. The persistence of multiple consensus statements over time underscores that this is an evolving field rather than a settled one. The introduction of commercially prepared polidocanol endovenous microfoam has added a new dimension to this debate. While standardized foam offers reproducibility and regulatory reassurance, it also raises questions about access, cost, and whether its evidence base can be generalized to all foam sclerotherapy practices worldwide [13, 14]. Moreover, different production methods for foam sclerotherapy might suggest an adaptation of the concentrations and volumes for the same targeted vein, yet no documents specifying this aspect can be found in the solid literature on the topic. The management of neurologic risk represents one of the most philosophically charged controversies in sclerotherapy guidelines. Serious neurologic events after foam sclerotherapy are rare, but their severity ensures that they loom large in both clinical memory and guideline discussions. Systematic reviews confirm a low overall incidence of neurologic complications, with some association between transient events and right-to-left shunts such as patent foramen ovale [15]. Despite this, no major guideline recommends routine patent foramen ovale screening prior to foam sclerotherapy. This restraint reflects a judgment that the prevalence of asymptomatic patent foramen ovale, combined with the low absolute risk of serious events, does not justify widespread screening. Yet many experienced clinicians adopt more conservative practices than guidelines require, tailoring foam volume and technique based on migraine history or prior neurologic symptoms. This divergence highlights the gap between population-level recommendations and individual risk management [16, 17]. Guidelines uniformly acknowledge thrombotic complications as a potential risk of sclerotherapy, but they diverge in definitions, surveillance strategies and prophylaxis recommendations. Some emphasize early duplex surveillance, others prioritize clinical assessment and few provide explicit anticoagulation algorithms applicable to all sclerotherapy scenarios. This heterogeneity reflects the wide spectrum of procedures encompassed by the term "sclerotherapy," from small-volume cosmetic injections to extensive foam treatment of axial veins. Compression after sclerotherapy exemplifies how small differences in evidence interpretation can produce lasting guideline variability. Randomized studies in telangiectatic disease suggest that prolonged compression improves cosmetic outcomes, yet adherence is variable and patient tolerance limited. Other guidelines recommend compression without specifying duration or strength, implicitly acknowledging the limits of available data and the influence of real-world compliance [1, 18, 19].

4 Absolute and Relative Contraindications

A review of contraindications across existing documents of different scientific societies and nations reveals considerable variability rather than a unified approach. While there is a general agreement on absolute contraindications, heterogeneity can be found in the relative contraindications (Table 17.2). Among the most evident discrepancies, acute superficial thrombophlebitis is an example. The Indian guidelines published in 2011 and the 2014 American Society for Dermatologic Surgery guidelines define it as an absolute contraindication, whereas the 2014 European consensus and the 2016 Australian guidelines categorize it as a relative one. The American Society for Dermatologic Surgery guidelines stand out as the only source identifying leg edema and poorly controlled diabetes as relative contraindications. In contrast, the Indian guidelines merely note that both conditions may impair circulation, without formally listing them as contraindications. The Australian recommendations include oral contraceptive use, hormonal therapy, recent travel exceeding four hours and poor patient compliance among relative contrain-

Table 17.2 Comparison among different guidelines absolute and relative contraindications

Comparison among international recommendations on sclerotherapy	
Similarities	Discrepancies
1. Ultrasound use (for scanning and for guidance)	1. Different outcome measures (anatomical recurrence, quality of life, disease severity, aesthetic satisfaction, etc.)
2. Absolute contraindications	2. Different positioning of sclerotherapy compared to varicose vein surgery
3. General consideration of sclerotherapy as safe	3. Different limits and recommendation strength for sclerotherapy in the saphenous trunks treatment
4. No routing patent foramen ovale screening	4. Elative contraindications
	5. Thrombotic complication definitions, surveillance strategies and prophylaxis recommendations
	6. Maximum volume per session
	7. Follow-up timing
	8. Post-procedural compression use
	9. Post-procedural venous active drugs use

dications. An asymptomatic right-to-left shunt is considered a relative contraindication in the 2014 American and 2016 Latin American guidelines, a position not reflected in other documents. Pregnancy is treated as an absolute contraindication solely in the Indian guideline, whereas other documents regard it as relative. Notably, the same Indian guideline also lists saphenofemoral junction incompetence as a relative contraindication. With respect to complications, there is broad consensus among guidelines regarding serious adverse events. However, greater divergence emerges in the reporting of minor or benign complications. Few documents provide estimates of complication rates and even among these sources; the reported incidences vary considerably [1].

5 Methodological Underpinnings: Why Guideline Panels Disagree Even When Reading the Same Studies

A recurring reason for divergence is that guideline panels often evaluate different implicit interventions under the same label. "Foam sclerotherapy" in one trial may involve small volumes, fractionated injections and strict ultrasound guidance, while in another it may represent a very different technical approach. This heterogeneity undermines meta-analytic certainty and forces guideline authors to rely on expert judgment when grading recommendations. Differences in methodology, stakeholder involvement and health-system context play a major role in shaping recommendations, sometimes as much as the underlying evidence itself. For the vascular expert, reconciling international guidelines on sclerotherapy requires moving beyond literalism. A useful mental model is to view guidelines as defining zones of certainty and zones of discretion. In zones of certainty, such as the role of sclerotherapy in tributary disease or the need for ultrasound guidance, practice can align closely with recommendations. In zones of discretion, such as foam volume limits, compression duration or neurologic risk mitigation, experienced clinicians must integrate guideline principles with individual patient factors and technical judgment. Seen in this light, the persistence of controversy is not a failure of guideline development but an honest reflection of the complexity of sclerotherapy as a therapeutic modality. The similarities across international guidelines affirm its enduring value: the controversies remind us that sclerotherapy remains, at its core, a procedure where expertise matters. International guidelines on sclerotherapy converge on broad principles: the legitimacy of sclerotherapy as a core venous intervention, the importance of ultrasound guidance, the centrality of patient-centered outcomes, and the rarity, but seriousness, of major complications. They diverge on technical details, risk thresholds, and algorithmic positioning, reflecting differences in evidence interpretation, healthcare systems and professional culture. For vascular specialists, the challenge is not to choose one guideline over another, but to understand the assumptions and values that underlie each. When read with this perspective, the similarities provide reassurance and the controversies become an invitation to thoughtful, individualized practice rather than a source of confusion. At the same time, it must be crystal clear to the practitioner how the almost totality of the so-called guidelines are lacking either the methodology or the clinical governance requirements to be considered as legally binding documents in the different single countries. In this sense, a collaboration with both real experts in methodology as well as with governmental institutions is urged. Indeed, the typical example is provided by the current Italian authorization only for 3% polidocanol foam sclerotherapy, exclusively for the great saphenous vein in between 4 mm and 8 mm [20]. Independently by the evidence other publications are reporting, in Italy, whatever is outside that indication is to be considered off-label. Yet, every single day in the same Italy sclerotherapy is performed using off-label sclerotherapy: a situation that demands a prompt clinical governance evaluation. Indeed, for safety and liability reasons, the use of unapproved substances or any modification of the original formulation of medicinal products is generally discouraged. Such changes may affect the product's safety profile and are undertaken at the physician's own discretion and risk, falling outside the responsibility of the pharmaceutical manufacturer. This principle also extends to the use of sclerosant foam created by combining detergent-based sclerosants with air or other gases. Although sclerotherapy is well-established and considered safe in several countries, it is nevertheless advisable to follow a standardized method, aware of all the nuances.

6 National Clinical Governance Versus International Guidance in Sclerotherapy

For the vascular specialist, sclerotherapy sits at the intersection of pharmacology, device-like technique and regulatory interpretation. Unlike many endovascular procedures, the "what" and the "how much" in sclerotherapy are not defined solely by physiology or evidence, but by a complex overlay of national licensing, professional governance and international consensus documents. As a result, there is often a substantial gap between what international guidelines describe as acceptable or effective practice and what is formally permitted within a given country under product labeling and clinical governance frameworks. International guidelines in venous disease are, by design, descriptive and aspirational. They synthesize available evidence, expert consensus and long-standing clinical practice across multiple jurisdictions. Their primary purpose is to guide clinical decision-making, not to define regulatory compliance. By contrast, national authorities, such as the Food and Drug Administration in the United States or the Medicines and Healthcare products Regulatory Agency in the United Kingdom, license products, not techniques. A detergent sclerosant is approved at specific concentrations, for specific vein sizes or indications, sometimes with explicit limits on injected volume or total dose. Anything outside that frame becomes off-label or unlicensed, even if it is widely described in international literature. Clinical governance then determines how far clinicians may reasonably deviate from the label, under what conditions and with what level of documentation and patient consent. European and international venous documents are remarkably consistent in tone: they acknowledge the long-standing use of both liquid and foam sclerotherapy, recognize the lack of high-level evidence for strict dose ceilings and therefore rely heavily on expert consensus.

The European Guidelines for Sclerotherapy in Chronic Venous Disorders describe concentration selection primarily according to vein diameter and wall thickness, rather than rigid numerical limits. For foam, they explicitly note that no evidence-based maximum volume exists, while referencing conservative expert-opinion thresholds that historically clustered around 10 mL of foam per session [6]. More recently, the 2022 Clinical Practice Guidelines of the European Society for Vascular Surgery adopt a slightly more permissive and pragmatic tone. They acknowledge that contemporary practice in many European centers routinely exceeds earlier conservative thresholds and describe a consensus range of approximately 10–20 mL of foam per treatment session [5]. Crucially, these documents treat physician-compounded foam as a legitimate technique, discuss foam use in tributary and truncal veins, emphasize technique, ultrasound guidance and patient selection over strict numerical caps. What they do not do is resolve how these recommendations interact with national product licenses. In the United States, the regulatory environment is strongly product-centric. The FDA licenses specific sclerosants with narrow, indication-based labeling. Liquid polidocanol, marketed as Asclera™, is approved only in 0.5% and 1.0% concentrations and specifically for spider veins and reticular veins up to 3 mm in diameter. The label emphasizes small injection volumes and, in practice, a 10 mL maximum per session has become a commonly cited ceiling. From a regulatory standpoint, the use of liquid polidocanol for truncal veins or larger varicosities is therefore off-label, regardless of what international guidelines describe. The introduction of proprietary polidocanol endovenous microfoam (Varithena™) created a parallel, on-label pathway for foam treatment. This product is licensed with explicit constraints, typically no more than 5 mL per injection and no more than 15 mL per session and is allowed for the treatment of the great and anterior saphenous vein, together with visible varicosities. For the American vascular specialist, the discrepancy is clear: international guidelines may describe foam sclerotherapy for truncal reflux as established practice, but the FDA-compliant route depends heavily on whether a specific foam product is used rather than the foam technique itself. The UK represents a different model. Here, product licenses coexist with an explicit and mature framework for off-label and unlicensed use. Sodium tetradecyl sulfate is licensed in multiple concentrations, with the Summary of Product Characteristics (SmPC) directly linking concentration choice to vein type, from very low concentrations for telangiectasia to 3% for larger varicosities [21]. Polidocanol is similarly licensed in a wide range of concentrations, with a clearly stated maximum dose of 2 mg/kg per day. Some UK SmPCs also include explicit statements on foam, often recommending that microfoam volumes should not exceed 10 mL per session, irrespective of patient weight. Importantly, these statements are product-specific and do not necessarily reflect broader professional consensus. National bodies such as National Institute for Health and Care Excellence endorse ultrasound-guided foam sclerotherapy as a treatment option for varicose veins, particularly when endothermal ablation is unsuitable. However, NICE guidance addresses clinical effectiveness, not dosing limits or formulation legality. In practice, UK clinicians operate within a governance framework that allows deviation from the SmPC, provided it is justified, documented and explained to the patient. As a result, there is often closer alignment between international guideline recommendations and real-world UK practice than in more label-restrictive systems, even though the legal responsibility remains squarely with the treating physician. Worth of notice is the example of Canada, where sodium tetra decyl sulfate is licensed for "small (1%, 0.5–2 mL), medium and large (3%, 0.5–2 mL)" veins: indeed, the definition of small/medium and large is present in different licensing documents around the world, yet not specifying what the exact precision is, therefore generating possible confusion. It's also interesting how the same Canadian document mention a 5 cm distance between the injection sites: this is usually not found in other nations documentation and it is not associated with the vein network wideness and/or tortuosity [22]. Across continental Europe, detergent sclerosants are widely available, but the regulatory interpretation of foam varies substantially between countries. Polidocanol and sodium tetradecyl sulfate are generally licensed in liquid form. Foam is frequently described in SmPCs not as a separate formulation, but as a method of preparation, often with explicit constraints. In some countries, foam preparation is restricted to certain concentrations or specific liquid-to-gas ratios. In others, foam is not mentioned at all, effectively placing physician-compounded foam in a gray zone between licensed use and accepted practice. This heterogeneity explains why European guidelines tend to speak in general terms about foam volumes and concentrations, while simultaneously acknowledging that "national regulations may differ." For the vascular expert working across borders, this is not a theoretical concern but a practical one: the same technique may be fully routine in one country and technically off-label in another. Australia provides an instructive contrast. Here, professional college standards play a dominant role in defining acceptable practice. Guidance from specialist phlebology bodies sets explicit numerical ceilings: a maximum polidocanol dose of 2 mg/kg per day, a total foam volume not usually exceeding 20 mL per day, and more conservative sub-limits for truncal veins (often around 10 mL per leg). These figures sit comfortably within the upper range described by European guidelines, yet are formalized in a way that provides clinicians with defensible boundaries. In this context, international guidelines do not so much conflict with national governance as they are absorbed into it, with local expert consensus translating broad recommendations into concrete limits. Three recurring areas generate the most friction between international guidance and national governance:

1. Foam Volume Limits
International documents acknowledge 10–20 mL as common contemporary practice, whereas some product labels still cite 10 mL or less.
2. Truncal Vein Treatment
Guidelines discuss foam as an option for truncal reflux, but several liquid sclerosant licenses remain formally restricted to small veins.
3. Physician-Compounded Foam
Widely described and supported in the literature, yet variably treated as off-label, unlicensed, or conditionally acceptable depending on jurisdiction.

For the experienced clinician, the key is not to choose between national governance and international guidelines, but to understand their different purposes. International guidelines describe what works and what is widely accepted by the expert community. National licenses and governance define what is formally authorized and where responsibility lies. Safe, defensible practice emerges where the two are consciously reconciled, through informed consent, meticulous documentation and an explicit understanding of when one is practicing within or deliberately beyond the product label.

In this sense, the divergence between "allowed" and "recommended" in sclerotherapy is not a flaw of the system, but a reflection of the field's evolution: a mature technique advancing faster than the regulatory frameworks that attempt to contain it. Interestingly, in some USA states and UK, as well as in other countries, sclerotherapy injections can be performed also by nurses, opening another large debate on the technical, strategical and medical culture requirements for appropriate performance. Such consideration includes also the medical specialty eventually required to practice sclerotherapy as heterogeneity is found also for this aspect around the world [23]. In the end, the common aspects linking all sclerotherapy proper scientific and regulatory documents together with the real-world scenario is the need to consider sclerotherapy surely not just an injection of some product inside some vein, rather the final act of a longlasting and deep learning process that can allow this technique to be applied in the safest and most effective way possible.

References

1. Gianesini S, Obi A, Onida S, et al. Global guidelines trends and controversies in lower limb venous and lymphatic disease: narrative literature revision and experts' opinions following the vWINter international meeting in phlebology. Lymphol Aesthet Phlebol. 2019;34(1 Suppl):4–66.
2. Gianesini S, Danese M, AlQedrah D, et al. Multispecialty recommendations for the appropriate and affordable lower limb vein-lymphatic disorders management. Int Angiol. 2026;45(1):1–64.
3. Gloviczki P, Lawrence P, Wasan S, et al. The 2022 Society for Vascular Surgery, American Venous Forum, and American Vein and Lymphatic Society clinical practice guidelines for the management of varicose veins of the lower extremities. Part I. Duplex Scanning and Treatment of Superficial Truncal Reflux, MD
4. Gloviczki P, Lawrence PF, Wasan SM, et al. The 2023 Society for Vascular Surgery, American Venous Forum, and American Vein and Lymphatic Society clinical practice guidelines for the management of varicose veins of the lower extremities. Part II: Endorsed by the Society of Interventional Radiology and the Society for Vascular Medicine. J Vasc Surg Venous Lymphat Disord. 2024;12(1):101670.
5. De Maeseneer MG, Kakkos SK, Aherne T, et al. Editor's choice – European Society for Vascular Surgery (ESVS) 2022 Clinical Practice Guidelines on the Management of Chronic Venous Disease of the Lower Limbs. Eur J Vasc Endovasc Surg. 2022;63(2):184–267. https://doi.org/10.1016/j.ejvs.2021.12.024. Epub 2022 Jan 11. Erratum in: Eur J Vasc Endovasc Surg 2022;64(2–3):284–5
6. Rabe E, Pannier F, Guideline Group. Indications, contraindications and performance: European guidelines for sclerotherapy in chronic venous disorders. Phlebology. 2014;29(1 suppl):26–33.
7. Australasian College of Phlebology. Diagnose venous disease and treat superficial venous incompetence with injected sclerosants under ultrasound guidance. 2016 ACP Standards Guidelines, www.phlebology.com.au/.
8. https://www.accessdata.fda.gov/drugsatfda_docs/nda/2013/205098orig1s000toc.cfm.
9. Darke SG, Baker SJ. Ultrasound-guided foam sclerotherapy for the treatment of varicose veins. Br J Surg. 2006;93(8):969–74.
10. Gianesini S, Chi YW, Agüero C, et al. Fake-news-free evidence-based communication for proper vein-lymphatic disease management. Int Angiol. 2023;42(2):89–189.
11. Surveillance report 2016—varicose veins in the legs (2013) NICE guideline CG168 [internet]. London: National Institute for Health and Care Excellence (NICE); 2016. PMID: 31891464.
12. https://www.nice.org.uk/guidance/cg168/resources/varicose-veins-diagnosis-and-management-pdf-35109698485957.
13. King JT, O'Byrne M, Vasquez M, et al. Treatment of truncal incompetence and varicose veins with a single administration of a new polidocanol endovenous microfoam preparation improves symptoms and appearance. Eur J Vasc Endovasc Surg. 2015;50(6):784–93.
14. Kabnick LS, Jimenez JC, Coogan SM, et al. Comparative effectiveness of non-compounded polidocanol 1% endovenous microfoam (Varithena) ablation versus endovenous thermal ablation utilizing a systematic review and network meta-analysis. J Vasc Surg Venous Lymphat Disord. 2024;12(6):101896.
15. Sarvananthan T, Shepherd AC, Willenberg T, Davies AH. Neurological complications of sclerotherapy for varicose veins. J Vasc Surg. 2012;55(1):243–51.
16. Raymond-Martimbeau P. Transient adverse events positively associated with patent foramen ovale after ultrasound-guided foam sclerotherapy. Phlebology 2009;24(3):114–9.
17. Bush RG, Derrick M, Manjoney D. Major neurological events following foam sclerotherapy. Phlebology. 2008;23(4):189–92.
18. El-Sheikha J, Carradice D, Nandhra S, et al. Systematic review of compression following treatment for varicose veins. Br J Surg. 2015;102(7):719–25.
19. Lurie F, Lal BK, Antignani PL, Blebea J, et al. Compression therapy after invasive treatment of superficial veins of the lower extremities: clinical practice guidelines of the American Venous Forum, Society for Vascular Surgery, American College of Phlebology, Society for Vascular Medicine, and International Union of Phlebology. J Vasc Surg Venous Lymphat Disord. 2019;7(1):17–28.
20. https://www.aifa.gov.it/en/-/nota-informativa-importante-su-atossisclerol.
21. https://www.medicines.org.uk/emc/product/1199/smpc?utm_source=chatgpt.com.
22. https://pdf.hres.ca/dpd_pm/00063198.PDF.
23. https://www.nmbi.ie/NMBI/media/NMBI/Guidance-for-Registered-General-Nurses-Who-Perform-Non-Surgical-Aesthetic-and-Cosmetic-Procedures.pdf?ext=.pdf.

GPSR Compliance

The European Union's (EU) General Product Safety Regulation (GPSR) is a set of rules that requires consumer products to be safe and our obligations to ensure this.

If you have any concerns about our products, you can contact us on ProductSafety@springernature.com

In case Publisher is established outside the EU, the EU authorized representative is:

Springer Nature Customer Service Center GmbH
Europaplatz 3
69115 Heidelberg, Germany

Batch number: 10731385

Printed by Printforce, the Netherlands